ADDICTIVE BEHAVIOUR: MOLECULES TO MANKIND

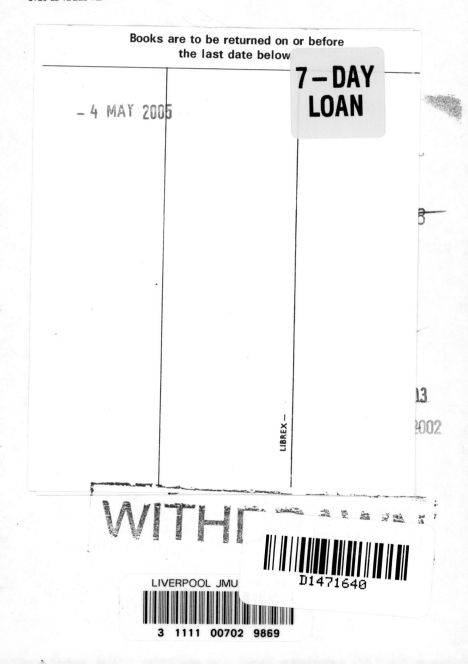

Books are to be returned on or before
the last date below

7-DAY LOAN

− 4 MAY 2005

LIBREX —

13

2002

Addictive Behaviour: Molecules to Mankind

Perspectives on the Nature of Addiction

Edited by

Adrian Bonner
Director
Addictive Behaviour Centre
Roehampton Institute
London

and

James Waterhouse
Senior Research Fellow
School of Biological Sciences
University of Manchester
and
Lecturer in Physiology
School of Human Biology

Foreword by

Timothy J. Peters

First published in Great Britain 1996 by
MACMILLAN PRESS LTD
Houndmills, Basingstoke, Hampshire RG21 6XS
and London
Companies and representatives
throughout the world

A catalogue record for this book is available
from the British Library.

ISBN 0–333–64555–3 (hardcover)
ISBN 0–333–64556–1 (paperback)

First published in the United States of America 1996 by
ST. MARTIN'S PRESS, INC.,
Scholarly and Reference Division,
175 Fifth Avenue,
New York, N.Y. 10010

ISBN 0–312–16046–1

Library of Congress Cataloging-in-Publication Data
Addictive behaviour : molecules to mankind : perspectives on the
nature of addiction / edited by Adrian Bonner and James Waterhouse.
p.   cm.
Includes bibliographical references and index.
ISBN 0–312–16046–1 (cloth)
1. Substance abuse.   I. Bonner, Adrian.   II. Waterhouse, J. M.
(James M.)
RC564.A3235   1996
616.86—dc20   95–53928
                                                          CIP

10   9   8   7   6   5   4   3   2   1
05   04   03   02   01   00   99   98   97   96

Printed and bound in Great Britain by
Antony Rowe Ltd, Chippenham, Wiltshire

To Gill, Adam and Kirsten for their patience

Contents

PART III   ADDICTIONS AND THE STUDY OF MIND

PART IV   MOLECULES, MOOD AND ADDICTIVE BEHAVIOUR

PART V   ALCOHOL ABUSE IN SOCIETY

List of Tables

Foreword

Timothy J. Peters

King's College School of Medicine and Dentistry

The challenges of addiction remain one of the major unresolved problems of the twentieth century in western society. It is a problem consequent upon increasing affluence and, as such, is fast spreading to developing countries. In the past, monoaddictions, i.e. alcohol, tobacco or illicit drugs, were the order of the day. Increasingly, however, polydrug misuse and multiple cross-addictions are presenting us with additional difficult clinical problems.

It is against this background that this study has been presented, largely reflecting the principal interests of the well-established Addictive Behaviour Centre at the Roehampton Institute in south-west London. The chapters reflect a spectrum of concern from the molecule to the community with emphasis on the latter hues. This is much in keeping with current thinking on optimal clinical practice, i.e. prevention, detection and treatment, where possible in a primary care setting. This emphasis also reflects the long-standing philanthropic philosophy of the Roehampton Institute and its constituent colleges.

This volume guides us through the biological, psychological, medical, forensic and clinical challenges of this fascinating group of addictions, explaining both the individuality and the thematic aspects of the various addictive processes. Thought-provoking challenges to the reader, specific case studies, pragmatic advice and the distillation of the latest research make this study an essential requirement for the undergraduate and postgraduate student and for their teacher. In addition, the research worker will find much of interest. The editors are to be warmly congratulated on this invaluable contribution to the literature.

Acknowledgements

The editors would like to thank all those involved in the development of this text. It provides a review of the objectives of the Addictive Behaviour Centre, Roehampton. The Centre is concerned with research into the nature of the addictions and the application of such academic studies into the minimisation of harm in individuals and society by education and prevention. Particular thanks are addressed to the Rector and staff of Roehampton Institute, London, for enthusiastically supporting the establishment of the Centre.

We are indebted to Professor Hamid Ghodse (Division of Addictive Behaviour, St George's Medical School, London) and Professor Timothy Peters (Department of Clinical Biochemistry, King's College School of Medicine and Dentistry, London) for their moral and academic support of the Addictive Behaviour Centre.

Thanks must also go to the teaching team of the MSc Behavioural Biology and Healthcare programme, at Roehampton, who have helped in the academic supervision of some contributors to this compilation and continue to provide a stimulating academic environment in which these and other activities flourish.

Notes on the Contributors

Abdulla A.-B. Badawy, Research Scientist, Biomedical Research Laboratory, Cardiff Community Healthcare NHS Trust, Whitchurch Hospital, Cardiff, Wales.

Adrian Bonner, Director of the Addictive Behaviour Centre, Roehampton Institute, London.

Sarah Brien, Researcher, Addictive Behaviour Centre, Roehampton Institute, London.

Woody Caan, Director of Research & Development, Lifespan Healthcare, Douglas House, Cambridge.

Mary Chad, Senior Lecturer, School of Health Studies, University of Portsmouth.

Margaret Cooksey, Course Director, Kingston and St Georges NHS College of Health Studies, London.

Paul E. Davis, Consultant Clinical Psychologist, SW Thames Regional Drug and Alcohol Team.

Chris Eberhardie, Reader in Neuroscience Nursing, Atkinson Morley's Hospital, Wimbledon.

Gwen Hewitt, Director of Health Studies, Roehampton Institute, London.

Colin Martin, Researcher, Addictive Behaviour Centre, Roehampton Institute, London.

Margaret Millar, Senior Lecturer in Health Studies, North East Surrey College of Technology, Ewell.

Catherine Otter, Research Officer, Addictive Behaviour Centre, Roehampton Institute, London.

Vinood Patel, Research Scientist, Department of Clinical Biochemistry, King's College School of Medicine and Dentistry, London.

J. J. Payne-James, police surgeon with the Metropolitan Police, London.

David Peers, Senior Lecturer, London School of Fashion, London.

Victor R. Preedy, Senior Lecturer, Department of Clinical Biochemistry, King's College School of Medicine and Dentistry and Reader in Tissue Pathology, Roehampton Institute, London.

Peter Richardson, Senior Lecturer, King's College School of Medicine and Dentistry and Consultant Cardiologist, King's College Hospital, London.

Penny Simpson, Senior Lecturer, School of Health Studies, University of Portsmouth.

Deborah Stanbury, Research Officer, Addictive Behaviour Centre, Roehampton Institute, London and Inner London Probation Service.

Gerry Waldron, Senior Registrar, Department of Public Health Medicine, Dumfries and Galloway Health Board, Scotland.

James Waterhouse, Addictive Behaviour Centre, London, and Universities of Manchester and Liverpool (John Moores).

Howard Why, Research Fellow in Cardiology, King's College Hospital, London.

Introduction

Adrian Bonner and James Waterhouse

In previous generations, dependence on alcohol, other drugs, and excessive behaviours, such as compulsive gambling, were regarded as personal issues. The fate of the individual was regarded as unfortunate, caused by a combination of a failure of personal circumstances and was possibly self induced. Whilst drug use has been common in human society for many centuries, societal control by peers, families, the Church and legislative means has been important. Those individuals whose maladapted behaviour was not contained dropped out of society either becoming 'mentally ill' and/or homeless.

In the 1990s public awareness, in Europe and the United States, of the links between infected drug-users and the human immune deficiency virus (HIV), and the increasing number of reports of drug-related crimes, have put what was previously a personal issue onto the main public agenda. HIV and crime-related factors are only part of the threat to public health and to the fabric of society. Modern working environments depend increasingly on high technology and a reduced workforce. This new industrial organisation has generated stress-related conditions in individuals in the working and non-working populations. The need for a high level of vigilance by key workers, such as those supervising the safe operation of an industrial chemical plant or driving a train, is vital: human failure can be catastrophic. The conclusion, therefore, is that individuals whose behaviours become excessive and out of control are the concern of society as a whole.

The response to problems of addiction arises from governmental and non-governmental agencies. In the UK, at a governmental level the Home Office has produced an agenda on the social, socio-medical and epidemiological aspects of drug misuse. The Department of Health's total spending for combating drug misuse has increased from £15.5 million in 1990–1 to more than £25 million in 1994–5. In April 1993 local authorities in the UK were given responsibility by the Department of Social Security for assessing the needs of client groups and for purchasing services and resources. In the Government's strategy for Health set out in *Health of the Nation*[1] a key target is to reduce the percentage of drug misusers who report sharing needles from 20 per cent (1990) to 10 per cent in 1997 and 5 per cent by 2000. Approximately £526 million was spent combating drug misuse by the UK government in 1993–4.

As far as research is concerned, the Medical Research Council (MRC) spent £2.7 million on research relating to addiction, including smoking and alcohol in 1992–3 and in 1994 published MRC *Field Review: The Basis of Drug Dependence.*[2] In the USA most research is provided by the National Institute on Drug Abuse (NIDA), with funding of $550 million in 1992. In Europe the Federal Ministry for Research and Technology has a budget of DM4 million in 1994 for drug related activities.

In addition to government-funded agencies, non-governmental agencies such as the Salvation Army, the Alcohol Recovery Project and Alcoholics Anonymous make a significant contribution to minimising the harm caused to individuals by their addictive life-styles. Additionally, an increasing number of counselling services, residential detoxification and rehabilitation, needle- and syringe-exchange schemes, advice and aftercare services are being developed in the community by statutory and independent agencies. These approaches to alcohol and drug-abuse and eating disorders are focused on individuals and families: it is these local issues which are the concern of this book. A brief insight into accessing data on the extent of alcohol abuse in society is provided in Section V.

Although national resources are limited in this aspect of healthcare, in comparison with the acute services, there is increasing funding and activity, by Western governments, into the research and treatment in specific areas of substance misuse. Unfortunately, research into addiction is fragmented: in the UK, the *MRC Field Review: The Basis of Drug Dependence* in 1994 has recommended that 'the disparate disciplines with an interest in addiction research need to be brought together to allow ideas to spread both between clinical and basic scientists and between basic scientists with different approaches'. 'An area of high priority . . . includes . . . multidisciplinary research that integrates:

  (i) basic and clinical studies;
 (ii) social and biological approaches;
(iii) findings from animal studies with work with humans.'

Undoubtedly, biological, psychological and social factors are important in the development and maintenance of addictive behaviours in individuals. However, because of the highly specialised nature of these disciplines and the variety of methodologies employed by researchers working in these areas, a multidisciplinary approach is not easy. There is a need for training and improved communication between disciplines.

As a contribution to facilitating this communication a conference was organised at Roehampton Institute, London, in 1993 in order to bring together representatives, from various disciplines, for discussions on the nature of addiction. Contributions to this compilation have developed from the discussions following the conference and are aimed at providing reviews of developments in psychology and the biomedical sciences where insights into the nature of addiction are resulting from an increasingly multidisciplinary perspective.

This developing view of addictive behaviours is considered within a biopsychological and social perspective. Major advances in technology and the development of research strategies in these fields of study are producing data and an increasing amount of information on brain and behaviour. However, the research approaches used by these disparate disciplines are not always compatible and are open to interpretive difficulties. The problems of inappropriate methodology are addressed in the last chapter.

Included in the Roehampton conference were presentations from healthcare professionals who had completed MSc dissertations in related areas to the addictions. Although these research projects were conducted within the relatively short time-span of six months and so need more data and analysis before achieving autonomous scientific status, they do indicate the potential value of such pilot studies into unique populations. Four of these projects are presented as case studies in this volume.

It is hoped that this volume will not only summarise the current state of knowledge in some important areas of the study of addictions but also point the way forward for more interdisciplinary communication and better designed investigations.

NOTES

1. *Health of the Nation* (London: HMSO, White Paper, July 1992).
2. *MRC Field Review: The Basis of Drug Dependence* (London: Medical Research Council, 1994) pp. 1–96.

Part I
Addictions in Society

1 From Toads to Toddies: An Overview of Addictive Behaviour

Paul E. Davis

Addictive behaviour concerns behaviours which are appetitive (i.e. characterised by a desire to satisfy an 'appetite') and excessive. The 'excessive appetite'[1] may be for consumption of drugs, alcohol, chocolate or any number of other substances; or it may be a behaviour such as gambling , eating, golf, fishing, playing computer games, stealing, or even working – you name it, it can become an addiction. Given this diversity, it seems likely that our search for a common understanding of the addictions will have to take account of more than one theoretical approach, and will probably include a combination of biological, sociological and psychological factors. The remainder of this chapter attempts to give a 'taste' of these combined factors.

Firstly, and particularly with respect to substances, it is important to recognise that not all are used in a dependent way, substances can be used in an **experimental** way (the vast majority of aerosol/ glue sniffers are young people who try it out only a few times). And they can be used in a **recreational** way (most cannabis smokers and gamblers would describe their behaviours as such). Of course **dependent** use is the one most likely to create medical, psychological and social problems but **problem** use can occur at all three levels (many glue sniffing deaths occur amongst people trying it out for the first time; and many road traffic accidents are related to alcohol consumed 'recreationally').

HISTORICAL AND CULTURAL COMPONENTS

Chemicals which are necessary to sustain normal bodily functions are not 'drugs'. Chemicals which, on the other hand, are taken to produce pleasant feelings, an altered state of consciousness or for whatever other desired effect, are, and have been sought after throughout the history

3

of mankind and throughout every extant culture. There is evidence of the fermentation of cereals by Neolithic Man, and Stone Age beer jugs have been found.[2] Hallucinogenic drugs, which include many naturally occurring substances, have been used by many different cultures in religious ceremonies (for example mescaline, which is obtained from a cactus in Central America was used by ancient civilisations there). The association of hallucinogenics with witchcraft is well known – the witch's toad secretes bufotenine and 'magic' mushrooms, were no doubt also dropped into the cauldron. 'Toad licking', literally, has recently been rediscovered (an article reporting this practice in England appeared recently in the national press) which demonstrates the lengths people will go to for an 'experience'.

Opium use also has its place in world history, including a long history of use in Britain. It is well known that many famous authors and poets were users, including Byron, Coleridge, Keats, Shelley, and Scott. And of course the famous Sherlock Holmes character regularly injected himself with cocaine without any apparent fear of legal or other ill consequences. The use of opium has been influenced by political and economic factors – wars between nations have been fought over the supplies of opium, and the fall of the Shah of Iran in the late 1970s had a major influence on the production and supply of opium in the USA and Europe, contributing in part to the increased prevalence of heroin misuse in this country in the 1980s.

Ghodse[3] describes the history of another drug, now known as a food, in order to show how social, cultural and economic forces have influenced drug use. The story of coffee has parallels with virtually every other drug. As was the case with cannabis, amphetamines, LSD, etc., coffee at one time was used in religious ceremonies and as a medicine in the Arabic countries where the plant is indigenous. It was first consumed by chewing the beans or infusing the leaves, but in the fourteenth century the techniques of roasting and grinding the beans were developed which then led to its widespread use as a **recreational** drug. Technological innovations with other drugs have similarly had major influences in their use – for example, the discovery of how to distil alcohol in the Middle Ages in Britain to produce 'spirits' altered the pattern of alcohol use, as did the technology for refining coca leaves, modifying opium into its derivatives, and the acquisition of the chemical 'know-how' for producing amphetamines and LSD.

Coffee drinking further increased in Islamic countries with the banning of alcohol by the Koran – an example of how the banning of one drug is often compensated for by the increased use of another. The fashion to drink in coffee houses became associated with people thought of as dissidents and anti-establishment figures. Coffee houses became centres of dissent which then led to State control – attempts at banning coffee were made, and once prohibition failed coffee was instead heavily taxed. The coffee houses then became valuable sources of revenue for the authorities. Once part of the economy of a country is 'institutionalised' and it becomes difficult for the national budget to do without this source of revenue – the parallels with the banning of alcohol in the USA and the status of alcohol in the UK economy are obvious.

During the seventeenth century coffee drinking spread to Europe and a similar history was repeated there. The spread of drugs today is much more rapid, partly because of the rapid changes in transport seen in this century, partly because of the movement of large numbers of people around the world, and partly because the media today is more global and influential. These factors have resulted in many more people than ever being exposed to drug-taking practices of another culture. Out of their traditional and cultural constraints, drugs which in one country are relatively harmless can have devastating effects (the introduction of alcohol for example to the Indian cultures of America and the introduction of cocaine use to cultures outside South America).

Returning to coffee, it is interesting that its popularity declined for reasons beyond State control or any 'demand reduction strategies' of the time – the clientele of the coffee houses in England started to frequent clubs as 'the meeting place', and the heyday of the coffee house was over, hastened as well by the importation of tea and its emergence as the 'national beverage'.

Another parallel between coffee and other drugs is in its use as a reason for a social gathering – the coffee morning shares much with the sherry reception, the cocktail party, etc. Many cannabis smokers only smoke in social situations, the same for solvent abusers; and injecting drug users often report the importance of injecting in a communal setting (although with the increased awareness most injectors have about the risks of HIV transmission, the habit of sharing injecting equipment is now, one hopes, decreasing). The drug then, in part, becomes a focus for group identity and a reason for the group coming together, and this 'group' influence is clearly often one of the important factors in how and why a drug is used. Where a drug is banned, these social groups sometimes develop into sub-cultures with the possible consequent production of numerous new problems.

The point has been made that there are many parts of the world which can be used for the cultivation of drugs: vineyards in Europe, cannabis crops in Africa, opium poppies in many parts of Asia, coca plantations in South America, and tobacco in North America, to name some of the more obvious examples. This is not to say that the whole world and its inhabitants are consumed with drugs. The point is that we are all drug users to some extent, it is statistically abnormal **not** to use a drug. The term 'drug-taker' is sometimes used as a pejorative term, as a way of identifying someone who is involved in a deviant form of behaviour; to some extent this distinction between 'acceptable' drug use (alcohol, 'over the counter' medicines, caffeine and, to a decreasing extent, tobacco smoking) and unacceptable is arbitrary, and in part serves to make drinkers etc. feel more comfortable about their own drug use. The factors which distinguish the acceptability of different drugs are these social, cultural and historical factors rather than the chemical properties of the drug.

THE NATURE OF DEPENDENCY

Some of the problems involved in defining the state of dependency may be illustrated by a clinical example – take the case of a young man who works very successfully in the City, drives a Porsche, carries a mobile 'phone, and who 'snorts' (i.e. inhales a powder into a nostril where the drug is rapidly absorbed by the numerous small blood vessels) anything from $\frac{1}{2}$ to 5g of cocaine every day, and has done so for the last two years. Whilst using cocaine he is energetic, fun to be with, and capable at work; any interruption of his habit, on the other hand, leads to sleep problems, poor concentration, irritability, lethargy and depression, and so he has learned not to be left without a supply of his drug for anything longer than half a day. We can assume he is dependent on cocaine, yet it is likely that he does not have a tolerance to the drug nor that he has any other signs of a physical dependency. The expression and severity of psychological dependency will be shaped by a variety of internal and external factors, including his employment and financial circumstances, his relationships and social support, his personality characteristics and other social and psychological factors. For these reasons a description of dependence needs to draw on physical, psychological, and sociological factors, as shown in the World Health Organisation's description: 'a state, psychic and sometimes physical, resulting from the interaction between the living organism and the drug, characterised by behavioural and other responses that always include a compulsion to take the drug on a continuous or periodic basis in order to experience its psychic effects and sometimes to avoid the discomfort of its absence'.[3]

The relationship between the physical and psychological aspects of dependence described in the WHO definitions is often misunderstood. The two are not opposites – for example the severity of withdrawal is often strongly influenced by psychological factors and, conversely, the psychological consequences of withdrawal may be entirely a feature of physical changes (for example, depression following cocaine withdrawal in the case above). Physical and psychological dependence are perhaps better thought of as different views of the same phenomenon, one expressed in terms of cellular functioning, the other in terms of thoughts, feelings and drives. With this in mind, the concept of drug dependence may be examined in the light of the contribution of physical, psychological, and social factors.

Physical and Biological Factors

Signs of tolerance and withdrawal symptoms are the two main biological features of dependency. Most drugs are used because they have an effect on the central nervous system (CNS). For some drugs tolerance develops, that is the CNS responds in such a way as to reduce the effects of repeated drug administration, meaning that the drug user has to take more of the drug in order to get the same effect. Many people dependent on benzodiazepines, for example, consume many times the normal dose without getting the same tranquillising effect they used to get with much smaller doses. If the drug use is interrupted then there is a loss of tolerance and previously safe doses become lethal (which is why lapses after a period of abstinence can prove fatal).

Tolerance does not develop equally to all of the effects of a drug; for example tolerance to the euphoric and analgesic effects of opiates develops rapidly, whilst there is little or no tolerance to the action of opiates on the bowel. Ceiling effects occur for some actions of a drug but not for others; for example, with barbiturates there is a ceiling of tolerance beyond which a dose will be fatal. This is different from the ceiling effects of a drug's dosage – seen, for example, in a cigarette smoker who never goes above 25 per day, or the tranquilliser user who seems to reach an upper limit of, for example, 50 mg of diazepam, daily; consequences of over-consumption (in terms of physical/toxic effects or possibly also the financial, or social costs, etc.) outweighing for the user the desirable effects.

There are many mechanisms proposed to explain the development of tolerance, and most are described in terms of physical responses at the neuronal level. **Neuroadaptation** (the ability of brain cells to adapt to the presence of a drug) is an important concept in explaining the build-up of tolerance and the presence of a characteristic **withdrawal** syndrome if drug use ceases (see Chapter 12). When the drug is discontinued, the neuroadaptation leads to decompensation or rebound symptoms. These withdrawal symptoms typically have characteristics which tend to counterbalance the effects produced by the drug itself – withdrawal from stimulants such as cocaine and amphetamines leads to lethargy, sleepiness and low mood; while depressant drugs such as alcohol produce excitatory withdrawal symptoms such as agitation, tremor, etc.

Although the physical and biological factors are important influences on drug-taking behaviour, they are only a part of the overall picture and by themselves they are insufficient as an explanation or description of dependence. For example, people with severe pain may be prescribed opiates at doses which, after several months, will undoubtedly produce physical signs of dependency, particularly tolerance. As will be described later, there is, however, an absence of psychological and behavioural signs and symptoms of dependency, and in the absence of a social and cultural context the overall experience is not one of 'dependency'. Moreover, the relationship between the different physical features is poorly understood; for example, tolerance and withdrawal are in many ways related but do not always go together. Some drugs produce little tolerance yet a clear withdrawal syndrome is present (for example, cocaine); while for others the reverse is true (for example, pentazocine). Clearly the physical symptoms are not the sole basis of dependence; it is only when they are set in the context of psychological and social factors that the full meaning of dependence can be appreciated.

Psychological Factors

The acquisition and maintenance of dependence are markedly influenced by a range of psychological factors such as learning and personal characteristics. These learning factors may follow the rules of **operant conditioning** (i.e. the behaviour is controlled by the stimuli preceding it and the reinforcing consequences following it). These consequences may be positive reinforcers (never forget that many people use drugs because they enjoy the effects) or negative reinforcers (they may, for example, get rid of unpleasant withdrawal effects created by the drug in the first place; alcohol, tobacco, and opiates, for example, can produce strongly aversive withdrawal states and anything which reduces these, usually further drug taking, becomes a powerful reinforcer).

The sensations produced by a drug will vary between different people, at different times and in different settings. Expectancy also plays a large role in the effects obtained, and greatly influences the enjoyment of the drug as well as the severity of craving. Expectancy will be affected by the person's previous experiences, group and peer influences, the personality of the individual and many other psychological factors. Environmental stimuli can also become conditioned by the drug's effects so that they themselves become cues or triggers for craving or the desire to perform the addictive behaviour. The mechanism for this kind of learning is that of **classical conditioning**. The strong associations formed may not be so obvious: good news, certain settings, or taking the silver foil wrapping (in the case of injectors) off a chocolate biscuit! These cues, relating to the psychological and physical aspects of drug taking and its paraphernalia, are important aspects of learning. These factors are considered in therapy as discussed in Chapter 10.

Although individual personality characteristics undoubtedly contribute to the onset and maintenance of dependence, there is no evidence for an 'addictive personality'. People differ in their desire to experiment, their need for stimulation and their responses to problems, and some people will be more vulnerable than others. It is important to remember that some of the best childhood predictors of later substance use[4] have nothing to do with personality, but relate to the sex of the person (males tend to be more frequent and heavier users of most categories of substances other than prescribed anxiolytics), the availability of a drug and opportunities to try it out, and whether or not you have siblings or friends who are using a drug. It is known that people who try drugs, including legal ones, at an early age are more likely to try other, more illicit drugs later on. For dependent drug users, early childhood problems of **any** kind, including conduct disorders, truancy, childhood abuse, and emotional problems, is a predictor of their later drug use. Similarly, a family history of drug misuse is predictive. The mechanism for this relationship may be environmental or genetic; certainly in the case of alcohol dependency there is strong evidence, at least for men, of an inherited predisposition which then interacts with environmental and other factors.[5]

Sociological Factors

Both the acceptance of drug use by an individual and the immediate availability of drugs are predominantly determined by peer groups and other social factors. Roles such as those of 'skaghead', 'dealer', 'smoker', 'drinker', etc. may be rewarding for some people in that they contribute to a sense of personal identity or identification with the sub-group; and the various roles adopted may themselves perpetuate the substance misuse.

There are numerous social factors involved in 'fashions' for drugs, the need for a drug sub-culture, and how and why certain drugs are used in different groups. In addition, there are large cultural variables in the drugs used around the world (see Gossop, 1993, for an account of these).

IDENTIFYING A DEPENDENCY SYNDROME

What counts as addictive behaviour? In 1981 the WHO gave a checklist of the main criteria necessary for the assessment of the dependence syndrome:

1. Subjective awareness of a compulsion to take the drug or engage in the particular behaviour. This is sometimes referred to as 'craving' for the drug, a term which disguises what is a complex, personal and often intensely unpleasant experience. Craving includes ruminations about the activity or drug and where there are strong 'positive outcome expectancies' (i.e. an expectation that it will be fun or will reduce distress, etc.) the craving will intensify. Paradoxically, this may be particularly so if the drug or activity is unavailable and also when a small 'taster' or priming dose is experienced. Sometimes craving is described in terms of pleasurable anticipation; interestingly, for some the experience becomes aversive, which makes stopping much easier! This will be more fully explored in Chapter 11.

2. Increased tolerance to the drug/habituation of the reinforcing effects of the activity unless performed at greater frequency and/or intensity.

3. Increased salience of drug-seeking or other behaviour – as depen-

dency develops, simply obtaining the drug or the opportunity to engage in the addictive behaviour assumes increasing importance. Thus in our cocaine user example, obtaining and using the drug may start to take precedence over previously important activities, even to the extent of risking losing job, family and health.

4. Narrowing of the repertoire of the addictive behaviour – the pattern of the excessive behaviour becomes increasingly stereotyped, as evidenced, for example, by the smoker who develops a daily routine of when and where cigarettes are smoked, and having a preferred brand.

5. Repeated withdrawal symptoms – when the behaviour is prevented or stops, discomfort and distress are experienced and these may continue for several weeks if not months, varying, of course, with the substance and addictive behaviour.

6. Rapid reinstatement of the syndrome following a period of abstinence – this is more the case with substances than other addictions; tolerance and withdrawal symptoms can reappear within a few days of relapse even after long periods of abstinence.

7. Relief or avoidance of withdrawal symptoms – using the drug or activity to relieve the unpleasantness of withdrawal can become a strong reinforcer of the addiction and, once learned as a solution, is difficult to replace. Avoiding withdrawal in this way can become increasingly important to the extent that, for example, the severely dependent drinker will save some alcohol in order to relieve withdrawal the next morning, even when this means curtailing drinking the night before.

Not all of these need to be present in every instance of addictive behaviour, but most of them are usually evident to a greater or lesser extent. Evidence of any single criterion such as neuroadaptation is insufficient, which is why it is incorrect to describe someone who has developed tolerance to opiates prescribed for the management of pain as having an addictive behaviour. The key features of the syndrome are: a **compulsion** or strong desire to engage in the behaviour; an overwhelming priority or **salience** being given to the behaviour; an impaired capacity to **control** the behaviour; and **distress** if prevented from carrying out the behaviour. The whole picture has to be taken into account, and the relative contribution of the severity of each criterion considered before labelling a behaviour as an 'addiction'.

CONCLUSIONS

Possible aetiological factors range from the level of neurotransmitters and nerve plate endings, through psychological explanations which derive from learning theory, theories of drive, motivation, and personality, to social and cultural influences. Given that dependence and addictive behaviours are described in these sociological biological and psychological terms, it is unlikely that any **one** cause or explanation will ever be found. Rather, research which will advance our knowledge and understanding of the nature, causes and treatments of 'excessive appetites' is likely to draw on several different branches of science and professional disciplines. Addictive behaviour is not unique in this respect; it is, however, one of the reasons why our understanding and knowledge remain relatively underdeveloped.

NOTES

1. J. Orford, *Excessive Appetites: A Psychological View of Addictions* (Chichester: John Wiley, 1985).
2. M. Gossop, *Living with Drugs*, 3rd edn (Aldershot: Arena-Ashgate, 1993).
3. A. H. Ghodse, *Drugs and Addictive Behaviour: A Guide to Treatment* (Oxford: Blackwell, 1989).
4. B. Segal, *Drugs and Behaviour: Cause, Effects and Treatment* (Lake Worth: Gardner Press, 1988).
5. D. W. Goodwin, 'Biological Factors in Alcohol Use and Abuse: Implications for Recognising and Preventing Alcohol Problems in Adolescence', *International Review of Psychiatry*, 1 (1/2) (1989):41–50.

2 Addictions in Industrialised Society

Adrian Bonner

In the previous chapter the nature of addictive behaviour has been shown to be complex. There are many factors involved which lead to **compulsion, salience, impaired control** of behaviour, and **distress** if the individual is prevented from carrying out the behaviour. Although biological and psychological factors are involved in the origins and maintenance of the behaviour, social factors are also important. Reference has already been made to the legal, economic and social aspects of substances which are associated with addictive behaviours. In the twentieth century the rise and changing nature of industrialised societies have influenced the nature and importance of a range of addictions. In an industrialised society some addictive behaviours are thought to result from affluence (resulting in increasing availability of alcohol and other substances which might become addictive), frustration (due to unobtainable expectations generated by the global advertising), job stress (modern management strategies demand more commitment from the declining number of individuals in work, with consequences for their families), and the stress of unemployment. These manifestations in industrialised groups become important when their economic consequences are considered; the occupational health aspects of substance misuse are, therefore, becoming increasingly an issue in personnel management.

In the last decade of the twentieth century the links between *substance misuse* and crime, promiscuous sexual behaviour and the spread of HIV have become high profile news items in the media. Few sections of the community are unaffected by the growing problem of drug taking in young people and drug-related crime. Law enforcement agencies appear to be having limited success in reducing the amount of drug material available for sale in the community. The police, health promotion organisations and other agencies are now putting considerable energies into various initiatives aimed at changing the behaviour of young people. Addictions to alcohol and drugs provide a very significant threat to the fabric of society and the commercial world will not

13

be unaffected by this growing set of problems. Other addictions, including *gambling and smoking*, are also frequently encountered. However, *addictions to love, sexuality* and *work* [1, 2, 3] are less well known but are perhaps as equally devastating to the affected individuals as other addictions. All of these addictions will be manifested either directly or indirectly in the workplace. There are many myths, but it is patently clear that alcohol, drugs and perhaps other addictions exact a crippling cost at work in the form of accidents and absenteeism, poor decision making, poor concentration and disciplinary problems.[4]

Workaholism suggests a great capacity and passion for work and is a term often used to applaud a person's commitment and zeal. Conversely, the label also implies an addictive dependence on work. Whilst an individual would not particularly worry about being described as a workaholic, the same person would desperately avoid being classified as an alcoholic, drug addict, or compulsive gambler.

Workaholism is the acceptable face of addiction compared to other behaviours, or is it? The employed members of our society spend approximately 50 per cent of their waking hours at work. It is not surprising, therefore, that the working environment has a potentially major influence on attitudes to health behaviours.

ALCOHOL

The importance of alcohol and drug misuse by employees has been recognised for some time. It has been estimated that alcohol misuse in industry results in over £964.4 million of losses due to sickness absence each year.[5] The annual value of industrial days lost through alcohol consumption in the UK in 1987 was estimated to be over £1.7 billion, excluding the value of lost productivity, accidents and injury.[6] In 1991 8.4 million working days were lost during the year.[7] The trends are not encouraging, as various indicators point to escalating problems ahead. A report from the Royal College of Psychiatrists (1986) reviewed the changes between 1970 and 1985:

Percentage increases in alcohol consumption	+38%
Hospital admissions for alcohol dependence	+97%
Cirrhosis deaths	+80%
Drinking and driving convictions	+184%

This view is supported by the General Household Survey in 1989 which found increased consumption of alcohol per head: '1960 . . . 4.3 litres; 1988 . . . 7.6 litres'. The survey also found that 27 per cent of men in the UK drank more than the medically recommended 'sensible limits' of 21 units per week.

In an analysis of the 1984 General Household, Jeoman[8] found higher rates of sickness absence in male heavy drinkers in all three main industrial sectors and in the major occupational groups. An exception to this was in young heavy drinkers who appeared to be no more likely to take sickness absence than their young colleagues who drank more moderately. Heavy drinkers who smoke as well are even more likely to be away from work. This was true of all age groups. The data did not reveal any association between drinking patterns and sickness absence in female employees. This is probably explained by the small sample size. There was considerable variation between different sectors and occupations. No generalisation can be made from the data without more detailed information on patterns of alcohol consumption and sickness absence for different types of individuals.

The financial costs to industry have been reviewed by Maynard:[5]

	*£million**
Sickness absence	964.37
Housework services	64.78
Unemployment	222.23
Premature deaths	870.76
Total	2122.14

* England and Wales 1990 prices.

Other costs to society include costs to the National Health Service: £146 000 000; material damage (e.g. road accident damage): £138 000 000; and costs of criminal activities (policing and legal costs): £50 000 000.

A less well-publicised issue is that of premature deaths. Alcoholic groups have death rates which are double that of the normal population. There are considerable losses to industry caused by the loss of key executives or highly trained and experienced management. Company directors have the highest death rate from liver cirrhosis (22 times the general population). The damaging effects of alcohol in the workplace have been reviewed by Pratt.[9]

Recent research suggests that moderate drinking results in increased sickness absence and lack of promotion in men[10] and that alcohol consumption was strongly related to grade of employment – relatively high levels of alcohol consumption being common among top administrators.[11] There appears to be a mismatch between the perceptions of senior directors and personnel directors with regard to the importance of health of the workforce and the management of problems such as excessive alcohol consumption. Smoking, stress, back problems and heart disease are viewed by both sets of managers as the major concerns to their organisations. Alcohol consumption was thought to be only moderately serious. The larger the company, the more likely alcohol consumption was recognised as a concern. Personnel directors were concerned about the effect of alcohol on team morale and employee relations, in contrast to senior directors who were more concerned about discipline.[12]

SMOKING

The addiction to smoking has a wide range of direct and indirect consequences for the health of employees. Smoking is the principle cause of several debilitating and often fatal diseases: chronic obstructive lung disease (COLD),bronchitis, small airways disease, emphysema, pulmonary fibrosis, cancer, and cardiovascular disease. The World Health Organisation[13] has investigated the potentially harmful interaction of smoking with materials encountered in the workplace. There is also growing concern regarding the health consequences of passive smoking and this occupational stressor is being addressed by an increasing number of organisations. A MORI survey[14] revealed that four out of five workers would agree to some form of restriction. Support for a restriction of smoking areas is higher in non-manual workers (85 per cent) than manual groups (79 per cent). Women and white collar workers strongly believe that companies and organisations should have set policies on smoking.

Estimates of the economic and social consequences of excessive alcohol consumption and smoking can only be imprecise at best. Such studies take no account of the alcohol-related illnesses which lead to high healthcare and staffing costs. Auditing the commercial consequences of the range of addictions is fraught with difficulties but, nevertheless, this component of a nation's economy must be addressed.

THE DEVELOPMENT OF ADDICTIVE BEHAVIOURS

Paul Davis, in the first chapter, discussed the problems of identifying **dependency** as a syndrome and, at first sight, there might appear to be little apparent similarity between the various addictions. However, there are some common underlying factors which are important in addressing the problem of addictive behaviours as human-resource-management issues, an increasingly important question in the commercial world of the 1990s. There is a growing awareness that the traditional medical model is not always the most useful context in which to identify and manage the problem. From a psychological perspective, addictions are considered to be motivational problems.[15] Various pieces of evidence suggest that dependence results from problems in early development of self-image. Drugs increase self-esteem and make one feel less inadequate, more accomplished, less insecure. From the perspective of occupational psychology, three main approaches to understanding motivation as applied to addiction include *decision theory*, which considers addicts to be individuals who work out the costs and benefits of their behaviour and make decisions that lead to the continuation of their addiction. *Drive theory* asserts that addicts are subject to powerful forces that energise and direct behaviour. These forces may result from the addiction tapping into existing drive mechanisms, creating disturbances in these drive mechanisms, or resulting from the acquisition of new drives. The *behaviourist approach* focuses on directly observable associations between behaviour and environmental events.

In workaholism, as in other addictions, success itself becomes a reward. The satisfaction of one set of needs creates an equally powerful set of secondary drives. These ideas can be used to explore the motivation of particular types of individuals such as Type A personalities. Pace *et al.*[15] suggests that managers who persist in a Type A behaviour pattern (marked by impatience, irritation, anger, aggression) do so to the detriment of employee involvement. Extreme Type A behaviour is seen as addictive and related to other addictive behaviours; compared to Type B managers, Type A managers are more likely to be workaholics and stress-prone. The need to change dysfunctional or extreme Type A behaviour on a personal and organisational level should be an important personnel management objective. More recent discussions on the consistency of Type A behaviour include issues such as why these individuals present themselves as Type A in their occupational setting and display Type B characteristics at home. The nature of *hostility* in these behavioural types and the wider range of mental health problems such as eating disorders (see Chapter 11) are presently being explored.

Addictions have an underlying biological basis,[16] knowledge of which is important for understanding the natural forces which are imprisoning individuals in particular addictive behaviours. There is substantial evidence that some individuals are genetically predisposed to addictive behaviours such as alcohol-seeking. During recent years, advances in the biological sciences have begun to open up the Pandora's box of genetic markers which could lead to the early detection of individuals who are genetically more prone to becoming addicted to pharmacologically active compounds and perhaps situational stimuli important in priming and maintaining addictive behaviours (see Chapter 12).

THE MANAGEMENT OF ADDICTIONS IN THE WORKPLACE

There are some indicators that an employee has a problem. These include increased sick leave, loss of efficiency, increasing numbers of mistakes, interpersonal problems and accidents. Alcohol intake affects a wide range of physiological variables; the risk factors associated with a particular type of job will obviously depend upon the skills utilised by the employee.[14] Heavy drinking in salesmen and marketing executives (and similar occupations) occurs with separation from normal social and sexual relationships. Some occupations are more vulnerable than others as assessed in terms of liver cirrhosis mortality. The industrial response to these issues is two fold: *alcohol education*, including educating the workforce about potential alcohol problems should be complemented with *dealing with the individual who develops an alcohol problem*.

A systematic way of managing such problems is addressed by the extensive and well-developed 'Employee Assistance Programs' in the United States, now being taken up by an increasing number of UK companies. There is considerable agreement on the need for and type of assistance required to deal with alcohol and drug problems among workers. One area of great contention, however, is *drug testing*. The National Association of Manufacturers in the United States, for example, suggests that drug testing 'should be done in a fair and equitable manner with due concern for the employee's privacy'. It opposes any legislation that would prohibit employers from testing applicants and employees for substance abuse, believing that 'testing policy' should be left to the company. The United States Government Drug-Free Federal Workplace Executive Order (1986) instructs each federal agency to establish its own policy and programme to test for the use of illegal drugs by employees. There are many objections to this approach.[17] Fear of abuse of the information by employers, inaccuracy of the screening and the metabolic breakdown of misused substance in the body are often cited by opponents of drug testing such as AFL–CIO (the US federation of trade unions) and the Canadian Labour Congress. There are obvious benefits to a company in pre-employment screening. To safeguard its generous sick leave benefits and pension scheme investments, a company may wish to avoid recruiting an 'at risk' employee. However, unless testing is carried out at frequent intervals and the method is well validated the exercise will be pointless.

Random drug testing is becoming more common in UK companies. The 1992 Transport and Works Act obliges employers in the transport sector to prevent employees from working under the influence of alcohol and drugs. The majority of British Rail employees are instructed not to consume alcohol eight hours prior to commencing work and a maximum of four pints of beer (or equivalent) in the previous sixteen hours. Random testing for drugs and alcohol is also carried out on the 80 000 British Rail and 14 000 London Underground employees who have been designated as 'safety critical'. Other organisations such as Nuclear Electric and Shell carry out tests after incidents where there is cause for suspicion.[18]

Employers are faced with three specific areas of law in relation to addictions in the workplace. At *common law* an employer may be guilty of negligence where a person has suffered personal injuries or economic loss as a result of an act of negligence committed in the course of employment. Employers may also be guilty of a *criminal offence* for breach of statutory duty, such as not ensuring a 'safe system of work'. Thirdly, the employer may be in breach of *contract law* if, for example, an employee were suspended from duty or had his or her company car withdrawn as a result of an addiction problem.[18] The combination of profitability and legal liabilities relating to recent health and safety regulations is increasing the pressure on employers to consider alcohol and drug issues in their corporate planning.

The caring professions are not exempt from alcohol abuse and smoking. The paradox of nursing, one the best health-educated occupational groups, having high levels of alcohol abuse and smoking (see Chapter 16) suggests the importance of these activities as a response to job stress. The United Kingdom Central Council for Nursing (UKCC) has indicated that the number of nurses and midwives brought before its health committee for dependency problems has increased 146 per cent in 1992–3. In that year the number of alcoholics considered by the council tripled and those believed to have a drug-dependency problem rose by 50 per cent. In response to this developing problem the UKCC is presently considering the recommendation of alcohol/drug testing for staff suspected of being under the influence of drink and drugs while on duty.

Whilst policies on drugs and alcohol need not include testing, programmes established to drug-test employers should be set within the context of a clearly stated and comprehensive policy. Validation and quality control of the analytical testing procedures are important in drug and alcohol monitoring. However, in view of the legal liabilities referred to above, if such data are to have any value in law, the whole procedure of collection, storage, analysis, and interpretation of sample data must be tightly controlled. An example of this is given in Figure 1, in which a *chain of custody* involves a high level of security of the samples and reporting.

The effectiveness of pre-employment drug screening has been investigated by mathematical modelling techniques for decision making in the selection of policies on testing for drug use[19, 20] in 2537 US employees. Screening for marijuana or cocaine predicts a number of adverse employment outcomes. Marijuana-positive and cocaine-positive urines predicted increased employee turnover, injuries, disciplinary problems, and absences. This effect was lower in the second year after testing for marijuana-positive cases, suggesting that elevated risks may decrease after the first year of employment. Despite the experimental validity of this 'blinded' postal survey, there remains the problem of false positives and false negatives both of which have organisational costs (i.e. legal claims) and social costs. Additionally, proper comparison of the economic benefits and costs of drug screening requires more than simple comparisons of employed drug users and employed drug abstainers; for example, the true cost of any activity should be measured against the next best available alternative, i.e. why was the drug user selected in the first instance?

The moral, ethical and legal issues of drug and alcohol testing in the work have been reviewed by Raskin.[21]

Some of the problems of testing arise from a 'unitary' approach. That is the addiction is viewed from a solely physiological/toxicological perspective. As indicated above, addictions are primed and devel-

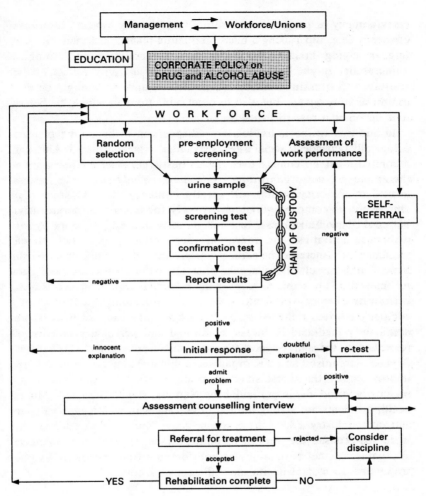

Figure 2.1 Flow diagram summarising the implementation of a workplace policy (courtesy MEDSCREEN Ltd, London).

oped by a number of factors which could be summarised as: biological, psychological and sociological. On this basis an 'at risk' employee or potential employee (in the case of pre-employment screening) perhaps should be considered in a more global framework. If objective testing is required, then surely psychological–biological profiling would be appropriate for particular situations. Where a particular job will carry a heavy responsibility for safety (e.g. driving a train), high level efficiency (e.g. supervising a mass production plant), or decision making (e.g. managing director) the individual's psychological and biological vulnerability might be assessed. This would not only reflect his/her resistance to stressful work, in which alcohol and drugs might be used as anti-anxiety agents, but also to other addictions in which the behaviour becomes a reward in itself.

In addition to the individual's predisposition to becoming pharmacologically dependent, social aspects should also be considered. Although, a company has no control over the domestic/personal environment of the employee, the *organisation itself might be addictive*. The 'mental health' of the organisation will greatly influence the behaviour of its employees. A company which is narrowly focused on corporate survival could become ruthless, lose all morality and ethics, adopt overtly dishonest activities, and focus on short term 'fixes'. Such an environment will increase the addictive tendencies of its workforce. Wilson Scheaf and Fassel[22] have argued that once the indicators have been recognised it is possible to recover the *addictive organisation* and bring it from its illusory world into reality. The philosophy and culture of a company is often reflected in its rate of absenteeism, and this is predominantly mediated by stress, emotional and personal problems experienced by the staff. Support for this comes from comparisons between Japanese-organised and UK-organised companies operating in the UK. In this survey the worst sickness-absence rate was found in public sector organisations, in particular the National Health Service.[23] Mental health problems are among the top three causes of sick leave in Britain and cost industry £3.7 billion every year. The need to address this issue has aroused the interest of both business and political agencies. The nature of the motivations of both organisation and the individual are central to mental health and efficiency of both.

PROFILING OF POTENTIAL ADDICTS

Age and gender are important factors in the development of particular addictions. In the case of alcohol abuse, young people drink differently from older people and traditional models of addiction and treatment work better with older populations than with younger ones. It is therefore important when developing approaches to early interventions to include tailoring the interventions to the specific problems of this age group, matching treatment according to individual responses to alcohol. By determining the specific function of alcohol for the individual it should be possible to change his/her life-style towards a lower risk strategy. The interplay between psychological and biological forces at different ages and across the sexes provides an enormous variation between individuals. In studying any addictive process it is, therefore, important to collect a wide range of data which could be integrated into the design of the treatment package. Profiling techniques might possibly be developed which integrate both psychological and biological assessments. Aspects of personality such as novelty seeking, reward dependence, and harm avoidance are reviewed in Section III of this book. From a biological perspective, metabolic approaches which relate not only to the genetic liability of certain individuals but also provide an insight into the physiological basis of **excessive appetites** are beginning to focus on the importance of tryptophan metabolism (see Chapters 4 and 12). Tryptophan is the dietary precursor of the important brain neurotransmitter, serotonin, which is implicated in the central modulation of a range of consummatory behaviours including eating, drinking and sexual behaviour. A combination of psychological and metabolic assessments, based on tryptophan biochemistry, might provide a useful profile. Profiling would, perhaps, require a response to a questionnaire and a small urine sample. The development of markers and profiles should permit the early detection of substance misusers and therapeutic interventions are more likely to lead to a positive outcome. How this might be applied to personnel selection and management in commercial organisations would depend on a range of factors including level of risk and ethos of the organisation.

FOR THE FUTURE

In the workplace the development of Employee Assistance Programmes should include a more detailed assessment of the needs of the individual. It is unlikely that this can be adequately achieved by a narrow medical model approach. The psychological–biological profiling outlined above will hopefully provide more useful indications as to the best way to help an employee. Profiling might also be applied to the recruitment of candidates to specific 'at risk' jobs.

Employee Assistance Programmes should also contain preventative education strategies. Individuals identified as being at risk require information about the nature of their addiction. Appropriate packaging of that information is essential in order that the individual will be enabled to modify his or her behaviour.

The commercial world has a very important part to play in the minimisation of addictive behaviours in the community. Although there are a number of support agencies in the community these have been shown to be primarily taken up by women. Employment-based strategies appear to be the most effective for men.

NOTES

1. T. C. Timmreck, 'Overcoming the Loss of a Love: Preventing Love Addiction and Promoting Positive Emotional Health', *Psychological Reports*, 66(2) (1990):515–28.
2. R. H. Earle, 'Sexual Addiction: Understanding and Treating the Phenomenon', *Contemporary Family Therapy: An International Journal*, 12(2) (1990):89–104.
3. M. C. Helldorfer, 'Church Professionals and Work Addiction', *Studies in Formative Spirituality*, 8(2) (1987):199–210.
4. F. Dickenson, *Drink and Drugs at Work: The Consuming Problem* (Institute of Personnel Management, 1988) VI, p. 133.
5. A. Maynard, 'Is It Helpful to Measure the Social Costs of Alcohol Misuse?' (Research Training information, Yorkshire Addictions Research, Training and Information Consortium, May 1992).
6. M. Powell, *Reducing the Cost of Alcohol in the Workplace: The Case for Employer Policies* (1990).
7. Editorial, 'Alcohol: Days Lost from Work', *The Times*, 18 November 1991.
8. L. M. Joeman, 'Alcohol Consumption and Sickness Absence: Analysis of the 1984 General Household Survey Data', Research Series Report 4 (1992).
9. O. Pratt, 'Review: Approaches to the Alcohol Problem in the Workplace', *Alcohol and Alcoholism*, 24 (5) (1989):453–64.
10. R. Jenkins, 'A Six-Year Longitudinal Study of the Occupation Consequences of Drinking over "Safe Limits" of Alcohol', *British Journal of Industrial Medicine*, 49 (1992):369–74.
11. M. G. Marmot, 'Alcohol Consumption and Sickness Absence: From Whitehall II Study', *Addiction*, 88 (1993):369–82.
12. *Attitudes Towards Alcohol in the Workplace* (1994), summary of the key findings of the research study conducted by MORI for the Health Education Authority, March 1994.
13. K. Rothwel, *The Interaction of Smoking and Workplace Hazards* (1992), Office of Occupational Health and Tobacco: Health Programme (World Health Organization, Geneva).
14. B. Hore, 'Alcohol and Work', *British Journal of Alcohol and Alcoholism*, 17 (2) (1982):72–9.

15. L. Pace, 'Addictive Type A Behavior Undermines Employee Involvement', *Personnel Journal*, 67(6) (1988):36–42.
16. D. W. Goodwin, 'Biological Factors in Alcohol Use and Abuse: Implications for Recognizing and Preventing Alcohol Problems in Adolescence', *Special Issue: Psychiatry and the Addictions: International Review of Psychiatry*, 1(1–2) (1989):41–9.
17. *Conditions of Work Digest: Alcohol and Drugs* (Geneva: International Labour Office, 1987).
18. 'British Companies Start to Test the Water', press release, 13 May 1994, London Incomes/Data Services Ltd.
19. H. Correa, 'An Application of Mathematical Models for Decision Making to the Selection of Policies on Testing for Drug Use', *International Journal of Addictions*, 26 (6) (1991):697–712.
20. J. Ryan, 'The Effectiveness of Preemployment Drug Screening in the Prediction of Employment Outcome', *Journal of Occupational Medicine*, 34 (11) (1992):1057–62.
21. C. Raskin, 'Drug and Alcohol Testing in the Workplace: Moral, Ethical and Legal Issues', *Bulletin on Narcotics*, XLV (2) (1993):45–83.
22. A. Wilson Schaef, *The Addictive Organisation* (New York: Harper & Row, 1988).
23. B. Clement, 'Staff of Japanese Firms in UK Take Less Sick Leave', *The Independent*, 11 March 1993, p. 5.

3 Aspects of Illegal Drug Misuse

Deborah Stanbury

INTRODUCTION

The relationship between drug use and the law is one which at first glance may appear obvious and clearly defined. Certainly the media often portray this relationship in simplistic and misleading terms: drugs are illegal and cause people who use them to behave in dishonest and violent ways. Such behaviours often constitute breaking the law in their own right. However, as was highlighted in the opening chapter of this book, the acceptability of certain drugs is influenced by social, cultural and historical factors and this acceptability therefore influences how the law deals with drug use. Until recently cannabis use was not considered to be harmful (NB: more recent opinion in Chapter 5) and on the whole was only used recreationally, despite the fact that it is a controlled drug under the law of this country. Alcohol and tobacco, however, are probably the two most harmful drugs used, yet their use is not prohibited by the law.

This chapter will therefore try to unravel some of the complex issues involved in trying to understand how illegal drug use in the United Kingdom relates to the law, in particular the criminal law, and then go on to discuss what further information and understanding crime-related statistics can teach us about the extent of drug use in general.

DRUG USE AND THE LAW

The first obvious statement that must be made is that not all drugs that have the potential to harm an individual are completely controlled under the law. Thus, for instance, many people have suffered the negative consequences of long-term tranquilliser use but, provided these drugs are properly prescribed, their use is not illegal. Or, for another example, solvent abuse is not in itself against the law but, as is well documented, can lead to serious injury or even death.

26

The two main laws concerning drugs are the Medicines Act (1968) and the Misuse of Drugs Act (1971). The former controls the way medicines are made and distributed. The Misuse of Drugs Act prohibits the non-medical use of certain drugs and places them in different classes. The penalties for offences involving a drug is dictated by the class it is in. Thus Class 'A' drugs such as heroin, cocaine and ecstasy carry the highest penalties, and Class 'C' drugs such as benzodiazapines and some amphetamines, the lowest. Official statistics for 1993 demonstrated that heroin and cocaine offenders were more likely to be imprisoned than to be fined or cautioned. On the other hand, LSD and ecstasy offenders (also Class 'A' drugs) were more likely to be cautioned first, then fined, with imprisonment being almost the last resort in terms of punishment. This differential treatment would appear to be influenced by popular and judicial perception of the seriousness and dangerousness of certain drugs as compared to others.

In addition to the class system for categorising drugs, the law also makes a distinction between the various illegal acts of possessing, manufacturing and trafficking controlled drugs. Thus an individual found in possession of a small quantity of illegal drugs, which in all likelihood is for personal use, will be dealt with under the law more leniently than a person believed to be involved in supplying that same drug. In fact, a regular dealer of a Class 'A' drug could ultimately be sentenced to life imprisonment under current British law.

The Misuse of Drugs Act also makes it an offence to allow anyone on one's premises to produce, give away or sell illegal drugs or even to offer to supply a controlled drug free of charge. Therefore, if a landlord or parent is aware that drugs are being used on their property and does nothing to stop it, they can be prosecuted. The law states that if a person finds what they believe to be an illegal drug they must immediately hand it over to someone allowed to possess controlled drugs such as a police officer, or alternatively destroy it. As well as legislating for the punishment of the offender, the law as contained in the 1986 Drug Trafficking Offences Act allows for the destruction of drugs seized by the authorities and the confiscation of any profit derived from drug dealing or importation.

DRUG USE AND OFFENDING

The above explanation in many ways represents the simplistic perception of the relationship between drug use and the law, i.e. drug use is illegal, and therefore those involved in it are breaking the law. However, in order to try to understand this relationship in greater depth, it must be acknowledged that the links do not end there. The types of criminal behaviour outlined above are what have been called 'drug-defined offences'.[1] These include offences that are defined by law in terms of the illegal use of a specific substance in various ways such as possession, supply and importation. The most common offence of this type is possession of cannabis which is extremely widespread and, as already indicated, not perceived as a criminal offence by a large number of the population. However, many other crimes are committed that involve the use of drugs but are not defined under either the Medicines Act or the Misuse of Drugs Act. Such offences can be divided into the further two categories of 'drug-inspired offences' including those of a dishonest nature committed to finance the purchasing of a supply of the desired substance and 'drug-induced offences' – those that occur as a result of the effect a substance can have on behaviour. The particular offences believed to be inspired by drug use include shoplifting, cheque-book fraud, theft and burglary, and self report studies would seem to indicate that only a fraction of this type of offence ever comes to light. An example of the drug-induced offences could be violence, although it would be wrong to assume that illegal drug use automatically leads to aggression. This could be the case with some stimulant drugs, but would be an unlikely result of a depressant such as heroin, despite, again, common popular perception of the automatically assumed relationship between drugs and violence.

It must be acknowledged, however, that the above categorisation of drug-related offences is in itself too simplistic. After all, is a drug-using woman convicted of prostitution committing a drug-inspired or a drug-induced offence? Or is the small time drug dealer only committing a drug-defined offence? Or could he (and most drug dealers are male) be dealing in illegal drugs as a way of supplementing his income to buy his own personal supply as well? Nevertheless, such a classification does help to point out something of the complex relationship between drug use and offending and does provide a starting point for a discussion as to how and why drug use and criminal behaviour are so closely linked.

Drugs and Offending: Statistics

Despite the illegal nature of drug misuse, many statistics are available that add to the overall picture of drug use in the United Kingdom. However, they cannot in themselves provide a total picture as the illegal nature of drugs means that much drug use and related crime goes unreported. Therefore whilst it may be justifiably assumed that some car thefts may well be linked to drug use, and although this type of crime is very likely to be reported due to the need for insurance claims to be made, its relationship to drugs will be unknown. Other offences that are considered to be 'victimless' crimes may also be missing from official statistics. Additionally, it is known that the clear-up rate for drug offences by the enforcement authorities must be very small. It is generally accepted that on average about one-quarter of all crimes are recorded; this figure for drug-related offences only is likely to be far lower. The British Crime Survey suggests that in 1991 about two million residents in the United Kingdom used cannabis, but only 2 per cent [approximately 40 000 people] were sentenced or cautioned for an offence related to its use.

However, attempts to obtain more accurate statistics regarding drug use and crime are being made. For instance, in the 1992 British Crime Survey, a sample of over 7000 people aged between twelve and 59 years living in England and Wales were asked about their use of twelve drugs which are controlled by law. The questions asked related to use of these drugs at any time during their lives and also to use of them during 1991. The results obtained showed that only 17 per cent of the sample had ever taken any of the included drugs at all and only 6 per cent admitted to using them during 1991. Perhaps not surprisingly, cannabis was the most commonly used drug; 5 per cent had taken it during 1991 and 14 per cent had used it during their past. With regard to age, the people most likely to have used illegal drugs fell into the 16–29 age bracket; 28 per cent of this group had used drugs, 14 per cent during 1991. This last statistic would therefore seem to confirm the widely held view that drugs are a 'young' problem. A recent study by Howard Parker of 776 14th and 15th year-olds from eight schools demonstrated that 36 per cent of the sample had tried illicit drugs.[2] Whether the conventional expectation that many young people will actually grow out of drug use and crime is correct is a further question related to this issue. Possibly the greatest indicator that this expectation is, in fact, correct comes from the knowledge that few known, i.e. registered, addicts are over the age of 40. The reasons for this are varied, but a major factor appears to be the wearing-down process of long-term involvement with drugs; people therefore could be said to grow out of drugs and crime. Alternatively, the incarceration or even death of long-term addicts may mean that they do not appear in official statistics.

Other statistics available on drug use and crime include those provided by the enforcement agencies. These records mainly cover the outcomes, in terms of convictions and seizures, of the police or Customs official's action taken against people who have committed drug offences as defined by the law.

Quantities of drugs seized by the Customs authorities are an example of such statistics. Customs and Excise officers intercept drugs being illegally imported into Britain and therefore can be seen to reflect trends in the overall drugs market, i.e. which drugs are in greatest demand. Thus, for example, the number of seizures of cocaine increased from 385 to 440 between 1989 and 1992 and MDMA (ecstasy) increased from 1 to 38 seizures during 1989 and 1991. Such figures appear to reflect an overall trend in the increasing popularity of these two drugs. However, it cannot be assumed that if seizures of a particular drug decrease, this reflects diminished use, as it may simply mean that the drug is being manufactured on a larger scale in the United Kingdom, and therefore external sources are no longer as necessary. Alternatively, a large increase in seizures without a corresponding escalation in use may suggest that Customs are now intercepting a higher proportion of this drug, possibly as a result of changes in enforcement policy.

It is therefore very useful to consider Customs and Excise statistics in the light of figures provided by the police which reflect seizures of drugs that have already entered, or been manufactured in, Britain. Such internal statistics may more readily reflect trends in street availability of controlled drugs as is suggested by the increase in the numbers of seizures of crack cocaine from 140 in 1989 to 864 in 1992, and, in the case of LSD, from 876 in 1989 to 2404 in 1992. However, again such figures must be treated with caution as, between 1987 and 1991, nearly three times as many people were stopped and searched for drugs, thus increasing the likelihood of seizure and conviction. The overall picture is once again, however, supported by crime statistics that show the numbers of people found guilty, cautioned or dealt with by compounding for drug offences. Again, convictions relating to cocaine use rose from 591 in 1988 to 913 in 1992. LSD and MDMA offences have increased even more. However, given the process through which a person who is found to have committed a drug-related criminal offence must pass, it is perhaps not surprising that each stage of this process supports the previous and the next one. And again, the statistics will also reflect changes in policing policies and strategies. However, they are able to add other information about the types of people involved in these offences, thus telling us that in 1991, 90.8 per cent of the known drug offenders in the United Kingdom were male, as compared to 9.2 per cent females.

Again though, it has been suggested that enforcement policies may be discriminatory. For instance, research carried out by NACRO, The National Association For the Care and Resettlement of Offenders[3] has suggested that young males from ethnic minorities are more likely to be stopped and searched by police than their white male counterparts. Equally, if large numbers of older people were using illegal drugs, it is unlikely that the enforcement agencies would become aware of this so readily.

Enforcement statistics generally are therefore filtered versions that reflect, only imperfectly, the prevalence and pattern of drug misuse in Britain. Their main contribution is in the consistency and regularity with which such statistics are collected and recorded, which can help to provide indications of trends in drug use that are unavailable from other sources. Therefore the apparent increase in all the statistics pertaining to LSD and ecstasy in all likelihood reflects the increased popularity of the 'dance drug' culture and obviously contributes to the overall increase in abuse of Class A drugs.

More specialised statistics concerning drug use and the prison population have recently been provided in a report published in 1994 by The Centre For Research on Drugs and Health Behaviour.[4] This study demonstrated that drugs are readily available in the prison system, given that all of the sample of 44 drug users had been able to use drugs whilst serving their last sentence of imprisonment. The picture that emerges is one of a range of drugs being regularly available in prisons; if the first drug of preference is not available, then users substitute this with a drug that can be purchased. The report concluded that drug use in prison cannot be separated from the drug scene outside, or as Her Majesty's' Chief Inspector of Prisons, Judge Tumin, commented in 1992, 'society can no more expect total control over the presence of drugs in prisons than elsewhere'.

Drug Use and Crime

That there is a connection between illegal drug use and crime is now
generally acknowledged by academics, the medical profession and
politicians. Indeed, there is now a considerable amount of statistical
information available to prove that these activities are related. The first
studies to produce data on this issue were carried out in America[5]
during the 1930s and produced a mixture of results, some suggesting
that criminal activity preceded drug misuse, others demonstrating that
drug use led on to other types of offending. The earliest research studies
in Britain[6] tended to be based on the heroin-using population and
also reported significant offending behaviour both prior and subsequent
to drug use. Pre-drug conviction rates varied between 30 per cent and
50 per cent and subsequent conviction rates after drug use had com-
menced were over 90 per cent. All of these surveys therefore indicated the high incidence of a criminal record in established drug users. In
fact, one recent study carried out in America of 354 drug addicts reported that criminal activity was admitted by every member of the
sample group.

The debate today is therefore mainly concerned with whether drug
use causes other criminal behaviour or whether involvement in crime
and a criminal subculture can cause a greater likelihood of involvement in the drug scene. Alternatively, could drug use and offending
both be independently caused by a third factor? The dominant lay-
explanation of drug use and crime is probably a causal one; i.e. drug
use leads to other criminal behaviour. After the 1960s when drug use
first became acknowledged as a problem in Britain, Bean[7] suggested
that heroin users fell into two very different groups. On the one hand
there were addicts from the middle classes who tended not to have
convictions prior to their drug use. Such users became involved in
drugs as part of an ideology of the world and humankind and any
involvement in crime was caused by their drug misuse. The other group,
usually from the working classes, already had criminal convictions before
starting to use heroin. Their offending could therefore be viewed in
terms of the criminal model, that is their offending was merely an
extension of an already deviant lifestyle. Alternatively, such users were
perceived as offending because of the economic-necessity model, meaning
they offended to support their habit financially.

Nurco[8] from his research suggested that during heavy periods of
heroin use, users commit more crimes. Addiction in this study is therefore
viewed as a pharmacologically caused state that cannot be controlled

by the user – neither the use itself or any resulting behaviour. However, another analysis of the criminal records of users who were first notified by doctors as addicts between 1979 and 1981 found much the same pattern of offending, no matter how heavy the heroin use at the time.

Whether the availability of a drug further influences criminal activity is another consideration. By the beginning of the 1980s there is no doubt that supplies of illicitly imported heroin were cheaply and readily available and the number of regular users was increasing in certain parts of the country, particularly in Southern Scotland and the North West of England. Research carried out on Merseyside[9] at the time demonstrated a considerable rise in household burglaries between 1981 and 1985 at the same time as increasing numbers of unemployed young people became involved with heroin (usually by smoking it). This study also found that more of these young people were convicted of offences of dishonesty (theft and burglary in particular) than would be expected and as compared with their non-delinquent peers.

Most explanations of the relationship between drug use and crime have important influences on policy and treatment considerations. For instance, if, as suggested by Nurco, heroin use leads to criminal activity, then treating drug users and making drugs less available should in turn reduce crime. Or if the economic-necessity model was accepted as most clearly explaining how drug use and offending are related, then increased legal prescribing would be expected to reduce levels of criminal behaviour.

A further theory, put forward by Hammersley *et al.* has suggested that the need for opioids does not simply cause crime, rather crime and opioid use tend to influence each other: 'Drug users do not need to commit crimes; that they do so is because they are and have been criminal before drug use.'[10] If this theory is correct, then criminal behaviour will be a good predictor of future drug use and treatment should be aimed at the offending not the drug use.

An even more recent study by Collinson[11] looked closely at the drug-use, criminal record, treatment and institutional careers of young male offenders, mainly from the North West of England. This research found high levels of offending before the onset of drug use (64 per cent) and although 45 per cent admitted to drug dealing during recent years, only 9 per cent had been convicted of a drug-defined offence. The study therefore concluded that chaotic forms of drug use and chaotic crime usually co-exist. Often young people become involved in both for the same reasons: the 'buzz', the excitement. From this point, young people may well progress to different types of offending that not only provide the same 'buzz', but also provide an income to enable increased consumption of the many commodities in the market place for the young – including drugs, but also clothes and 'leisure'. In turn, the individual's appetite to consume drugs may well develop, just as consumers wish to move on to better cars or designer clothes.

In addition, because crime and drug 'economies' are frequently linked, involvement in both is widespread and promises a whole range of products and experiences to try. The only problem for most young drug users therefore tends to be the cost of financing their drug use. The consumption of drugs is therefore just one aspect of delinquency rather than its defining core. Drug consumption is enabled by crime as certain kinds of drugs enable crime. This study also went on to show that the subjects of the research viewed 'expert' help for their 'drug problem' as irrelevant; their information about the legal and health implications of drug use comes from street and peer knowledge, which is not necessarily correct.

The wide variety of research can therefore be seen to have led to many different explanations as to the relationship between drugs and crime, none of which conclusively support one theory to the exclusion of all the others. Bean and Wilkinson[12] therefore tried to find a different type of explanation suggesting that the link between drug taking and crime had less to do with the origins of the user's offending than with their current situations. Thus whilst many drug-using offenders are also involved in the supply of drugs, those more heavily involved use violence to enforce their position and crimes such as burglary as a debt-collecting mechanism. Others who are less involved may become violent when out of control or use the profits from dishonest offences to support their habit. Such an explanation means that an individual drug user's offending will depend on how involved s/he is in the dealing scene.

A further group of explanations looks at the issue from the standpoint of a supply-and-demand model. Therefore if there are only a few drug users in an area, the supply of drugs is likely to come via a network of friends and acquaintances. When the market increases, however, the structure of supply is likely to become more sophisticated. Bean and Pearson[13] in a recent study described a localised crack market in terms of larger-scale dealers who then employed runners equipped with mobile telephones to distribute the drugs, with other employees carrying out the debt-collecting function, using violence as and when needed.

In addition, it may be true to suggest that trends in drug use could have an impact on the types and numbers of crimes being committed. Therefore a link may be established between the increased use of crack cocaine and offending as a result of the influence of the drug on behaviour. Alternatively, increased offending may reflect the cost incurred in feeding a drug habit. A policy response to this type of explanation would therefore focus on the need to control and police the drugs market so as to prevent illegal substances becoming widely available. However, such steps if successful could in turn increase the cost of purchasing illegal drugs which could either deter people from using them or increase the need for people to commit crime to support their habit.

Given the wide-ranging theories of the link between drug use and crime as discussed above, it is extremely difficult to find any one of them that can adequately explain why so many drug users are also involved in offending. None the less, the fact this issue has been widely researched has provided a significant amount of quantitative and qualitative information that has helped to inform government policy relating to both enforcement and treatment.

CONCLUSION

Despite the many difficulties in establishing both the extent and nature of drug use and related crime in Britain, what is clear is that both exist and do relate to each other. Therefore, unless drugs were to be decriminalised and so allow for more open examination of the issue, it is likely that the extent of both activities will never be accurately recorded. Changing attitudes in recent years within the criminal justice system is allowing for agencies such as The Probation Service to be more explicit in its work with drug-using offenders. Thus, in theory at least, Pre-Sentence Reports prepared for the criminal courts on offenders awaiting sentence should realistically explore the extent and nature of the individual's drug use as it relates to his/her offending without the defendant being penalised any further. Such a practice in theory allows for a more honest approach to these issues in the hope that the individual may feel more able to seek appropriate help. Additionally, it would be hoped that such a policy which fits in well with the 'harm minimisation' model would also influence the social and healthcare provision for all drug users. However, it would be naive not to recognise that drug users and offenders are not always receptive to the suggestions and help seen to be offered by the authorities.

It is inevitable that drug use and offending will both continue and that the ways in which they develop will be influenced as much by the criminal activities of those supplying drugs to the market as by enforcement trends. Additionally, as new drugs come on to the scene, our understanding of the relationship between drugs and crime will have to be re-examined, as has been highlighted by the recent increase in the supply and use of crack cocaine. It is also inevitable that fashions will continue to exist on the drugs scene and that research will always, in a sense, be behind current practices. None the less, as I hope has been demonstrated in this brief overview of drug use and crime, continued research and the regular collection of relevant statistics are crucial in illuminating the relationship between drug use and criminal behaviour.

The biomedical and social consequences of this behaviour are diverse and depend upon a wide range of factors. The relative contribution of biological, psychological, and sociological factors is not only important in terms of the individual's response to substances which might be abused but also important in the origination of an addictive life style. The following chapters attempt to review some of the data which accounts for differences between individuals.

NOTES

1. Inner London Probation Service, 'Drug and Alcohol Misuse: A Summary of Demonstration Unit Interviews' (Inner London Probation Service, London, 1990).
2. H. Parker, 'The New Drug Users', *Criminal Justice Matters*, no. 12 (Summer 1993), Institute for the Study of Drug Dependence, London.
3. NACRO, *Race and Crime: A Basic Briefing* (NACRO, 1988).
4. P. J. Turnbull, G. V. Stimson and G. Stillwell, *Drug Use in Prisons* (AVERT, 1994).
5. Dai Bingham, *Opium Addiction in Chicago* (1937; reprinted New Jersey: Patterson Smith, 1970).
6. J. Willis, 'Drug Dependency: Some Demographic and Psychiactric Aspects in U.K. and U.S. Subjects', *British Journal of Addiction*, 64(1)(1969): 135–46.
7. P. T. Bean, 'Report to the Home Office on the Means by which Agencies deal with the Drug Problem in Nottingham', mimeo.
8. D. N. Nurco, 'Drug Addiction and Crime: A Complicated Issue', *British Journal of Addiction*, 82, (1987):7–9.
9. H. Parker, K. Bakx and R. Newcom, *Living with Heroin* (Milton Keynes: Open University Press, 1987).

10. R. Hammersley, A. Forsyth, V. Morrison and J. Davies, 'The Relationship between Crime and Opioid Use', *British Journal of Addiction*, 84 (1989):1029–43.
11. M. Collinson, 'Drugs and Delinquency: A Non Treatment Paradigm', *Probation Journal*, (December 1994):203–7.
12. P. T. Bean and C. K. Wilkinson, 'Drug Taking, Crime and the Illicit Supply System', *British Journal of Addiction*, 83 (1988):533–9.
13. P. T. Bean and Y. Pearson, 'Cocaine and Crack in Nottingham 1989/ 1990', 1991/1992, London Home Office Unit Paper no. 70.

Part II
Biochemical Aspects of the Addictions

4 The Neurobiological Background to the Study of Addiction

Abdulla A.-B. Badawy

INTRODUCTION

In this article, a general but brief account of the neurobiology of drug dependence will be presented and followed by a more specific review of work from this and other laboratories concerning the possible role of the brain monoamine 5-hydroxytryptamine (5-HT, serotonin) in alcohol dependence and alcoholism.

Dr Paul Davis has clearly demonstrated in the introduction to this book that, as a consequence of the complex nature of addiction, our understanding of the basis of dependence is more likely to be advanced through multidimensional clinical and laboratory studies combining the psychological, behavioural and pharmacological approaches. This should provide a wider biological, sociological and psychological understanding of the basis of drug dependence and thereby enable specific, rational and more effective therapeutic and preventative strategies in the field of drug dependence to be developed.

GENERAL BACKGROUND

Drug-seeking Behaviour

Drug-seeking behaviour appears to be a central phenomenon in drug dependence. The behavioural model proposed by Stolerman[1] suggests that drug-seeking behaviour will be influenced by several factors, the most important of which are the positive reinforcing effects of the drug, because these cause the person to continue to pursue his/her drug-taking habit. This behaviour is negatively influenced by the aversive effects of the drug. Discriminative effects of the drug are also important. A series of modulating variables such as the social context, genetic factors, behavioural, pharmacological and medical history will also influence the individual's behaviour towards drug seeking and, hence, intake.

Reward Mechanisms

There appear to be three major reward systems in the brain through which the positive reinforcing effects of drugs of dependence are achieved.[2] These three reward systems are associated generally with the brain chemicals dopamine, opioids and GABA (gamma-aminobutyric acid). From neuroanatomical and pharmacological evidence, the nucleus accumbens area of a midbrain–forebrain–extrapyramidal circuit appears to be the focus of the reward process. In general, it is thought that reward in the case of psychomotor stimulants, such as amphetamine and cocaine, is linked mainly to dopamine,[2,3] whereas that for opiates is related to both dopamine and endogenous opioids.[4] Reward in the case of alcohol may be associated with the transmitter GABA as well as with dopamine.[5] It should, however, be emphasised here that these are only broad outlines of the major effects of these three drug categories as far as the reward systems are concerned, and that other brain chemicals may also play important roles. Thus, for example, there is also good evidence that: (1) modulation of metabolism and/or function of the brain indolylamine 5-HT can increase the reward activity for cocaine and amphetamine; (2) the ethanol reward mechanism may be dopamine-independent; (3) opiates can exert their reinforcing effects independently of dopamine in the nucleus accumbens and the ventral–tegmental area. It is thus difficult to assign to a particular behaviour or function only a single neurochemical and it is, therefore, more likely that the outcome of any particular physiological process is the result of interaction between all neurochemical systems present at the particular site of such a process. The same also applies in the case of sedatives and hypnotics. Another group of mood-altering drugs, the cannabinoids, appears to be an exception in that they exert no effects on the reward mechanisms and, although they cause tolerance, they do not induce physical dependence.[6] However, the recent discovery of the cannabinoid receptor (for references, see note 6 and for endogenous cannabinoids, see note 7) may provide some interesting explanations of the behavioural and other biological effects of this class of drugs. Another drug of dependence that does not have any specific receptors mediating its actions, which are exerted at the level of many neurotransmitter systems, is ethanol.[5]

ACTIONS OF DRUGS OF DEPENDENCE

In addition to the reinforcing, aversive, discriminative and other related effects, drugs of dependence exert a variety of actions at many levels. In general, these actions are classified broadly under three headings based on pharmacological principles, namely tolerance (and cross-tolerance), dependence and the withdrawal syndrome. These actions vary both within and between the different groups of drugs of dependence in many respects, e.g. speed of onset and of acquisition of tolerance, dosage and duration of intake, and severity of dependence and consequently of the ensuing withdrawal syndrome upon cessation of intake. Whereas withdrawal of an addictive drug reflects the severity of dependence on it, the phenomenon of tolerance can be separated entirely from that of dependence, and the best example illustrating this point is that of the cannabinoids, which, as stated above, produce tolerance, but not dependence. Tolerance can in some cases be explained in metabolic, rather than neuronal, terms. The best example of metabolic tolerance is that of ethanol, where an enhanced rate of its metabolism following chronic intake leads to a decrease of its availability to the central nervous system. The following is a brief account of the main effects of different classes of addictive drugs in relation to the above main pharmacological actions (see Table 4.1)

CNS Stimulants

The main effect of this group of addictive drugs is that of facilitation of release and/or blockade of reuptake of dopamine and noradrenaline, and this seems to be particularly important in relation to their positive reinforcing action. Another important effect of this group of addictive drugs is their induction of sensitisation (the opposite of tolerance) upon repeated intake, at least in experimental animals. Cocaine, unlike other drugs of dependence, does not cause a strong withdrawal syndrome, yet it induces in humans a strong dysphoric state and intense craving, which render it perhaps the most powerful drug of dependence known. The biological basis of these effects is not fully understood at present. Additionally, this group of addictive agents are also known to exert serious behavioural and toxic effects, notably homicidal aggression and cardiovascular dysfunction.

TABLE 4.1   *Comparison of the general effects of drugs of dependence*

Type of drug	Major reward receptors	Other action receptors	Tolerance	Dependence and withdrawal
CNS stimulants	DA	5-HT	+	+
Opiates	Opioid, DA	5-HT, GABA, G.protein	+	+
Other sedatives/ hypnotics	GABA/ BNZD	?	+	+
Nicotine	DA	Nicotinic	+	+
Cannabinoids	–	Cannabinoid	+	–

Abbreviations: DA, Dopamine; 5-HT, Serotonin; BNZD, Benzodiazopens.

Opiates

Opiates, such as heroin, morphine and related compounds, produce tolerance, physical dependence and a strong withdrawal syndrome. Opiates are generally thought to exert their actions at specific opiate receptors, of which there are three major classes, with possible subtypes. The major CNS effects of opiates are inhibitory. Opiates exert a variety of effects on many neurotransmitter and other brain systems, notably dopamine, 5-HT, GABA and G proteins, but the precise sites of their action in relation to their tolerance, dependence, withdrawal and euphoric effects remain to be identified.

Ethanol

As stated above, this most commonly abused drug of dependence has no specific receptors to which modulation of its effects can be ascribed. Ethanol, in common with most other drugs of dependence, causes tolerance, dependence and a withdrawal syndrome and also exhibits cross-tolerance with other sedative/hypnotic addictive drugs. Metabolic tolerance to ethanol following its chronic intake can be explained by induction of the (cytochrome P-450-dependent) microsomal ethanol-oxidising system (MEOS) and, in particular, the CYP-450 2El isoenzyme, and this induction process may also have other implications in ethanol–drug interactions and the resultant toxicity potentiation. As stated earlier, ethanol influences a large number of neurochemical and neuronal processes in the brain, the most important of which are 5-HT, dopamine the *N*-methyl-D-aspartate (NMDA) receptor, voltage-sensitive calcium channels and the GABA-A receptor. The importance of dopamine is mainly in relation to the positive reinforcing effects of ethanol, whereas that of 5-HT is mainly in connection with the behavioural and psychological changes associated with alcohol consumption (e.g. aggressive behaviour and depression) and also in relation to genetic predisposition to alcohol consumption and, hence, dependence. These aspects will be discussed later. The actions of ethanol on the NMDA and GABA-A receptors and voltage-sensitive calcium channels are of particular interest in relation to possible mechanisms of alcohol tolerance, dependence and withdrawal.[5] Thus acute exposure to ethanol inhibits the excitatory action of glutamate at the NMDA and kainate receptors and voltage-sensitive (dihydropyridine-sensitive) calcium channels, and stimulates the actions of GABA at its A receptors. By contrast, chronic exposure to ethanol does not influence kainate receptors, but increases the numbers of NMDA receptors and voltage-sensitive calcium channels and decreases GABA-A receptor function. It is thought that these chronic effects of ethanol result in the hyperexcitability symptoms associated with alcohol withdrawal.

Other Sedatives/Hypnotics

Benzodiazepines are commonly prescribed as anxiolytic agents and are also used as anticonvulsants during acute alcohol withdrawal. Barbiturates are rarely prescribed nowadays. Both groups, like alcohol, cause tolerance, dependence and a withdrawal syndrome and there is also cross-tolerance between them. The major pharmacological effects of this group of sedatives/hypnotics, leading to euphoria, disinhibition, anxiety reduction, sedation and hypnosis, appear to be related to their ability to modulate the GABA/benzodiazepine/chloride ionophore complex.[8] Apart from these correlates, very little work has been done to address the neurochemical basis of dependence on this group of addictive drugs.

Nicotine

It is clear that nicotine is the addictive constituent of tobacco products and, in common with other addictive agents, it induces tolerance, dependence and a withdrawal syndrome. Less appears to be known about the neuronal mechanisms of nicotine addiction, other than the possible involvement of the mesolimbic dopamine system and other neurochemical processes in its positive reinforcing action, and that nicotine binds to specific nicotinic cholinergic receptors.[9, 10] Much work is required to ascertain the functional significance of these effects in relation to the above major pharmacological actions of nicotine and its other behavioural and psychological effects in man.

THE ROLE OF GENETICS IN THE STUDY OF DRUG DEPENDENCE

Familial, twin and adoption studies have shown clearly that there is a genetic component to alcohol dependence.[11] It is generally thought that about 20–25 per cent of chronic alcoholics may inherit a genetic predisposition to drinking. The neuronal mechanisms likely to explain this genetic predisposition are currently receiving much interest. Two potential mediators of such predisposition are the dopamine D2 receptor and 5-HT. Additionally, genetic difference in the alcohol-metabolising enzymes alcohol dehydrogenase (ADH) and aldehyde dehydrogenase (AlDH) among different human races have been shown to explain the differences in sensitivity towards alcohol (for review, see Hodgkinson *et al.*[14]) and are therefore important determinants of the ability of populations to handle, and therefore continue to use or abuse, alcohol. By contrast, very little work has been done to address the question of genetic predisposition to dependence on other drugs. As regards alcohol, the dopamine D2 receptor studies have yielded mixed results,[12] whereas with 5-HT, although no genetic evidence is available as yet from human studies other than the implication of the tryptophan pyrrolase gene,[13] evidence from studies with animal strains and lines known to prefer alcohol strongly implicates a central 5-HT deficiency as an important biological determinant of alcohol consumption. These aspects will be discussed later. Genetically different animal models are important not only in relation to the 5-HT deficiency of alcoholism, but also many other aspects of the actions of alcohol and also other drugs of dependence.[14] Thus, in the case of mice, there are withdrawal seizure-prone and resistant lines, severe and mild withdrawal-exhibiting lines and high and low addictability lines, in addition to the well-known alcohol-preferring C57BL strain. With rats, there are a number of alcohol-preferring lines, including the Sardinian SP from Cagliari, the P and the HAD from the USA, the ALKO AA from Finland and the UChA from Chile. Other rat lines of a wider distribution, such as the Maudsley reactive and Fawn-hooded rats, also prefer alcohol. Rat lines with differing sensitivities towards the pharmacological effects of alcohol include ALKO tolerant and non-tolerant (AT/ANT) and the high- or low-alcohol-sensitive (HAS/LAS). As regards other drugs of dependence, a variety of mouse lines are available for the following functions: high and low analgesic responses, high and low stress-induced analgesia, diazepam-sensitive and -resistant responses, high and low diazepam-sensitive responses, and nicotine-activated or -depressed responses. The availability of all these animal models should facilitate the search for the biological determinants of predisposition to dependence on alcohol and other addictive drugs, as well as for the various pharmacological effects of these drugs. As stated above, the brain 5-HT deficiency has already been demonstrated in a number of alcohol-preferring animal lines/strains.

COMMONALITIES BETWEEN DRUGS OF DEPENDENCE

If there is a common basis of drug dependence, our understanding of its nature and mechanism(s) is more likely to be advanced by examining what actions or features drugs of dependence exhibit in common, rather than by attempting to differentiate between them. In general, there are three major features common to various drugs of dependence: (1) their positive reinforcing properties leading to drug-seeking behaviour; (2) their ability to induce dependence; (3) their ability to alter mood. It is therefore not unreasonable to try to find out if the mechanisms underlying these three major actions are, or include elements, common to all drugs of dependence. Much work is needed to examine this possibility. However, as stated 'earlier, already some commonalities exist between drugs of dependence in terms of their effects on the reward mechanisms. Perhaps once all the elements of the reward system become fully identified, some of the differences between drugs of dependence, currently differentiating them in this respect, may be seen as constituent parts of the same wider process.

The same could be said of the mechanisms of dependence and the behavioural and clinical differences between the different withdrawal syndromes that characterise the different classes of addictive drugs. As regards mood, very few clinical studies, mainly in relation to alcohol dependence, have addressed this issue and hardly at the neurochemical level. There is strong evidence that the cerebral indolylamine 5-HT plays an important role in the regulation of mood (for review, see van Praag[15]) and it is also known that modulation of 5-HT is a common

TABLE 4.2 *Common effects of drugs of dependence on tryptophan metabolism and disposition in the rat*

Treatment	Effect	Ethanol	Morphine	Nicotine	Phenobarbitone
Acute	Increase in liver Trp pyrrolase	(+++)	(++)	(++)	(+)
	Mechanism	Substrate	Substrate	Hormonal	Hormonal
	Increased brain 5-HT	+,−	+	?	?
Chronic	Inhibition of liver Trp pyrrolase	+	+	+	+
	Mechanism	NAD(P)H	NADPH	NADPH	NADPH
	Increased brain 5-HT	+	+	+	+
Withdrawal	Increase in liver Trp pyrrolase	+	+	+	+
	Mechanism	Hormonal	Hormonal	Hormonal	Hormonal
	Increased serum corticosterone	+	+	+	+
	Decreased Brain 5-HT	+	+	+	+
	Peak of all withdrawal changes (day)	8	1	3	2

Symbols: +, positive effect or increase; (+) to (+++), arbitrary scale of increase; −, decrease; ?, effect unknown. *Abbreviations*: 5-HT, 5-hydroxytryptamine; NAD(P)H, reduced nicotinamide-adenine dinucleotide (phosphate); Trp, tryptophan. For details, see Badawy *et al.* (1981)[16] and Badawy and Evans (1983).[17]

action of drugs of dependence[16, 17] (see Table 4.2). Thus chronic administration to rats of ethanol, morphine, nicotine or phenobarbitone causes an enhancement of cerebral 5-HT synthesis, whereas subsequent withdrawal leads to an inhibition. These opposite effects are achieved through corresponding changes in circulating tryptophan (Trp) availability to the brain caused respectively by inhibition and induction of activity of the major Trp-degrading enzyme, hepatic tryptophan pyrrolase (tryptophan 2,3-dioxygenase, EC 1.13.11.11). These effects may be of importance in relation to the mood disorders, particularly depression, frequently associated with drug dependence and withdrawal, but examination of these aspects in humans remains to be performed. Also of equal importance is the need to elucidate the biological nature of anxiety states associated with drug dependence and the relationship between affective disorders in general and drug dependence.

ALCOHOL AND 5-HT

Of all biogenic amines and neurotransmitter systems, 5-HT is the most intensively studied brain chemical in relation to alcohol and alcoholism. This is almost certainly because of the role of this indolylamine in the regulation of mood and certain other behaviours. In recent years, however, the interest in 5-HT metabolism and function has focused on aspects related to alcohol consumption in both man and experimental animals, where there is a large body of evidence suggesting that modulation of 5-HT metabolism and function can influence the extent of alcohol consumption (for recent reviews, see LeMarquand *et al.*[18]), and, as stated earlier, evidence also exists for an important role of a 5-HT deficit in alcohol preference in experimental animals. Thus in relation to genetic aspects of alcoholism other than those involving alcohol-metabolising enzymes, metabolic and pharmacological studies on 5-HT have occupied centre stage, with molecular biological and other genetic aspects sure to follow. It is therefore appropriate at this stage to summarise briefly the 5-HT metabolic status in relation to pharmacological and genetic aspects of alcohol and alcoholism.

5-HT Metabolism

Cerebral 5-HT synthesis is controlled mainly by brain tryptophan (Trp) concentration, because the rate-limiting enzyme of the 5-HT-biosynthetic pathway, Trp hydroxylase, exists unsaturated with its Trp substrate (see Figure 4.1). It follows therefore that peripheral factors influencing circulating Trp availability to the brain must play important roles in the control of cerebral 5-HT synthesis. These peripheral factors are: (1) Trp binding to albumin; (2) extent of competition between Trp and the other five amino acids (Val, Leu, Ile, Phe and Tyr) known to share the same cerebral uptake mechanism; (3) activity of the major Trp-degrading enzyme, liver Trp pyrrolase (for references, see Badawy[19]). In studies in humans, because of methodological limitations, the status of brain 5-HT has to be assessed by indirect methods. One of these involves measuring changes in the ratio of circulating Trp concentration to the sum of those of its five competitors, or the [Trp]/[CAA] ratio. An increase in this ratio can almost certainly predict an enhancement of cerebral 5-HT synthesis, and vice versa.

    The effects of alcohol on tryptophan and 5-HT metabolism in experimental animals have been reviewed briefly by the author[20] and more recently in greater detail by LeMarquand *et al.*[21] The ethanol effects

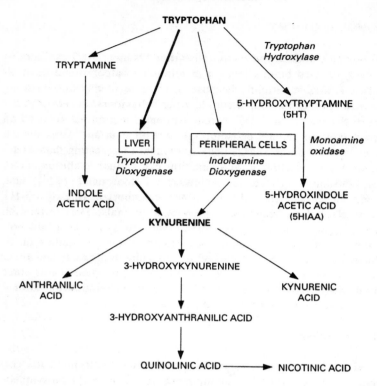

Figure 4.1 Metabolic pathways of tryptophan showing principal enzymes (*in italics*) and the most quantitatively significant pathway (**bold lines**).

are complex and varied, and depend in part on whether the drug has been administered acutely or chronically and whether measurements were made during the chronic administration period or after subsequent withdrawal. Compounding variables include factors such as the dose(s) of ethanol and route of its administration, duration of treatment, methods of assessment of some of the parameters tested (e.g. 5-HT turnover rate), choice of species and/or strain and the nutritional status of animals tested. In general, however, it is recognised that, in the rat, whose Trp metabolism resembles closely that of man, acute ethanol administration exerts a biphasic effect on cerebral 5-HT synthesis, an early enhancement and a later inhibition. Both effects are mediated by corresponding alterations in circulating Trp availability to the brain, caused respectively by a lipolysis-dependent non-esterified fatty-acid-mediated increase in circulating free [Trp] and a later decrease in circulating

Trp levels secondarily to activation of liver Trp pyrrolase following the earlier increase in Trp availability (to the liver). Brain 5-HT synthesis is also enhanced by chronic ethanol administration, but is inhibited during subsequent withdrawal. Here again, appropriate changes in circulating Trp availability to the brain are responsible for these opposite effects, with these latter changes being caused respectively by inhibition and induction of liver Trp pyrrolase activity. From this account, it appears that the activity of liver Trp pyrrolase plays an important role in the effects of ethanol on brain 5-HT in experimental animals.

As regards the effects of ethanol on 5-HT receptor function, less work has been done (for a review, see LeMarquand et al.[21]. In general, ligand binding to 5-HT receptor subtypes is only moderately inhibited after administration acutely of pharmacologically high doses of ethanol. The chronic and withdrawal effects are even less clear and more controversial; available evidence suggests that changes are secondary to 5-HT hypoactivity during the withdrawal phase.

Effects of Alcohol on Tryptophan and 5-HT Metabolism in Man

These effects have also been reviewed.[20, 21] The best known effects of ethanol consumption in man are those concerning the ability of the drug to divert the metabolism of 5-HT from the major oxidative route leading to the formation of 5-hydroxy-3-indole-acetic acid (5-HIAA) to the minor reductive pathway producing 5-hydroxytryptophol (for review and references, see Hunt and Majchrowicz).[22] In fact, determination of the ratio of concentrations of 5-hydroxytryptophol/5-HIAA in urine is being developed as a very promising laboratory marker of recent alcohol intake.[23] Less is known about the effects of acute and chronic ethanol consumption and subsequent withdrawal on other aspects of 5-HT metabolism, particularly synthetic ones and the possible role of the Trp precursor. For ethical reasons, the acute or chronic effects of ethanol could not be studied in abstinent chronic alcoholics, and have therefore to be examined either in control or non-abstinent subjects. In controls, acute ethanol intake has been shown[20] to decrease circulating Trp availability to the brain, as assessed by the [Trp]/[CAA] ratio. The decrease in this ratio is due only to a decrease in circulating [Trp], because [CAA] is not altered. The decrease in [Trp] is not associated with altered Trp binding to albumin and must therefore be assumed to be caused by an enhancement of liver Trp pyrrolase activity, though this latter possibility requires further assessment. This decrease in circulating Trp availability to the brain caused by acute alcohol consumption

may provide a biological explanation of the incidence of aggressive
behaviour in certain subjects following alcohol consumption, and may
also have important implications in relation to the incidence of depression in alcoholism. These possibilities clearly merit further investigation. The effects of acute ethanol consumption on Trp availability
to the brain in non-abstinent alcoholics is currently under investigation
in the authors' laboratory and available evidence so far suggests that
the ability of acute ethanol consumption to lower circulating Trp availability to the brain may be impaired, almost certainly because of a possible
inhibition of liver Trp pyrrolase activity by chronic alcohol intake.

That liver Trp pyrrolase activity may be inhibited by chronic alcohol consumption in chronic alcoholic subjects was first suggested
by results from the study by Walsh *et al.*,[24] in which the urinary excretion of kynurenine metabolites, following a Trp load was impaired
in subjects within 24 hours following cessation of alcohol intake. In
more recent Trp loading studies, it was shown (Friedman *et al.*, 1988)[25]
that chronic alcoholics form kynurenine from Trp at a higher rate at 1
month after abstinence compared to the immediate post-detoxification
phase and that kynurenine formation from Trp remains higher at 3
months of abstinence, but reverts back to the lower rate if subjects
relapse into drinking, thus suggesting pyrrolase inhibition by chronic
alcohol intake. A higher rate of hepatic Trp degradation in recently
abstinent alcoholics is likely to cause a decrease in circulating Trp
availability to the brain and a consequent inhibition of cerebral 5-HT
synthesis. Such a decrease in Trp availability to the brain, as assessed
by the [Trp]/[CAA] ratio, has already been reported.[26]

The question then arises as to whether a higher rate of hepatic Trp
degradation is always present in chronic alcoholics, even after long-
term abstinence, or occurs only in recently abstinent subjects in contrast with the lower rate observed before abstinence. Much work including
control data is needed to address these questions and it is particularly
important to ascertain whether any likely enhancement of hepatic Trp
degradation in long-term abstinence is related to family and/or drinking history and whether such an enhancement and the associated likely
depletion of brain 5-HT are important biological determinants of predisposition to alcohol consumption and, hence, alcoholism.

Tryptophan and 5-HT Metabolism in Alcohol Preference

As stated earlier, there is evidence from studies in animal species and
strains known to prefer alcohol that preference is associated with a

brain 5-HT defect. Thus, the C57BL mouse strain, which prefers alcohol, shows a deficiency in cerebral 5-HT levels caused by a higher liver Trp pyrrolase activity due to a higher circulating concentration of the glucocorticoid inducer of this hepatic enzyme, corticosterone[27]. Two alcohol-preferring rat lines, the P from Indiana, USA,[28] and the Fawn-Hooded rat[29] also exhibit a central serotonin deficiency, which in the former is due to a low density of serotonergic fibres in cortex[30]. Experiments in progress in the author's laboratory also suggest that the alcohol-preferring Sardinian (SP) rat line also shows a central 5-HT defect, the mechanism of which is still unclear. Other alcohol-preferring rat lines are also currently under investigation. So far, only one alcohol-preferring rat line, the AA from Finland, has been reported[31] not to exhibit a 5-HT defect. There is no logical reason to assume that the central 5-HT deficiency of alcohol preference should be explained by only a single mechanism. It is perhaps more important to establish which animal model most resembles man in relation to the likelihood of the 5-HT deficiency being a potential genetic determinant of predisposition to alcohol consumption and, hence, dependence. Evidence so far, however preliminary, points to the C57BL mouse being such a possible animal model.

NOTES

1. I. Stolerman and I. P. Stolerman, 'Drugs of Abuse: Behavioural Principles, Methods and Terms: The Neurobiology of Tobacco Addiction', *Trends in Pharmacological Science*, 12 (1990):467–73.
2. G. F. Koob, 'Drugs of Abuse: Anatomy, Pharmacology and Function of Reward Pathways', *Trends in Pharmacological Science*, 13 (1992): 177–84.
3. W. L. Woolverton and K. M. Johnson, 'Neurobiology of Cocaine Abuse', *Trends in Pharmacological Science*, 13 (1992):193–200.
4. G. Di Chiara and R. A. North, 'Neurobiology of Opiate Abuse', *Trends in Pharmacological Science*, 13 (1992):185–92.
5. H. H. Samson and R. A. Harris, 'Neurobiology of Alcohol Abuse', *Trends in Pharmacological Science*, 13 (1992):206–11.
6. M. E. Abood and B. R. Martin, 'Neurobiology of Marijuana Abuse', *Trends in Pharmacological Science*, 13 (1992):201–5.
7. V. Di Marzo *et al.*, 'Formation and Inactivation of Endogenous Cannabinoid Anandamide in Central Neurons', *Nature*, 372 (1994):686–91.
8. J. H. Wood, J. Katz and G. Winger, 'Benzodiazepines: Use, Abuse and Consequences', *Pharmacology Review*, 44 (1992):151–347.

9. G. Bock and J. Marsh (eds), 'The Biology of Nicotine Dependence', 1990 (abstract), CIBA Foundation Symposium.
10. I. Stoleman and M. Shoaib, 'The Neurobiology of Tobacco Addiction', *Trends in Pharmacological Science*, 12 (1991):467–73.
11. S. Hodgkinson, M. Mullen and R. M. Murray, 'The Genetics of Vulnerability to Alcoholism', in *The New Genetics of Mental Illness*, ed. P. McGuffin and R. M. Murray (Massachusetts: Butterworth Heineman, 1991) pp. 182–97.
12. D. Goldman. 'The DRD2 Dopamine Receptor and the Candidate Gene Approach in Alcoholism', in P. V. Taberner and A. A. Badaway (eds), *Advances in Biomedical Alcohol Research* (Oxford: Pergamon Press, 1993) pp. 27–9.
13. Comings, D. E., 'Serotonin and the Biochemical Genetics of Alcoholism: Lessons from Studies of Attention Deficit Hyperactivity Disorder (ADHD) and Tourette Syndrome', in P. U. Taberner and A. A. Badawy (eds), *Advances in Biomedical Alcohol Research*, Alcohol Alcohol. suppl. 2 (Oxford: Pergamon Press, 1993) pp. 237–41.
14. J. C. Crabbe and Belknap, 'Genetic Approaches to Drug Dependence', *Trends in Pharmacological Science*, 13 (1992):212–6.
15. H. M. van Praag, 'Amine Hypothesis of Affective Disorders', *Handbook of Psychopharmacology*, 13 (1978):187–297.
16. A. A.-B. Badawy, N. F. Punjani and M. Evans, 'The Role of Liver Tryptophan Pyrrolase in the Opposite Effects of Chronic Administration and Subsequent Withdrawal of Drugs of Dependence on Rat Brain Tryptophan Metabolism', *Biochemical Journal*, 196 (1981):161–70.
17. A. A.-B. Badawy and M. Evans, 'Opposite Effects of Chronic Administration and Subsequent Withdrawal of Drugs of Dependence on Metabolism and Disposition of Endogenous and Exogenous Tryptophan in the Rat', *Alcohol and Alcoholism*, 18 (1983):369–82.
18. D. LeMarquand, R. O. Pihl and C. Benkelfat, 'Review Article: Serotonin and Alcohol Intake, Abuse, and Dependence: Findings of Animal Studies', *Biological Psychiatry*, 36 (1994):395–421.
19. A. A.-B. Badawy, *Liver Tryptophan Pyrrolase, Brain 5-Hydroxytryptamine and Alcohol Preference* (New York: Plenum Press, 1991).
20. A. A.-B. Badawy et al., 'Effects of Acute Ethanol Consumption on Tryptophan Metabolism and Disposition by Fasting Normal Male Volunteers', *Advances in Biosciences*, 71 (1988):275–9.
21. D. LeMarquand, R. O. Pihl and C. Benkelfat, 'Review Article: Serotonin and Alcohol Intake, Abuse, and Dependence: Clinical Evidence', *Biological Psychiatry*, 36 (1994):326–37.
22. W. A. Hunt and E. Majchrowicz, *Alterations in Neurotransmitter Function after Acute and Chronic Treatment with Ethanol* (New York: Plenum Press, 1979).
23. A. O. Voltaire et al., 'Urinary 5-Hydroxytryptophol: A Possible Marker of Recent Alcohol Consumption', *Alcoholism: Clinical and Experimental Report*, 16 (1992):281–5.
24. M. P. Walsh et al., 'Pyridoxine Deficiency and Tryptophan Metabolism in Chronic Alcoholics', *American Journal of Clinical Nutrition*, 19 (1966): 379–83.
25. M. J. Friedman et al., 'Altered Conversion of Tryptophan to Kynurenine

in Newly Abstinent Alcoholics', *Biol. Psychiat.*, 23 (1988):89–93.

26. L. M. Branchey *et al.*, 'Depression, Suicide and Aggression in Alcoholics and their Relationship to Plasma Amino Acids', *Psychiatry Research*, 12 (1984):219–26.

27. A. A.-B. Badawy *et al.*, 'Liver Tryptophan Pyrrolase: A Major Determinant of the Lower Brain 5-Hydroxytryptamine Concentration in Alcohol-Preferring C57BL Mice', *Biochemical Journal*, 264 (1989):597–9.

28. J. M. Murphy *et al.*, 'Contents of Monoamines in Forebrain Regions of Alcohol-Preferring (P) and Non-Preferring (NP) Lines of Rats', *Pharmacology Biochemical Behaviour*, 26 (1987):389–92.

29. A. H. Rezvani, D. H. Overstreet and D. S. Janowsky, 'Genetic Serotonin Deficiency and Alcohol Preference in the Fawn Hooded Rats', *Alcohol*, 7 (1990):573–5.

30. F. C. Zhou *et al.*, 'Immunostained Serotonergic Fibres are Decreased in Selected Brain Regions of Alcohol-preferring Rats', *Alcohol*, 8 (1991): 425–31.

31. E. R. Korpi *et al.*, 'Brain Regional and Adrenal Monoamine Concentrations and Behavioural Responses to Stress in Alcohol-Preferring AA and Alcohol-avoiding ANA Rats', *Alcohol*, 5 (1988):417–25.

5 Exogenous Drugs and Brain Damage

Woody Caan

BACKGROUND

The earliest known agricultural society cultivated *Vicia* (the 'tares' of the Bible), presumably in awareness of its psychoactive potential and in spite of the excitotoxic risks of fits or neurolathyrism. Throughout recorded history, harmful effects of ethanol on memory, orientation, co-ordination and reasoning have been apparent, long before a concept of dependence emerged. At present, in the USA, 'alcohol-related neurological disorders' constitute a particularly large subset of medical problems with alcohol, including a puzzling 'great variety of these disorders, which may involve virtually any level of the nervous system'.[1] A similarly great variety of damage is seen after use of other psychoactive drugs. The possibility arises that a drug like alcohol could contribute to neuropathology in five ways:

1. direct damage to neurones from any single dose;
2. non-specific damage associated with use (e.g. head injuries or malnutrition);
3. altered metabolism following short binges of heavy use;
4. cumulative irreversible changes associated with chronic use;
5. impaired foetal development after maternal use.

Alcohol-related deaths in England have risen sharply over the last two decades (for example, a 5-fold increase in deaths for men aged 25–44)[2] and alarm about the rising frequency and variety of drug-related problems led Prime Minister John Major to declare his 'Biggest ever war on drugs' on 22 April 1994. The 1992 British Crime Survey suggested around a third of males aged 16-29 take illegal drugs sometimes and recently the Chief Medical Officer (Kenneth Calman)[3] voiced major concern about proliferating fatalities from poisoning and injury related to alcohol and drugs among young people aged only 10–19. Against this background of rising toxic substance use, it is likely that we will encounter more and more of all the five types of neuropathology, above.

DAMAGE FROM A SINGLE DOSE

In animals and man, MPTP (methyl-phenyl-tetrahydropyridine) is the archetypal illicit neurotoxin, causing damage to specific cells (dopaminergic neurones) soon after use. Animal research suggests that the Ecstasy family of drugs have a specific risk of neurotoxicity after a single dose, in neurons containing serotonin (5-hydroxytryptamine, 5-HT) and a few cases in man of a residual psychosis after recreational Ecstasy use have recently emerged. One mental health nurse involved in caring for two of the early British cases was so struck by features of their psychosis that she subsequently initiated a review of other contemporary reports.[4] Psychotic phenomena related to Ecstasy have also been reviewed[5] using a detailed psychopharmacological comparison across different hallucinogenic drugs. Non-competitive *N*-methyl-*D*-aspartate (NMDA) antagonists ('Angel Dust' or 'Special K' in users' terminology) have often been associated with prolonged after-effects (e.g. seizures and flashback hallucinations) and cortical histology in animals reveals specific changes after even single doses of ketamine.[6] Following experimental exposure to hallucinogens by the US Army in chemical warfare studies, it was claimed that 24 per cent of the subjects reported long-term after-effects but the reliability and consistency of these observations remains uncertain.[7]

In general, any drug whose use is directly followed by damage is unlikely to promote chronic, dependent, use. My observations on patients' use of hallucinogens fits this pattern, but the injection of exotic mixtures including cyclizine (e.g. the 'Mad' mixture of cyclizine, buprenorphine and temazepam) may be an exception which is administered repeatedly.[8]

NON-SPECIFIC DAMAGE

Alcohol contributes to a large proportion of road traffic accidents, home accidents and accidents at work[9] including many accidents which involve head injuries. Non-specific brain injury is commonly associated with many intoxicated states, and strokes or fits are particular hazards of high-dose cocaine use.[10] Poor nutrition was a feature of our drug-dependent patients,[11] and alcoholics may have the dual problems of inadequate dietary intake and malabsorption of nutrients. Malnutrition can play a role in either the peripheral neuropathy or Korsakoff's psychosis sometimes associated with chronic alcoholism. A larger number of chronic alcoholics eventually develop an alcoholic dementia; however, Hopkins[12] suggests that repeated head injuries due to 'falls or brawls' when drunk often add to their cognitive decline.

It has been suggested that such factors which are not drug-specific may be at the root of many supposed cumulative toxicities or neonatal impairments, which have been reported in humans. For example, a number of abnormalities have been reported retrospectively in cannabis users or their children, but in the absence of human data on pharmacologically specific toxic effects of cannabinoids, such abnormalities may sometimes be attributed to coincidental, non-specific, hazards.[13] This gives a crucial importance to animal experiments, carried out under controlled conditions. A pioneer in this area was the late Sir William Paton: unfortunately, he was unable to complete a definitive picture of cannabis toxicology, although I recall a vivid personal demonstration by Paton of developmental abnormalities in the basal ganglia of rats that had been exposed to cannabinoids *in utero*.

'BINGES'

Beta-carbolines (like the Harmala alkaloids) are well known to have long-lasting proconvulsant effects after repeated, sub-convulsant doses. Relatively short periods of heavy substance use may result in prolonged impairment of brain metabolism, after 'binges' of several drugs. High-dose alcohol intake, producing substantial levels of brain acetaldehyde, leads to the transient production of two types of toxins, beta-carbolines (from dopamine) and isoquinolines (from 5-HT). These effect gamma-aminobutyric acid (GABA)-A and NMDA receptors, respectively. In studies of rats consuming high doses of alcohol, Caan[14, 15] found prolonged cognitive and behavioural deficits after withdrawal of alcohol. Rats were impaired in their 3-dimensional spatial memory and in their reasoning to find detours by swimming around obstacles, and also intrusive aggressive behaviour appeared when they tried to follow a well-learned trail if another rat was present. Probing around the time of withdrawal, with the benzodiazepine antagonist flumazenil, suggested some contribution of the GABAergic system to the rats' 'dementia'.[16] However, the most striking results came from comparing the ex-alcoholic rats with rats treated with sub-convulsant doses of the excitotoxin BMAA (beta-methyl-amino-alanine), which is associated with human dementia on Guam. Using Lumafluor tracing techniques, it was possible to demonstrate microscopic neuronal changes in the same animals demonstrated to have impaired performance in behavioural tests. The same neocortical systems (involving inputs from the corpus callosum, basal nucleus and raphe) were altered after alcohol or BMAA, and performance was impaired in the same ways.[17] During the iontophoretic study of Armstrong-James *et al.*,[18] it was observed that drugs acting on the NMDA receptor produced physiological after-effects on particular populations of cortical single units, but we little guessed that specific behavioural and anatomical changes might persist in rats for months, after exogenous tampering with this system. It now appears that spatial learning problems develop earlier in the history of young alcoholics (average age 26.7)[19] than we used to believe, and magnetic resonance studies show that human brain metabolism has not yet recovered from past heavy drinking after 3–6 months of abstinence.[20] Periods of heavy drinking in earlier life increase the risk for humans to develop either dementia or depression in old age.[21] If one can extrapolate from rats to humans, then individuals already exposed to some level of NMDA-type excitotoxicity, such as people with CNS HIV infection, may be at additional risk of dementia following binge drinking.[22]

CHRONIC HEAVY USE

There is little doubt that heavy alcohol use by humans can be followed by changes in both CT scans and psychometric performance and, fortunately, these changes can sometimes be reversible after about a year of abstinence.[23, 24] Cannabis is another widely used substance, but it is still hotly debated whether any CNS effects outlast the immediate period of intoxication with cannabinoids. However, observations on psychiatric cases suggests that recent[25] or frequent[26] cannabis use may predispose to subsequent psychotic illness.

The 'court is still out' (consider the UK mass action legal case brought by patients prescribed sedative-hypnotic drugs against the manufacturers) on whether or not residual deficits persist after heavy benzodiazepine use. If a 'benzodiazepine dementia' exists, the evidence of Baldwin[27] may be relevant: that repeated benzodiazepine administration eventually leads to synthesis of an inverse agonist having the opposite action on GABA-A receptors to the exogenous sedative–hypnotic drug, with similar unpleasant effects to the beta-carbolines mentioned, above. In all elderly patients who may already be showing signs of dementia, Hopkins[12] suggests stopping any sedative medication they have been taking.

Chronic alcohol use in association with thiamine deficiency, and other factors, can lead to Korsakoff's psychosis. Two typical case descriptions are detailed by Mayes.[28] Korsakoff's memory deficits seem to be irreversible, with present knowledge.[29] Focal lesions in the hypothalamus, thalamus and midbrain have been described in such patients, *post mortem*.

Research using trained monkeys[30] suggested that a small region of medial thalamus showed a unique pattern of activity in long-term recognition memory. Single neurones here showed a close correspondence between their electrical activity and the monkey's subsequent recognition of particular stimuli that were repeated a long time after their original appearance. This may be a critical site for the anterograde amnesia in Korsakoff's cases. More recent anatomical, physiological, pharmacological and behavioural experiments suggest that these thalamic neurones might play a strategic role in many cortical activities. They and their cortical targets are sensitive to NMDA agonists and antagonists.[31, 32] One might speculate that in some alcoholics a chronic exposure to excitotoxic isoquinolines associated with depressed levels of neuroprotective kynurenic acid might eventually precipitate a catastrophic failure of this memory system (see Chapter 9).

Wernicke–Korsakoff pathology usually presents to clinicians only at the tragic end of many years of accumulating alcohol-related deterioration. To observe chronic substance use producing damage more quickly and with fewer confounding variables, I recommend researching cocaine. Such stimulants raise extracellular dopamine concentrations to supraphysiological levels for prolonged periods, allowing toxic metabolites to accumulate, synthesis to become depressed, and receptor density to alter.[33] Furthermore, particular memory systems, involving the prefrontal cortex, seem to show specific abnormalities following chronic cocaine use. The brain shows longlasting 'priming' or 'kindling' effects after cocaine, so that even intermittent, low doses may contribute to the accumulating damage. Animals, and an increasing number of humans, readily self-administer the drug. Aspects of pharmacology, behaviour and cognition all offer new insights in the biology of healthcare – for example, those self-experimenting with illicit cocaine often self-medicate with benzodiazepines and many other CNS depressants in an attempt, it appears, to temper the ruinous effects of this stimulant. This then provides opportunities for researchers to model the preferred patterns of choices across different combinations of substances which these future addicts may be learning or to guide clinical decisions about future poisonings involving such drug combinations.[22]

FOETAL DAMAGE

It has taken decades for FAS (foetal alcohol syndrome)[34] to be acknowledged worldwide as a common and disabling problem affecting some children of mothers who drink heavily during pregnancy. With or without the characteristic dystrophic physical features of FAS, many babies of alcoholic mothers later show an intellectual and behavioural disorder as they grow up. Both the public health and the individual, developmental, aspects of FAS are now being extensively researched[35] and research with rat pups[36] suggests that a single day of alcohol exposure, at a critical stage of brain development, can eliminate many GABAergic Purkinje cells in the cerebellum. Neonates may show withdrawal fits after maternal use of opiates, barbiturates or benzodiazepines during pregnancy[13] but it is not known if longer-term problems are likely to follow. There is growing evidence that maternal cocaine use can become hazardous to the foetus,[33] although 'crack babies' are usually born to mothers taking their cocaine with a combination of substances.

So far, we have considered five possible routes by which using a substance like alcohol might lead to Cassidy's 'great variety' of nervous system disorders observed in individual cases. However, it has been clear since the time of Jellinek[37] that 'decadent drinkers' or 'tired . . . cocainists' may disclose a family history of problems which interact with the effects of substance use. To understand the neurochemistry of drugs of abuse, we will need to know if there are genetic factors which alter their impact on individuals.[38] One area of pressing clinical concern is the vulnerability of those individuals who develop certain combinations of mental disorder, such as alcoholism and schizophrenia.[39]

TREATMENT OF BRAIN DAMAGE

With regard to the scope for treatment of drug-induced brain damage, obviously prevention is better than cure. Also, within any one programme to restore lost neurological function, it is common for different individuals to respond in distinctly different ways.[18] With recovering addicts it is advisable to be modest and flexible about the goals of treatment, building on particular personal needs or strengths for each patient.[40] A gradual and spontaneous recovery, after damaging use of drugs as different as cannabis, amphetamines or alcohol, often happens. The World Health Organisation[41] has evaluated, in general terms, the treatments currently used for mental disorders due to brain damage. WHO is unconvinced of the value of existing pharmacological agents, such as the cholinergic drug tacrine or the metabolic activator piracetam, for treating most demented patients. Rehabilitative approaches combining behavioural, psychological and social interventions were observed to promote the independence of such patients. Rehabilitative programmes (such as these designed by clinical psychologists, occupational therapists or physiotherapists) have helped many former drug users overcome particular deficits in performing the 'activities of daily living'. As well as receiving care by professionals, many addicts also benefit from mutual aid, for example attending groups such as Narcotics Anonymous seems to enhance participants' self-esteem.[42] With former cocaine users, integration of professional rehabilitation with other resources to promote a balanced mix of physical, psychological, social, occupational and spiritual regeneration may be especially helpful.[17] Just on the horizon, is the possibility that functional magnetic resonance imaging could enormously advance rehabilitation after neurological disabilities 'because rehabilitation programmes could be tailored to maximise the use of areas that were known to have the potential of taking over functionally from damaged areas'.[43]

A number of short-term medical treatments of brain dysfunction have been tried. In particular, the B and C vitamin preparation Parentrovite has certainly helped some malnourished addicts. More exotic combinations of nutrients[44] have been tried in other countries. Chronic use of many drugs can lower the threshold for seizures, and anticonvulsants like diazepam have a short-term role in managing the after-effects of such toxins, until brain metabolism recovers a more healthy equilibrium free of fits. If current animal research[45] can be extrapolated to man, L-calcium channel blockers like nitrendipine may someday aid recovery from alcoholism.

The longer-term use of existing therapeutic drugs with recovering substance abusers is a more controversial practice, because of inconsistent reports of any effectiveness and fears of iatrogenic damage to patients. Lithium and bromocriptine seem to have dropped out of use, for these reasons. However, there is evidence that some people recovering from cocaine addiction benefit from the antidepressant drug desipramine or the mood stabilizer carbamazapine, over months. Kleber[46] has suggested a therapy for the dopamine depletion caused by cocaine, starting with the ant-Parkinson drug amantadine followed and gradually replaced by desipramine. At present, there is no equivalent therapy for the effects of chronic alcohol or benzodiazepines on the brain, but Hughes[47] proposes that certain peptides, like an antagonist of cholecystokinin, might bring neurological improvements in the future. Another promising family of drugs, unfortunately with some abuse potential of their own, are the 'cognitive enhancers' such as ondansetron. These appear to act at more specific sites in the brain than the older metabolic activator drugs.

Finally, during this 'Decade of the Brain' it is possible that various efforts at 'brain repair' being tested for other types of pathology (e.g. Parkinson's disease) may also bring benefits to the victims of drug-induced brain damage. Iversen[48] has been investigating neuroprotective agents, nerve growth factors and the surgical transplantation of foetal brain tissue. Here in Cambridge, a Brain Repair Centre opens this year, to study a range of interventions drawing on surgery, pharmacology, neural development and behavioural science for new approaches to neurorehabilitation.

ACKNOWLEDGEMENTS

This work was made possible by generous funding from the British Technology Group, the Medical Research Council and the Mental Health Foundation.

GLOSSARY OF TERMS

Families of drugs with similar actions are in	**bold**
Specific drugs are given in	CAPITALS
Street names are given in	*italics*
Clinical conditions are	<u>underlined</u>

Opioid painkillers like BUPRENORPHINE are synthetic equivalents of the **opiate** narcotics MORPHINE or HEROIN, which act on the brain's encephalin receptors. As well as the **opioids** for medicinal purposes, 'designer drug' **opioids** are produced illicitly to satisfy a similar black market as HEROIN imports. MPTP is an accidental contaminant of some designer *opioids*, which produces irreversible brain damage resembling Parkinson's disease.

Psychomotor stimulants include COCAINE and AMPHETAMINE, which act mainly on re-uptake sites for dopamine and noradrenaline. Some illicit 'designer drug' production involves **amphetamines** (stimulant drugs) modified to produce an additional dreamy, hallucinatory, *Ecstasy* effect, particularly the drugs MDA and 3, 4 methylenedioxy-methampheta mine (MDMA). Animal research has suggested that certain **antidepressant** drugs (specific serotonin re-uptake inhibitors) might protect against the toxic effects of *Ecstasy*, but human cases of poisoning with *Ecstasy* have only recently become apparent.

Many popular drugs have sedative–hypnotic actions (including ALCOHOL, **barbituates** and the **benzodiazpines** like TEMAZEPAM, DIAZEPAM or the recently-withdrawn drug TRIAZOLAM used by President George Bush before his famous Japanese dinner). These all increase the effects on neurones on the inhibitory transmitter Gamma-amino-butyric-acid (GABA) – the antidote to a benzodiazepine overdose is the antagonist FLUMAZENIL. Some drugs called **inverse agonists** have the opposite action to **benzodiazepines**, reducing the effect of GABA. The drug HARMALINE has this untranquil action (shown in rather romanticised terms in the film 'Emerald Forest' about native recreations in the Amazon). Acetaldehyde production in heavy drinkers can generate similar beta-carboline **inverse agonists** to the tranquillisers, which may account for the episodes of panic, insomnia, hallucinatory states and seizures common in alcoholism.

A number of excitatory receptors respond to the brain's own amino acids glutamic acid or aspartic acid. However, at the same receptors exogenous amino acids from various sources can act destructively and these are called excitotoxins. Neurolathyrism is an irreversible paralysis associated with toxic amino acids in some plants (*Lathyrus* = the sweet pea). The amino acid BMAA comes from the false sago palm, which grows on Guam and other Pacific islands, and can produce features of different degenerating neurological diseases (Alzheimer's dementia, Parkinson's disease or motor neurone disease) in different individuals who eat this excitotoxin. BMAA overstimulates the same excitatory receptor, the NMDA receptor, as the isoquinolines produced after abnormal metabolism of the transmitter 5-HT in alcoholics who have generated high levels of acetaldehyde. These damaging levels of acetaldehyde are produced by the enzymatic action of alcohol dehydrogenase on big doses of alcohol. The brain's own protection against too much excitation normally involves KYNURENIC ACID. Synthetic drugs like PHENCYCLIDINE (*Angel Dust*) or KETAMINE (*Special K*) which also damp down excitation via NMDA receptors, were once widely used as dissociative anaesthetics, but they were found to have toxic side effects themselves. A mental effect similar to KETAMINE can be produced by the anti-emetic drug CYCLIZINE if injected at several times the oral dose used to control seasickness. A more modern anti-emetic, ONDANSETRON, which binds selectively to the 5-HT3 receptor, may have therapeutic potential in recovery from addiction, but has illicit uses too which are related to a mild enhancement of cognitive processing.

Korsakoff's psychosis is an irreversible, profound, amnesia which occurs in some alcoholics with Wernicke's encephalopathy of the tissues around the 3rd ventricle of the brain. Multivitamin preparations containing THIAMINE can often prevent permanent disability after a sudden manifestation of Wernicke-type damage. The same vitamin preparations can aid recovery from an alcoholic neuropathy affecting peripheral sensory and motor nerves, leading to an improved gait when walking. Abstinence from alcohol is crucial for any such recovery. Because dependence on alcohol lowers the threshold for seizures, an **anticonvulsant** (usually a **benzodiazepine** like DIAZEPAM or CHLORDIAZEPOXIDE) is needed during the transitional period of detoxification, leading to sobriety, to prevent withdrawal fits. Dementias often have a gradual onset, associated with progressive shrinkage of the brain's cerebral cortex. Memory and orientation are disrupted early in dementia, but eventually many faculties may disintegrate. The psychoses associated with stimulant or hallucinogenic drugs often resemble a paranoid schizophrenic illness, with disordered thinking, fearful or suspicious delusions, hallucinations and bizarre behaviours. If patients maintain a drug-free state, however, many show a rapid and complete recovery.

NOTES

1. J. Cassidy, *Drugs and Alcohol: Proceedings of the Conference on 'The Human Mind'* (Vatican City: The Vatican, 1991), pp. 63–265.

2. 'Divorce, Alcohol Abuse Linked to Rise in Male Suicides', *Alcohol Alert*, June 1993, p. 13.
3. C. Hall, 'Teenagers Taking Risks with Health at an Earlier Age', *The Independent*, 22 September 1992.
4. T. Y. Black, 'An Informed Introduction to 3,4 Methylenedioxymethamphetamine (MDMA, "Ecstasy", "E")', unpublished, Department of Psychology, University of Hull, 1995.
5. L. Hermle, 'Zur bedeutung der historischen und aktuellen halluzinogenforschung in der psychiatrie', *Nervenarzt*, 64 (1993):562–71.
6. J. W. Olney, 'Pathological Changes Induced in Cerebrocortical Neurons by Phenyclidine and Related Drugs', *Science*, 244 (1989):1360–2.
7. A. Furnham, 'Mind Blowing or just another Swipe?', *British Medical Journal*, 306 (1993):660.
8. W. A. Caan, 'Deeply Designer Drugs', *European Journal of Neuroscience*, 1992 Supplement, no. 4, p. 322.
9. G. Lucas, 'Problem Drinking in the Workplace', *London Alcoholism*, no. 4, pp. 1–4 (newsletter of the Medical Council on Alcoholism).
10. N. L. Benowitz, 'How Toxic is Cocaine? Cocaine as a Biological and Medical Problem', CIBA Foundation Symposuim, London (1991).
11. W. A. Caan and J. Fenton, 'Self-catering during Rehabilitation', *British Journal of Psychiatry*, 157 (1990):780–1.
12. A. Hopkins, *Clinical Neurology: A Modern Approach* (Oxford: Oxford University Press, 1993).
13. H. Ghodse, *Drugs and Addictive Behaviour: A Guide to Treatment* (Oxford: Blackwell, 1989).
14. W. A. Caan, 'Chronic Alcohol Administration Leads to a Persistent Increase in Aggression in Rats after Withdrawal, in a New Behavioural Test', *Neuroscience Letters*, Supplement: 32 (1988) S32, S41.
15. W. A. Caan, 'Chronic Alcohol can Produce, in Rats, Persistent Disturbance of Certain Behaviours and CNS Neurones, after Withdrawal', *British Journal of Addiction*, 84 (1989):1392.
16. R. Armstrong, 'The Benzodiazepine Receptor Antagonist Flumazenil has Longlasting Effects on Alcoholic Rats', *British Journal of Pharmacology*, 95 (1989):881.
17. W. A. Caan, 'Crack – The Broken Promise', *Postgraduate Medical Journal*, 68 (1992):396.
18. R. Crisp, 'Personal Responses to Traumatic Brain Injury: A Qualitative Study', *Disability, Handicap & Society*, 8 (1993):393–404.
19. S. C. Bowden and W. A. Caan, 'Learning in Young Alcoholics: Chronic Alcohol Administration Leads to a Persistent Increase in Aggression in Rats, after Withdrawal, in a New Behavioural Test', *Journal of Clinical and Experimental Neuropsychology*, 1988: 10 (2) S32, S41, 157–168.
20. J. A. O. Besson, 'Magnetic Resonance Imaging and its Applications in Neuropsychiatry', *British Journal of Psychiatry*, 157 (1990):25–37.
21. P. A. Saunders, 'Heavy Drinking as a Risk Factor for Depression and Dementia in Elderly Men', *British Journal of Psychiatry*, 159 (1991): 213–216.
22. W. A. Caan, 'Crack – the Broken Promise', *Postgraduate Medical Journal*, 68 (1992):396.

23. M. A. Ron, 'The Brain of Alcoholics: An Overview', in *Neuropsychology of Alcoholism: Implications for Diagnosis and Treatment* (New York: Guilford, 1987) pp. 11–20.
24. R. E. Tarter, 'Neurobehavioral Disorders Associated with Chronic Alcohol Abuse', in A. M. Arria (ed.), *Alcoholism: Biomedical and Genetic Aspects* (New York: Pergamon, 1989), pp 113–29.
25. D. C. Mathers, 'Cannabis Use in a Large Sample of Acute Psychiatric Admissions', *British Journal of Addiction*, 86 (1991):779–84.
26. S. Andreasson, 'Cannabis and Schizophrenia', *Lancet*, ii (1987):1483–6.
27. H. A. Baldwin, 'Reversal of Increased Anxiety during Benzodiazepine Withdrawal: Evidence for an Anxiogenic Endogenous Ligand for the Benzodiazepine Receptor', *Brain Research Bulletin*, 20: (1989):603–6.
28. A. R. Mayes, 'Locations of Lesions in Korsakoff's Syndrome: Neuropsychological and Neuropathological Data on Two Patients', *Cortex*, 24 (1988):367–88.
29. R. E. O'Carroll, 'Korsakoff's Syndrome, Cognition and Clonidine', *Psychological Medicine*, 23 (1993):341–7.
30. E. T. Rolls, 'Neuronal Responses Related to Visual Recognition', *Brain* 105 (1982):611–46.
31. K. Fox, 'The Role of the Anterior Intralaminar Nuclei and *N*-Methyl D-Aspartate Receptors in the Generation of Spontaneous Bursts in Rat Neocortical Neurones', *Experimental Brain Research*, 63 (1986):505–18.
32. M. E. Diamond, 'Experience-dependent Plasticity in Adult Rat Barrel Cortex', *Proceedings of the National Academy of Science USA*, 90 (1993): 2082–6.
33. J. Strang, 'Cocaine in the UK – 1991', *British Journal of Psychiatry*, 162 (1993):1–13.
34. P. Lemoine, 'An Historical Note about the Foetal-Alcohol Syndrome', *Addiction*, 89 (1994):1021–3.
35. U. Rydberg, 'Addiction Research in Europe', *European Addiction Research*, (1995):26–31.
36. C. R. Goodlett, 'A Single Day of Alcohol Exposure during the Brain Growth Spurt Induces Brain Weight Restriction and Cerebellar Purkinje Cell Loss', *Alcohol*, 7 (1990):107–14.
37. E. M. Jellinek, *Alcohol Addiction and Chronic Alcoholism* (New Haven, Conn.: Yale University Press, 1942).
38. M. Rattray, 'Neurochemical Aspects of Drug Abuse', *The Biochemist*, 14 (1992):2.
39. W. A. Caan and M. Crowe, 'Using Readmission Rates as Indicators of Outcomes in Comparing Psychiatric Services', *Journal of Mental Health*, 3 (1994):521–24.
40. W, A. Caan, 'An Addict who Threatens the GP for a Prescription', *Prescriber*, 5 (1994):63–8.
41. World Health Organization, 1990.
42. G. Christo and S. Sutton, '*Anxiety and Self-Esteem as a Function of Abstinence Time among Recovering Addicts Attending Narcotics Anonymous*', *British Journal of Clinical Psychology*, 33 (1994):198–200.
43. S. J. Ellis, 'Functional Magnetic Resonance: Neurological Enlightenment?', *Lancet*, 342 (1993):882.

44. K. Blum, 'Neurogenetic Deficits Caused by Alcoholism: Restoration by SAAVE, a Neuronutrient Intervention Adjunct', *Journal of Psychoactive Drugs*, 20 (1992):297–313.
45. H. J. Little, 'Neuronal Calcium Channels and Ethanol Dependence', *European Journal of Neuroscience*, Supplement 4 (1991):323.
46. H. D. Kleber, 'Pharmacotherapy for Cocaine Addicts: Abstract in Cocaine as a Biological and Medical Problem', CIBA Foundation Symposium (1991).
47. J. Hughes, 'Brain Peptides May Hold Key to Severe Psychiatric Disease', *Viewpoint Depression Management* (1991) p. 2.
48. L. L. Iversen, 'The Neurobiology of Ageing', *Conquest*, 178 (1989):1–14.

6 Substance Misuse and Tissue Pathology with Special Reference to the Heart

Victor R. Preedy, Howard Why,
Vinood Patel, Adrian Bonner and
Peter Richardson

INTRODUCTION

Common drugs of misuse include alcohol, nicotine (and tobacco products), cannabis, cocaine and, to a certain extent, caffeine. Other lesser used drugs include amphetamines, opiates, sedatives/hypnotics, phencyclidines, hallucinogens and anabolic steroids. In Europe there are many millions of drug misusers and, similarly, the extent of drug misuse in North America is staggering. Thus, in the UK there are between 1 and 3 million alcohol abusers and a third of the adult population smoke tobacco products. The biomedical implications of this prevalence are considerable. In comparison with psychomotor, neuropsychiatric and cognitive reports on the above substances, investigations into organ damage are comparatively limited. This particularly relates to the biochemical mechanisms responsible for tissue specific lesions. It is a truism that virtually every single tissue system or organ in the mammalian body is adversely affected to some degree by one or more of the above drugs of misuse. At the extreme, there is organ failure and death. At the very least, there may arise compensatory mechanisms, that may be considered to be either *adaptive* or *destructive* but, nevertheless, impair organ function.

To embrace the entire spectrum of effects due to substance misuse in one review belittles the vast amount of scientific literature that has accumulated in the past three decades. To circumvent the interpretational problems that may arise from a survey of all the tissues affected, this review has focused on a single organ, namely the heart. The biochemical, morphological and functional injuries that arise in cardiac muscle are therefore reviewed. The overriding evidence suggests that cardiac defects due to substance misuse are extremely common and often under-diagnosed. Strategies to curtail substance misuse may be one avenue to avert end-organ damage but this direction has proved to be of limited efficiency. It is possible that, by understanding the biochemical mechanisms involved in organ dysfunction, novel therapeutic regimes that cure the damage *per se* may be devised.

A great deal of attention has focused on the mood-altering qualities of psychoactive drugs and other non-prescribed substances. The side-effects of these agents and social factors such as peer-pressure or a desire for peer-identification, that precipitate their self-administration or ingestion are well studied. However, the extra-CNS effects of substance misuse have received in comparison little attention. Defects in cell structure resulting from drug abuse may account for observed increases in mortality and morbidity. The available literature in the field is diverse, but one way of obtaining some sort of perspective can be achieved by focusing on a particular organ. The literature on the effects of drugs on the liver and non-hepatic tissues is vast. For example, these are reviewed in Lieber,[1] and Preedy *et al.*,[2] for liver and skeletal muscle, respectively. In this chapter the heart is selected. The rationale of this is that impairment in heart function will have profound implications for morbidity and mortality. Thus, Tunving[3] reviewed the cause of mortality in over 524 drug addicts over 10 years, during which 62 died, some of these due to overdoses. In the cases of overdose, there were signs of heart disease due to chronic drug abuse.

In order to give an overview of the deleterious effects of drugs, one prerequisite is necessary however: the use of animal models needs to be rationalised.

Whilst a number of studies have examined the effects of substance abuse on the human heart, the results and ensuing interpretations can be conflicting. This is due to the fact that other pathologies may co-exist.[4] For example, alcohol misuse may occur with thiamine deficiency and both induce specific lesions in heart muscle. In addition, substance abuse may involve a cohort of drugs (i.e. polydrug abuse) and a common example is combined alcohol and nicotine addiction.[5] Therefore, it may be difficult to dissect out the events or agents responsible for pathogenic alterations if no account is taken of subject variability or polydrug abuse.[6] To resolve this, animal models have been devised. It is important to reiterate that the ensuing pathways and processes elucidated from an analysis of drug-induced defects may be applicable to other metabolic processes. Understanding basic processes is a prerequisite for developing future strategies of treatment.

SUBSTANCE ABUSE

The classification of substance abuse is purely arbitrary but divisions used by the National Council on Alcoholism and Drug Dependence have been employed as follows:

1. Alcohol
2. Stimulants (including cocaine, amphetamines, caffeine and nicotine)
3. Opiates
4. Cannabis
5. Sedatives/hypnotics
6. Phencyclidines (PCP/Angel Dust)
7. Hallucinogens
8. Anabolic steroids
9. Solvents
10. Miscellaneous

These divisions are based largely on psychosocial factors and (to a lesser degree) a classification of physiological effects. They take no account of the basic biochemical mechanisms by which harmful effects are induced; neither are they in any way specific to the organs which may be affected by the abuse process. When considering the effects of substance abuse on the heart, the vast majority of problems encountered result from tobacco use which is firmly established as a major risk factor for the development of coronary artery disease.[7] Two other substances stand out with regard to cardiac morbidity; these are alcohol and cocaine. Detailed descriptions of their effects will be given below. Other agents with little known cardiovascular effect will not be discussed in detail.

TOBACCO

Between 50 and 150 μg of nicotine is absorbed into the circulation with each puff of tobacco. Tobacco smoke, however, is a complex entity of over 500 compounds containing a mixture of toxic substances including carbon monoxide. However, the precise toxins contributing to the development of coronary artery disease, and the mechanisms by which they act, are unclear. Several mechanisms have been invoked, including an alteration in the lipid profile (with a reduction in the high density lipoprotein (HDL) cholesterol and elevation of the low density lipoprotein (LDL) cholesterol) and an adverse effect on blood coagulation and platelets. The cardiovascular effects of smoking also include tachycardia, peripheral vasoconstriction and an elevation in the blood pressure of approximately 10–15 mm Hg. There is an increase in cardiac work with a concomitant coronary vasodilatation. Ventricular ectopic activity may be stimulated by smoking though sustained arrhythmias are rare. Smoking may induce myocardial ischaemia in individuals with atherosclerotic coronary artery disease. The mechanisms for this are unclear but may include the physiological changes indicated above and possibly further hypoxia in those with co-existing chronic lung disease and impaired oxygenation of the blood. In addition, the irreversible binding of carbon monoxide to haemoglobin reduces the effective oxygen carrying capacity of the blood.

Nicotine itself stimulates the release of catecholamines with a resultant tachycardia and generalised (including coronary) vasoconstriction.[8] In patients with pre-existing coronary atherosclerosis this process may lead to episodes of ischaemia. Smoking is associated with at least a 2-fold increase in the risk of myocardial infarction depending upon the patient's age. There is a positive correlation between the risk and the number of cigarettes smoked. Testament to the complexity of the relationship between smoking and coronary artery disease, however, is borne by the lack of variation of risk with the tar content of the cigarettes smoked. Thus neither nicotine nor carbon monoxide levels in the smoke inhaled directly influence the risk of developing coronary artery disease.[9]

ALCOHOL

Although acute ethanol may cause a fall in blood pressure, epidemiological studies show that hypertension is associated with chronic misuse. As many as 50 per cent of subjects in hypertension clinics may be classified as ethanol misusers.[10] Hypertension carries with it certain independent risk factors for heart disease including the development of left ventricular hypertrophy which is associated with changes in the heart muscle itself. Increases in blood pressure can be observed in subjects consuming as little as 20–40 g ethanol per day (approximately 10 g of alcohol is contained in half a pint of beer or one measure of wine or spirits). The actual mechanisms of this increase in blood pressure are unknown.[11, 12]

It is necessary to mention some of the findings that indicate moderate ethanol consumption may be cardioprotective in that it reduces the incidence of death due to coronary heart disease.[4, 13–15] These correlations have been observed in numerous studies and the finding of a U- or J-shaped curve (with increasing incidence of coronary artery disease in immoderate consumption) are now undisputed.[16] However, attention should be focused on two important points. Firstly, that alcohol misuse effects virtually every tissue system (for example, an increased incidence of cirrhosis is apparent at levels of consumption of 40 g ethanol/day). Secondly, there is a large number of people in the UK (1–3 million) who consume excessive quantities of alcohol. This approximates to about 2–6 per cent of the population and, as a good rule of thumb, similar proportions of ethanol abusers may be ascribed to other European or North American countries.

Heart-muscle damage may occur when the consumption rate is 80 g/day for 10 years or more, or the cumulative lifetime alcohol intake exceeds 250 kg ethanol. Strictly speaking, the term '*cardiomyopathy*' should not be used in relation to ethanol-induced heart-muscle damage because the cause of the pathology is known.[17] The term *alcoholic heart muscle disease* (AHMD) is more appropriate. The features of AHMD have been extensively reviewed and it is now accepted that the gross morphological changes are well defined and resemble those of dilated cardiomyopathy. The aetiological mechanisms at the cellular and biochemical level are not so well understood, though an important element is the change in protein synthesis, especially in the initial periods of ethanol exposure.[4, 12, 18]

Features of AHMD include dilatation of the left ventricle, cardiomegaly, dysrhythmias, sinus tachycardia, ventricular extrasystoles, atria fibrillation and fatigue. At the cellular level there may be lipid deposits, fibrosis, derangements in the myofibrillary architecture, abnormalities in the mitochondria or sarcoplasmic reticulum. Of course the exact nature of these lesions will vary with the course of the disease process.[12]

The biochemical basis for AHMD is not known, though defects in calcium homeostasis may be responsible and possibly account for effects on excitation–contraction coupling. Evidence to support this has been derived from the use of verapamil, a calcium-channel antagonist, which interacts with the phenylalkylamine recognition sites in the alpha subunit of the calcium channel.[19] Biopsies of heart muscle from chronic alcohol abusers have shown that there is an increased activity of some myocardial enzymes, including creatine kinase, alpha-hydroxybutyric dehydrogenase and lactate dehydrogenase. These raised enzyme activities may reflect a compensatory adaptation.[20]

There is little evidence to support the contention that AHMD is mediated by nutritional abnormalities (this is discussed in several reviews).[4, 12, 18] However, it is possible that free-radicals (biologically reactive oxygen species) may initiate some of the damage, especially inducing lipid peroxidation (see, for example, Reinke *et al.*[21] and other reviews[4, 12, 18]).

In animal models the synthesis of contractile proteins is reduced in response to acute ethanol treatment regimes and increased in response to chronic ethanol feeding regimens. The reasons for the contrasting changes are unknown. The inhibitory effects of acute ethanol dosage on the ventricles are also observed in the atria. It appears that acetaldehyde may be responsible for a component of the reduced synthesis rates.[4, 12, 18]

As mentioned above, consideration must be given to co-ingestion of other drugs. Cocaine and ethanol, for example, are frequently taken together. Apart from detrimental CNS effects, a combination of cocaine and ethanol induces the formation (in the liver) of cocaethylene. This product is toxic to myocardial cells in culture as determined by release of lactate dehydrogenase, depressed lysosomal neutral red retention, depressed contractility and morphological changes.[22] Cocaine alone also increases blood pressure and heart rate, an effect which is potentiated by alcohol.[23]

COCAINE

Whereas amphetamine abuse may be considered to be a social phenomenon of the 1970s, the abuse of cocaine has its roots in history. Sir Arthur Conan Doyle vividly describes its intravenous use as a cerebral stimulant by his famous detective hero Sherlock Holmes. The 1980s and 1990s, however, have seen a resurgence of the popularity of cocaine as a drug of abuse, fuelled by a belief that its use was safe and not addictive. Figures for the prevalence of cocaine use in Britain are lacking, but it is estimated that up to 30 million people in the United

States have experimented with cocaine use at some time and approximately 5 per cent of the American population are thought to be regular users.[24]

The potentially dangerous effects of cocaine abuse have been highlighted by an increasing number of reports detailing a relationship between cardiovascular illness and cocaine. Many forms of cardiac disease have been associated with both acute and chronic cocaine use but among the most common are ischaemic heart disease (acute ischaemic events and myocardial infarction), heart muscle disease, hypertension, cardiac arrhythmias and sudden cardiac death. These reports are confounded, however, by factors such as differences in cocaine purity and dose, varying routes of administration and the simultaneous use of other substances (not least of which may be the base substance used to 'cut' the cocaine). Consequently animal studies have been directed at the elucidation of the cardiovascular effects of cocaine.

The suggested cardiotoxic effects of cocaine may be explained by one or more of its pharmacological actions on the cardiovascular system. Perhaps, most importantly, cocaine stimulates the release of catecholamines both peripherally and centrally[25] and blocks their reuptake in both peripheral and central nervous systems.[26] This results in an increase in circulating catecholamines with consequent stimulation of both alpha and beta receptors. The former causes vasoconstriction and hypertension whilst the latter leads to tachycardia and an increase in cardiac arrhythmogenic potential. Cocaine also has so-called membrane-stabilising activity which is effected by blocking the fast myocardial sodium channel.[26] This results in depression of myocyte depolarisation and slowing of conduction of the myocardial action potential with prolongation of both atrial and ventricular refractory periods. This action may account for the negative inotropic effect of cocaine which is common to other local anaesthetic agents which possess class I antiarrhythmic activity (e.g. lignocaine). Other mechanisms of cocaine cardiotoxicity may include stimulation of natural killer cells and direct hypersensitivity of myocytes to cocaine. It has been suggested that the lack of tolerance may contribute to myocardial toxicity due to cocaine.[27]

In animal models, the acute administration of cocaine leads to an increased heart rate and sometimes blood pressure.[28] Despite this, the majority of studies show that left ventricular function is depressed by cocaine, especially in higher doses. In addition, most studies have documented a reduction in coronary artery diameter with a concomitant reduction in coronary blood flow shortly after cocaine administration.[29] Cocaine also has adverse effects on cardiac electrophysiology with prolongation of all phases of the action potential. It is proarrhythmogenic and animal studies have documented the induction of atrial tachyarrhythmias and ventricular tachycardia.

Very few animal studies of chronic cocaine administration have been performed. It appears to induce disorganisation of the cardiac cellular architecture with reductions in myocyte enzyme levels.[30] These changes may explain the myocardial alterations seen in some human cocaine abusers (see below). Possibly the most interesting and well-documented chronic effect of cocaine, however, is its ability to induce accelerated atherogenesis.[31] This has profound implications for harm in long-term human users.

The haemodynamic effects of acute cocaine usage in human subjects are similar to those in animals, with an increased heart rate and elevated blood pressure. When cocaine is administered during coronary angiography, acute reductions in coronary artery diameter are observed.[32] Interestingly, this vasoconstriction has been reported to be greater in atherosclerotic arteries than in non-diseased ones[33] although *in vitro* work with isolated human coronary artery rings did not support these findings.[34] An important sequela of coronary vasoconstriction may be myocardial infarction and the literature abounds with reports of acute coronary events in association with cocaine use. The actual incidence remains unknown but most reported cases appear to be in chronic abusers. The majority are young men and about one-third of the patients are subsequently shown to have anatomically normal coronary arteries, suggesting that spasms may be a pathogenic factor.[35] The induction of acute myocardial ischaemia without myocardial infarction has also been reported in cocaine users. Some reports also indicate that the accelerated atherogenesis in human cocaine abusers leads to an increased incidence of myocardial ischaemia and infarction. Dressler *et al.*[36] reported on a series of autopsies of cocaine addicts with a mean age of only 32 years. Over one-third had significant coronary artery stenosis. These findings have been confirmed by other researchers.

Several reports have highlighted the potential for cocaine to cause heart muscle disease in the absence of definable coronary artery disease. In one study, significant left ventricular dysfunction was detected in 7 per cent of cocaine addicts[37] while other reports have described reversible left ventricular dysfunction associated with congestive cardiac failure after cocaine use. In some patients the changes are irreversible and are identical to those found in dilated cardiomyopathy. The mechanisms underlying this dysfunction are unclear but two possible explanations are the negative inotropic properties of cocaine itself or an indirect effect via an excess of circulating catecholamines. It appears also that cocaine may have a direct toxic effect upon the heart muscle causing a myocarditis. Twenty per cent of patients undergoing autopsy in whom there were detectable blood cocaine levels were found to have a lymphocytic infiltrate of the myocardium associated with myocyte necrosis.[38] It has been postulated that excess circulating catecholamines may contribute to these appearances.[39]

Cardiac arrhythmias have also been reported in association with cocaine abuse. The majority of these have been episodes of ventricular tachycardia or ventricular fibrillation, the latter progressing occasionally to asystole. Such arrhythmias may occur as isolated events or may complicate cocaine-associated myocardial infarction.[40] In population studies, cardiac arrhythmias are more common in habitual cocaine users than their non-drug-dependant controls.[41]

CAFFEINE

In Western societies, caffeine is one of the most extensively used drugs. Like alcohol, it is distributed to virtually all tissue compartments.[42] Caffeine affects calcium channels in the same way as opiates[43] while high levels of caffeine (10 mmol/l or above) also cause myofilament and mitochondrial damage.[44, 45] Like the interaction with cocaine and alcohol, other drugs of misuse also have the potential to interact with caffeine. Smits *et al.*[46] examined the effects of either nicotine alone (4 mg), caffeine alone (250 mg) or a combination of both in healthy volunteers. A combination of the two raised blood pressure and was effectively the sum of the independent effects as was the effect on heart rate.[46] Arrhythmias may also develop in caffeine-naive subjects ingesting caffeine. This may be due to direct myocardial stimulation as well as an increase in circulating levels of catecholamines.[42] Myocardial contractility is also perturbed with an impairment in relaxation.[47]

Little information is available regarding the long-term cardiovascular risks of caffeine ingestion in practice. Despite its ability to increase both blood pressure and heart rate (thus increasing cardiac work), caffeine also causes coronary artery vasodilatation and therefore any direct link with myocardial ischaemia remains unproven. More interest has focused on the adverse effects of coffee on blood lipids and the potential for coffee consumption to be a long-term risk factor for the development of coronary artery disease. The relationship was examined in detail in a cohort of the Framingham study which demonstrated that total and LDL cholesterols were directly related to coffee consumption in women only.[48] In men the relationship was reversed. The overall conclusion from multivariate analysis was that coffee consumption was not an independent risk factor for the development of coronary disease.[48]

CANNABIS

Although cannabis is illegal in many European countries, the drug is legal is some Eastern countries. The usual method of abuse is by smoking (intravenous use is effectively prevented by the poor water solubility of cannabis resin) and, like tobacco, the smoke contains a large variety of compounds. The active ingredient is delta 9-tetrahydrocannabinol (THC) and during smoking between 25 and 50 per cent of the THC is delivered to the respiratory tract. This is rapidly absorbed into the blood and then taken up into the tissues. THC undergoes extensive biotransformation in the body. The majority of its metabolism takes place in the liver where it is converted into the psychoactive compound 11-hydroxy-THC and around 20 other derivatives.

Acute administration of THC produces marked bradycardia and hypothermia.[49] In contrast to these findings, most chronic cannabis users develop a tachycardia with generalised vasodilatation and, in higher doses, hypotension. In susceptible individuals these changes may produce angina and exercise-induced angina occurs more readily after cannabis use.[50]

AMPHETAMINES

The amphetamines are sympathomimetic amines which effect both the CNS and peripheral nervous system with side-effects which include enhancement of lipolysis with concomitant heat generation. They act by releasing noradrenaline thus elevating circulating catecholamine levels. Cardiovascular effects include tachycardia and vasoconstriction. In overdose, hyperpyrexia occurs and this may be associated with cardiac arrhythmias and subsequent cardiovascular collapse.

SOLVENTS

The abuse of solvents (also called *inhalants*) has markedly increased in the UK from the early 1970s, though in the last century there were sporadic reports on the misuse of chloroform and ether. The first recorded report on *glue-sniffing* in the UK appeared in 1962. It is estimated that up to 10 per cent of British adolescents have experimented with volatile organic solvent inhalation with between 0.5 and 1 per cent being established chronic abusers.[51] Currently, deaths due to solvent abuse in the UK exceed 100 per annum.[52] The effects of solvent abuse on the myocardium have been reviewed by Clayton.[53] Hydrocarbon-based substances exert varied effects upon the heart. Acute usage may induce cardiac arrhythmias either directly or due to anoxic damage. Sudden cardiac death frequently accompanies such episodes.[54] More chronic usage may induce cardiac damage resembling a dilated cardiomyopathy.[55] The mechanisms of damage remain unproven but it has been speculated that hydrocarbon exposure sensitises the myocytes to the effects of catecholamines. This sensitivity may, in turn, render the individual susceptible to arrhythmias or to the development of a catecholamine-mediated cardiomyopathy. The effects of solvent inhalation may be potentiated by hypoxaemia,[56] the concurrent consumption of catecholamine-releasing compounds and a direct vasospastic effect of the solvent itself. The last has been well demonstrated in several cases resulting in myocardial infarction with normal coronary arteries.[57–58]

CONCLUSIONS

Some substances taken in moderation do not induce deleterious effects on the heart or cardiovascular system, although they may cause subtle adaptive changes in function, perhaps via their pharmacological effects. A good example of this is alcohol, which, taken in moderation, may even reduce mortality due to coronary artery disease. However, the difficulty lies in determining the cut-off point when destructive changes occur. This concept is compounded by polydrug abuse and the ability of some individuals to show no adverse effects despite continued drug misuse. An example of this is the fact that some cocaine addicts show no signs of heart muscle disease despite chronic misuse. In contrast, a single bout of solvent abuse may precipitate heart failure in susceptible subjects. The moral issues of drug misuse are also entwined in the biology of the addiction process. This raises the issue of whether the toxicity of agents that are controlled drugs, or relatively bizarre agents such as solvents, should be a point for ethical debate. Although these questions may be rhetorical, it is our belief that attention should be focused on mechanistic actions in the ultimate belief that therapeutic strategies can be devised.

ACKNOWLEDGEMENTS

Part of the work described in this review was carried out by the Molecular and Metabolic Cardiology Group, in the Rayne Institute, Coldharbour Lane, London SE5 9PJ, UK. We acknowledge the support of Professor T. J. Peters and thank Dr T. Siddiq for his contribution to our studies and experimental programme. Vinood Patel is funded by The JRC Scheme, of King's College Hospital.

NOTES

1. C. S. Lieber, 'The Metabolism of Alcohol and its Implication for the Pathogenesis of Disease', in V. R. Preedy and R. R. Watson (eds), *Biological Mechanisms in Disease: Alcohol and the Gastrointestinal Tract* (Boca Raton: CRC Press, 1995).
2. V. R. Preedy, T. J. Peters, V. B. Patel and J. P. Miell, 'Chronic Alcoholic Myopathy: Transcription and Translational Alterations', *FASEB Journal*, 8 (1994):1146–51.
3. K. Tunving, 'Fatal Outcome in Drug Addiction', *Acta Psychiatrica Scandinavica*, 77 (1988):551–66.
4. V. R. Preedy, T. Siddiq, H. J. F. Why and P. J. Richardson, 'Ethanol Toxicity and Cardiac Protein Synthesis *in vivo*', *American Heart Journal*, 127 (1994):1432–9.
5. A. Rosengren, L. Wilhelmsen and H. Wedel, 'Separate and Combined Effects of Smoking and Alcohol Abuse in Middle-aged Men', *Acta Medica Scandinavica*, 223 (1988):111–8.
6. D. Lam and N. Goldschlager, 'Myocardial Injury Associated with Polysubstance Abuse', *American Heart Journal*, 115 (1988):675–80.
7. R. Doll, R. Peto, K. Wheatley, R. Gray and I. Sutherland, 'Mortality in Relation to Smoking: 40 years' Observation on Male British Doctors', *British Medical Journal*, 309 (1994):901–11.
8. M. D. Winniford, K. R. Wheelan, M. S. Kremers, V. Ugolini, E. Vanden-

Berg Jr, E. H. Niggermann, D. E. Jansen and L. D. Hillis, 'Smoking-Induced Coronary Vasoconstriction in Patients with Atherosclerotic Coronary Artery Disease: Evidence for Adrenergically Mediated Alterations in Coronary Artery Tone', *Circulation*, 73 (1986):662–7.

9. D. W. Kaufman, S. P. Helmrich, L. Rosenberg, O. S. Miettinen and S. Shapiro, 'Nicotine and Carbon Monoxide Content of Cigarette Smoke and the Risk of Myocardial Infarction in Young Men', *New England Journal of Medicine*, 308 (1983):409–13.

10. J. B. Saunders, D. G. Beevers and A. Paton, 'Factors Influencing Blood Pressure in Chronic Alcoholics', *Clinical Science*, 57 (1979):295S–298S.

11. J. A. Cauley, L. H. Kuller, R. E. LaPorte, W. S. Dai and J. A. D'Antonio, 'Studies on the Association Between Alcohol and High Density Lipoprotein Cholesterol: Possible Benefits and Risks', *Advances in Alcohol and Substance Abuse*, 6 (1987):53–67.

12. V. R. Preedy and P. J. Richardson, 'Ethanol-induced Cardiovascular Disease', *British Medical Bulletin*, 50 (1994):152–63.

13. H. S. Friedman, 'Cardiovascular Effects of Ethanol', in C. S. Lieber (ed.), *Medical and Nutritional Complications of Alcoholism. Mechanisms and Management* (New York: Plenum, 1992), pp. 359–401.

14. D. McCall, 'Alcohol and the Cardiovascular System', *Current Problems in Cardiology*, 12 (1987):353–401.

15. V. R. Preedy, T. Siddiq, H. J. F. Why and P. J. Richardson, 'The Deleterious Effects of Alcohol on the Heart: Involvement of Protein Turnover', *Alcohol and Alcoholism*, 29 (1994):141–7.

16. R. Doll, R. Peto, E. Hall, K. Wheatley and R. Gray, 'Mortality in Relation to Consumption of Alcohol: 13 years' Observations on Male British Doctors', *British Medical Journal*, 309 (1994):911–8.

17. P. J. Richardson, and A. D. Wodak, 'Alcohol-induced Heart Muscle Disease', in C. Symons, T. Evans and A. G. Mitchell (eds), *Specific Heart Muscle Disease* (Bristol: Wright PSG), 99–122.

18. V. R. Preedy, L. M. Atkinson, P. J. Richardson and T. J. Peters, 'Mechanisms of Ethanol-induced Cardiac Damage', *British Heart Journal*, 69 (1993):197–200.

19. J. L. Martinez and M. Penna, 'Influence of Changes in Calcium Concentration and Verapamil on the Cardiac Depressant Effect of Ethanol in Cat Papillary Muscle', *General Pharmacology*, 23 (1992):1051–6.

20. P. J. Richardson, A. D. Wodak, L. Atkinson, J. B. Saunders and D. E. Jewitt, 'Relation between Alcohol Intake, Myocardial Enzyme Activity, and Myocardial Function in Dilated Cardiomyopathy', *British Heart Journal*, 56 (1986):165–70.

21. L. A. Reinke, E. K. Lai, C. M. DuBose and P. B. McCay, 'Reactive Free Radical Generation *in vivo* in Heart and Liver of Ethanol-fed Rats: Correlation with Radical Formation *in vitro*', *Proceedings of the National Academy of Sciences USA*, 84 (1987):9223–7.

22. A. A. Welder, L. J. Dickson and R. B. Melchert, 'Cocaethylene Toxicity in Rat Primary Myocardial Cell Cultures', *Alcohol*, 10 (1993):285–90.

23. M. Farre, R. de-la-Torre, M. Llorente, X. Lamas, B. Ugena, J. Segura and J. Cami, 'Alcohol and Cocaine Interactions of Humans', *Journal of Pharmacology and Experimental Therapeutics*, 266 (1993):1364–73.

24. R. A. Kloner, S. Hale, K. Alker and S. Rezkalla, 'The Effects of Acute and Chronic Cocaine Use on the Heart', *Circulation*, 85 (1992):407–19.
25. G. Nahas, R. Trouve, W. Manger and C. Latour, 'Cocaine and Sympathoadrenal System', *Advances in Bioscience*, 80 (1991):151–64.
26. G. E. Billman, 'Mechanisms Responsible for the Cardiovascular Effects of Cocaine', *FASEB Journal*, 4 (1990):2469–75.
27. K. Kumor, M. Sherer, L. Thompson, E. Cone, J. Mahaffey and J. H. Jaffe, 'Lack of Cardiovascular Tolerance during Intravenous Cocaine Infusions in Human Volunteers', *Life-Sciences*, 42 (1988):2063–71.
28. T. D. Fraker, P. N. Temesy-Armos, P. S. Brewster and R. D. Wilkerson, 'Mechanism of Cocaine-induced Myocardial Depression in Dogs', *Circulation*, 81 (1990):1012–6.
29. S. L. Hale, K. J. Alker, S. Rezkalla, G. Figures and R. A. Kloner, 'Adverse Effects of Cocaine in Cardiovascular Dynamics, Myocardial Blood Flow, and Coronary Artery Diameter in an Experimental Model', *American Heart Journal*, 118 (1989):927–33.
30. M. E. Trulson, L. R. Epps, and J. C. Joe, 'Cocaine: Long term Administration Depletes Cardiac Cellular Enzymes in the Rat', *Acta Anatomica*, 129 (1987):165–8.
31. F. D. Kolodgie, R. Virmani, H. E. Rice, E. E. Hederick and W. J. Mergner, 'Intravenous Cocaine Accelerates Atherosclerosis in Cholesterol-fed New Zealand White Rabbits', *Journal of the American College of Cardiology*, 15 (1990):217A.
32. R. A. Lange, R. G. Cigarroa, C. W. Yancy, J. E. Willard, J. J. Popma, M. N. Sills, W. McBride, A. S. Kim and L. D. Hillis, 'Cocaine-induced Coronary-Artery Vasoconstriction', *New England Journal of Medicine*, 321 (1989):1557–62.
33. E. D. Flores, R. A. Lange, R. G. Cigarroa and L. D. Hillis, 'Effect of Cocaine on Coronary Artery Dimensions in Atherosclerotic Coronary Artery Disease: Enhanced Vasoconstriction at Sites of Significant Stenosis', *Journal of the American College of Cardiology*, 16 (1990):74–9.
34. S. K. Chokshi, D. Gal, S. DeJesus and J. M. Isner, 'Cocaine Produces Vasoconstriction of Human Coronary Arteries: *In Vitro* Studies using Coronary Arteries Obtained from Freshly Explanted Human Hearts', *Journal of the American College of Cardiology*, 15 (1990):215A.
35. F. H. Zimmerman, G. M. Gustafson and H. G. Kemp, 'Recurrent Myocardial Infarction Associated with Cocaine Abuse in a Young Man with Normal Coronary Arteries: Evidence for Coronary artery spasm culminating in thrombosis', *Journal of the American College of Cardiology*, 9 (1987):964–8.
36. F. A. Dressler, S. Malekzadeh and W. C. Roberts, 'Quantitative Analysis of Amounts of Coronary Arterial Narrowing in Cocaine Addicts', *American Journal of Cardiology*, 65 (1990):303–8.
37. B. D. Bertolet, G. Freund, C. A. Martin, D. L. Perchalski, C. M. Williams and C. J. Pepine, 'Unrecognised Left Ventricular Dysfunction in an Apparently Healthy Cocaine Abuse Population', *Clinical Cardiology*, 13 (1990):323–8.
38. R. Virmani, M. Robinowitz, J. E. Smialek and D. F. Smyth, 'Cardiovascular Effects of Cocaine: An Autopsy Study of 40 Patients', *American*

Heart Journal, 115 (1988):1068–76.
39. S. K. Peng, W. J. French and P. C. Pelikan, 'Direct Cocaine Cardiotoxicity Demonstrated by Endomyocardial Biopsy', *Archives of Pathology and Laboratory Medecine*, 113 (1989):842–5.
40. R. G. Stenberg, M. D. Winniford, L. D. Hillis, G. P. Dowling and L. M. Buja, 'Simultaneous Acute Thrombosis of Two Major Coronary Arteries Following Intravenous Cocaine Use', *Archives of Pathology and Laboratory Medecine*, 113 (1989):521–4.
41. K. R. Petronis and J. C. Anthony, 'An Epidemiologic Investigation of Marijuana and Cocaine-related Palpitations', *Drug and Alcohol Dependence*, 23 (1989):219–26.
42. T. K. Leonard, R. R. Watson and M. E. Mohs, 'The Effects of Caffeine on Various Body Systems: A Review', *Journal of the American Dietician Association*, 87 (1987):1048–53.
43. A. Varro, S. Hester and J. G. Papp, 'Caffeine-induced Decreases in the Inward Rectifier Potassium and the Inward Calcium Currents in Rat Ventricular Myocytes', *British Journal of Pharmacology*, 109 (1993):895–7.
44. C. J. Duncan, 'Role of Calcium in Triggering Rapid Ultrastructural Damage in Muscle: A Study with Chemically Skinned Fibres', *Journal of Cell Science*, 87 (1987):581–94.
45. S. Daniels and C. J. Duncan, 'Cellular Damage in the Rat Heart caused by Caffeine or Dinitrophenol', *Comparative Biochemistry and Physiology C*, 105 (1993):225–9.
46. P. Smits, L. Temme and T. Thien, 'The Cardiovascular Interaction between Caffeine and Nicotine in Humans', *Clinical Pharmacology and Therapeutics*, 54 (1993):194–204.
47. P. Bonazzola and J. E. Ponce-Hornos, 'Effects of Caffeine on Energy Output of Rabbit Heart Muscle', *Basic Research in Cardiology*, 82 (1987):428–36.
48. P. W. Wilson, R. J. Garrison, W. B. Kannel, *et al.*, 'Is Coffee Consumption a Contribution to Cardiovascular Disease? Insights from the Framingham Study', *Archives of Internal Medicine*, 149 (1989):1169–72.
49. M. Matsuzaki, G. A. Casella, and M. Ratner, 'Delta 9-Tetrahydrocannabinol: EEG Changes, Bradycardia and Hypothermia in the Rhesus Monkey', *Brain Research Bulletin*, 19 (1987):223–9.
50. J. G. Bernstein, 'Medical Consequences of Marijuana use', in N. K. Mello (ed.), *Advances in Substance Abuse, Behavioral and Biological Research* (Greenwich: JAI Press, 1980), pp. 255–88.
51. C. H. Ashton, 'Solvent Abuse: Little Progress after 20 Years', *British Medical Journal*, 300 (1990):135–6.
52. J. Ramsey, H. R. Anderson, K. Bloor and R. J. Flanagan, 'An Introduction to the Practice, Prevalence and Chemical Toxicology of Volatile Substance Abuse', *Human Toxicology*, 8 (1989):261–9.
53. S. M. Claydon, 'Myocardial Degeneration in Chronic Solvent Abuse', *Medicine Science and the Law*, 28 (1988):217–8.
54. M. Bass, 'Sudden Sniffing Death', *Journal of the American Medical Association*, 212 (1970):2075–9.
55. D. W. Nierenberg, M. B. Horowitz, K. M. Harris and D. H. James, 'Mineral Spirits Inhalation Associated with Hemolysis, Pulmonary Edema and Ven-

Addictive Behaviour

tricular Fibrillation', *Archives of Internal Medicine*, 151 (1991):1437–40.
56. C. F. Reinhardt, A. Azar, M. E. Maxfield, P. E. Smith and L. S. Mullin, 'Cardiac Arrhythmias and Aerosol "Sniffing"', *Archives of Environmental Health*, 22 (1971):265–79.
57. R. M. Wodka and E. W. Jeong, 'Cardiac Effects of Inhaled Typewriter Correction Fluid', *Annals of Internal Medicine*, 110 (1989):91–2.
58. S. R. Cunningham, G. W. N. Dalzell, P. McGirr and M. M. Khan, 'Myocardial Infarction and Primary Ventricular Fibrillation after Glue Sniffing', *British Medical Journal*, 294 (1987):739–40.

Part III
Addictions and the Study of Mind

7 Personality and Addictive Behaviours

Catherine Otter and Colin Martin

INTRODUCTION

The development and expression of addictive behaviours in relation to personality has been a topic of interest for several decades. Indeed, for a number of years personality was considered to be the primary, if not the exclusive, cause of addiction. However, it is now widely recognised that addictive behaviours are complex, multi-determined phenomena, involving the intricate interplay of biological, psychological and socio-cultural factors. Personality is therefore currently regarded as only one of a number of factors which interact together to determine an individual's vulnerability to such behaviours.

The purpose of this chapter is to give a brief review of some of the past and present research findings and theories regarding the links between personality and the onset and expression of addictive behaviours. No pretence of covering all the relevant literature is made as a comprehensive review would assume epic proportions. Furthermore, most of the studies selected for review are simply described and summarised, with little methodological critique or comment. Particular emphasis is placed on the relationships between personality and the abuse of alcohol and other drugs, since it is in these two areas that much of the research has been concentrated. Consideration is also given to some of the methodological approaches which have been used within this field of research. However, before proceeding with the main subject areas of this chapter the ground is first prepared by addressing the two preliminary questions 'what is personality?' and 'what are addictive behaviours?'.

WHAT IS PERSONALITY?

Personality is a term which is frequently used in everyday language, and one which has been defined in many different ways. Indeed, in his book *Concepts of Personality: Theories and Research* Levy[1] suggests that there are almost as many different definitions of the term as there are theorists who have written about the subject.

Personality as it is commonly understood is what makes one individual different from another. In its simplest sense personality can therefore be defined as:

the distinctive and characteristic patterns of thought, emotion, and behaviour that define an individuals personal style and influence his or her interactions with the environment.[2]

According to Nathan[3] most definitions of the term suggest that personality is internal, unique, enduring, active, causal and integrating. Numerous attempts have been made to define and explain what determines an individual's personality. Broadly speaking, most of these theories can be grouped into one of five classes: type theories, trait theories, social learning theories, psychoanalytic theories and phenomenological theories. It is beyond the scope of this chapter to describe in detail each of these different theories of personality, but it may be worth noting some of the main features of each approach.

The type theories are the oldest of the theoretical approaches. Type theories attempt to group people into discrete categories depending on whether or not they possess or display a particular characteristic. In 400 BC, Hippocrates suggested that there were four basic personality types: choleric (angry), sanguine (optimistic), melancholic (depressive) and phlegmatic (apathetic). Individuals were believed to be a representation of a particular balance of these four basic types. Another early type theory classified individuals into three categories on the basis of body type and related these body types to personality characteristics.[4] A short, plump person was said to be sociable, relaxed, and even tempered; a tall, thin person was characterised as restrained, self conscious and a 'loner'; a heavy-set muscular individual was described as noisy, aggressive and physically active. Although such type theories are appealing because they provide a simple way of looking at personality, it is now widely accepted that personality is far too complex for this kind of approach.

The trait theories are based on the assumption that personality is a compendium of traits or characteristic ways of thinking, behaving, feeling, and reacting: 'A trait refers to any characteristic that differs from person to person in a relatively permanent and consistent way' (Atkinson, *et al.*,[2] p. 389). Examples of traits include emotional stability, aggressiveness, creativity, intelligence, extraversion, excitability, nervousness, sociability and so on. Traits are assumed to predispose people to behave consistently across different situations. Although situations are recognised as having an influence on behaviour, trait theorists believe that it is the individual's personal characteristics or traits that have the greatest influence in determining his/her behaviour. Trait theorists are much more concerned with personality description than personality development, and the two main areas of interest for psychologists working in the area of trait theory are identifying the basic traits or dimensions of personality, and developing techniques and tools which can be used to measure these traits.

In contrast to the trait theorists, social learning theorists emphasise the importance of situational or environmental factors in determining behaviour. According to social learning theorists, an individual's personality is shaped through the way he or she learns to cope and interact with other people and situations. The role of observation, mimicking or imitating the behaviours observed in others, and the effects of situations and other people – the punishments and rewards – are believed to be the greatest determinants of personality and hence behaviour. For social learning theorists, an individual's behaviour in a given situation is very much dependent upon the specific characteristics of the situation, his/her previous experiences in similar situations and his/her appraisal of the situation.

The psychoanalytic theories differ considerably from the previous theories in that unconscious motives and conflicts rather than traits or situations are believed to be the key determinants of behaviour. Psychoanalytic theorists postulate that personality, in general, is a complex product of innate instincts or impulses whose expression is modified by early developmental processes, for example sexual drives, aggressive drives, inherited memories, the drive for power and superiority, and the drive for goals that contribute to a better society and quality of life. It is the interplay of these underlying instincts and motives which is presumed to be the primary determinant of personality and behaviour.

The phenomenological theories of personality share a common emphasis on subjective experience – 'the individual's private view of the world' (Atkinson *et al.*,[2] p. 399). They focus very much on how the individual perceives and interprets events and what a particular situation *means* to an individual. Some of the phenomenological theories have been labelled 'humanistic' because they focus on those qualities which distinguish humans from animals, for example freedom of choice, self-direction. Others are referred to as the 'self' theories because they emphasis the internal experiences that constitute a person's sense of being, for example his/her images, emotions, values and thoughts that characterise 'I' or 'me'.

WHAT IS ADDICTIVE BEHAVIOUR?

Behaviour is usually labelled addictive when it is excessive, appetitive, compulsive and beyond the control of the person who engages in it. As noted in the introductory chapter of this book the term 'addictive behaviour' can be used to refer to alcoholism, drug abuse, overeating, compulsive gambling, certain sexual deviations and compulsive working. Although these behaviours may seem quite diverse, Lang[5] points out that a number of authors have noted that:

> a distinguishing feature of addictive behaviours is that they all involve some form of immediate gratification or pleasure, but are accompanied by longer term adverse consequences. The short-term gratification may be referred to as a 'high', a 'rush', a 'trip', a 'release', a 'relief', or any variety of terms that describe an alteration in one's state of consciousness or affect. The long-term negative consequences typically involve a deterioration of functioning in important life areas such as health, vocation, and social relations. (Lang[5], p. 160)

THE ADDICTIVE PERSONALITY

During the middle part of this century, it was widely believed that individuals with addictive behaviours had a unique personality structure, or set of personality characteristics, that was both necessary and sufficient for the behaviours to occur. Although the exact origin of the concept of the 'addictive personality' is unclear, Cox[6] suggests that it may have arisen as a result of changing views on the causes of alcoholism.

Despite the fact that some early attempts were made to associate habitual drunkenness with a disease,[7, 8] during the seventeenth and eighteenth centuries excessive drinking was usually attributed to a personal vice or moral weakness. Individuals who drank excessively were considered to have little or no will power to resist alcohol, and although public drunkenness was not considered to be a serious social problem, the courts punished offenders, through fines, whippings, stocks, and occasional imprisonment. Punishments for recidivists were in fact often severe. However, during the early part of the nineteenth century as the Temperance Movement started to emerge, attitudes towards those who drank habitually began to change. The Temperance Movement advocated that the essence of alcoholism lay not in the vulnerability of some unfortunate individuals, but rather in the addicting nature of alcohol itself. Any person who consumed alcohol was considered to be at risk of becoming addicted to it, and it was therefore argued that the only way to eradicate alcoholism from society was to restrict the availability of alcohol altogether. Attempts to prohibit alcohol, particularly in America, nevertheless failed disastrously; for although prohibition did lead to a fall in alcohol consumption, which was accompanied by reductions in alcohol-related problems such as accidents, drunkenness arrests and admissions to hospital, it also led to an upsurge in black markets, gangsterism and a widespread lack of respect for the law.

Following prohibition, perceptions of drunkenness once again began to change. The disease concept of alcoholism re-emerged as the pivotal way of thinking about alcohol abuse, and it was argued that once a drinker had developed an appetite or craving for alcohol, he or she was powerless to resist it and lost control over his or her drinking. Drinking by the vast majority of individuals was not, however, believed to lead to addiction; only those individuals with some form of biological or psychological vulnerability were considered to be susceptible to the disease. It is interesting to note that the disease concept of alcoholism had become so dormant during prohibition that after its repeal the rediscovery of the theory was labelled 'the new approach to alcoholism'.[9]

Another significant change that occurred after the repeal of prohibition was the fact that psychiatrists began to utilise psychoanalytic theory to explain the aetiology of alcoholism and to treat alcoholic patients. The psychoanalysts Karl Abraham,[10] is believed to have been the first to have suggested that alcoholism might be linked to a deep-rooted personality disturbance.[11] Later, other psychoanalysts, including Freud himself, expressed similar views and proposed links between the aetiology of alcoholism and sexual difficulties or other forms of psychopathology that originated during early childhood.[12-15]

It is from the role which psychoanalysts assigned to personality in the development of alcoholism that the so-called 'addictive personality' is believed to have emerged.[11] Cox[11] also suggests that one of the reasons why the concept may have gained such widespread acceptance and popularity during the 1940s and 1950s was because it was fostered by members of the then newly established, and rapidly expanding, self-help organisation, Alcoholics Anonymous. Alcoholics Anonymous sub-scribed to the disease concept of alcoholism, and promoted the idea that 'alcoholics' had a special vulnerability to alcohol. Some of its members believed that the disease or vulnerability with which they were afflicted could be attributed to an underlying faulty personality structure.

As theories about the existence of an addictive personality began to emerge, investigations were undertaken to gain a greater understand-ing of its precise nature. Despite a great many studies however, no consensus has ever been reached. Within recent years the search for a specific addictive personality has therefore been more or less aban-doned. Nevertheless, research into the relationship between personality and the development and expression of addictive behaviours continues apace, but instead of considering personality to be the single cause of addiction, it is now widely recognised that personality characteristics interact with a number of other factors to determine a person's vulner-ability to such behaviours.

METHODOLOGICAL APPROACHES IN THE STUDY OF PERSONALITY AND ADDICTIVE BEHAVIOURS

In his review of the literature, Cox (1988) suggests that there are three different kinds of investigations which researchers who study the link between personality and addictive behaviours tend to undertake. The first approach is concerned with identifying the personality character-istics which may predict the development of such behaviours; the sec-ond approach is concerned with determining whether the personalities of individuals with addictive behaviours are distinctly different from those of non-addicts, and if so in what ways; and the third approach is concerned with both the acute and chronic effects of addictive behav-iours on personality. Investigators hope that by disentangling the causes of addictive behaviours from their effects they will not only be able better to explain why some people engage in behaviours or activities which are addictive, but will also be able to identify those who are at risk of developing such behaviours.

There are four basic procedures that are used in the identification of personality precursors of addictive behaviours: archival, archival longitudinal, retrospective and prospective longitudinal. Each methodological approach has its advantages and limitations. Some retrospective studies simply involve asking alcoholics, substance abusers or other addicts to describe what their personalities were like prior to the onset of their addictions. In some cases the respondents may also be asked to recall any significant life events that could be related to the development of their addictions. Obviously one of the major limitations of retrospective studies is the fact that they are highly subjective. They are also open to inaccurate recall, fantasy, purposeful exaggeration, and distortions in memory. Nevertheless, Cox[11] suggests that:

> the retrospective method has provided useful information, especially as it has generated hypotheses that could be more rigorously tested. (p. 152)

Archival studies utilise sources of information about addicts' personality characteristics before such individuals became addicted, and before they were identified as potential addicts. Information is usually gleaned from school reports of achievement, absenteeism and discipline, criminal records including court reports, clinical or hospital records of illness and psychological problems. When this information is gathered from more than one period of time in the addicts prior life, the methodological approach is called archival longitudinal. Although archival studies are more objective than retrospective studies, they are still beset with practical difficulties. For example, obtaining archival data can sometimes be a tedious and difficult task, and the information itself is often incomplete. Furthermore, archival data is often only available for a restricted number of addicts, and therefore how legitimate it is to generalise beyond the sample groups is questionable.[16]

In prospective longitudinal studies, individuals who are expected to develop such behaviours are tested and followed for a number of years, usually from an early age until some have developed problems with addiction. Typically individuals who participate in such studies are asked to complete various questionnaires including some personality tests on an annual basis. The data obtained from such questionnaires is then examined to determine whether there are any personality characteristics which predict the onset of addictive behaviours at a later date. Two of the obvious limitations of prospective longitudinal studies is that are usually expensive to conduct and are very time consuming. Therefore over recent years researchers have begun to expedite the approach by studying individuals at risk of developing addictive behaviours. High-risk individuals include children of addicts and children whose personality characteristics are similar to those of addicted adults. Comparisons are often made between those individuals at high risk and those at 'normal' or low risk. High-risk studies are advantageous because they not only help to identify the personality precursors of addictive behaviours, but also the factors that protect some people from developing such problems.

Much of the research which has been undertaken to examine the common personality characteristics of individuals with addictive behaviours has focused on individuals receiving treatment for alcohol or drug abuse. Initially, the characteristics of such individuals were studied through the case-study method. Clinicians working with addicts described their clients' personalities and suggested how their various addictions might be related to their personality characteristics. Later, as research evolved, it became the usual practice to administer standardised personality tests to groups of individuals with addictive behaviours, report on the findings in the form of group averages, and compare the results with those from other patients or individuals with no apparent addictions. However, this approach has been widely criticised on two main fronts. Firstly, it has been argued that individuals receiving treatment may not be representative of all addicts, and therefore it may not be legitimate to generalise beyond the sample groups; and, secondly, it has been argued that by averaging the responses for a large group of addicts and using the group-means, some important personality differences among the individuals may in fact be obscured. To try and overcome the first of these methodological difficulties some researchers have focused their studies on individuals whose use of alcohol or other drugs, for example, is excessive, but who have not been officially diagnosed as addicted or in need of formal treatment. College students, for example, have often been used in investigations regarding the relationship between alcohol use and personality.

With regard to the effects of addictive behaviours on personality, there are two kinds of investigation that researchers tend to undertake. One kind seeks to identify the immediate effects that such behaviours can have on personality, whereas the other seeks to determine the effects that such behaviours may have over time. The vast majority of studies which have been conducted within both of these areas have focused primarily on the effects of addictive substances particularly alcohol, caffeine and tobacco. The immediate effects of such substances on personality have usually been assessed by systematically monitoring personality changes that occur during either their acute or chronic administration. It is important to point out, however, that the maximum drug dosages which are administered in the research laboratory are usually considerably smaller than the dosages typically used by street drug abusers.[17] The longer-term effects of addictive behaviours on personality are usually assessed by studying how the habitual consumption of substances such as alcohol and other drugs effects personality during a period of sobriety. These studies typically focus on individuals who have undergone detoxification and, for a period of time at least, are abstinent from alcohol and other drugs. Unfortunately it is difficult to differentiate between the effects of withdrawal from such substances and confounding factors such as changes in life style or situation which may accompany the period of abstinence.

LINKS BETWEEN PERSONALITY AND ADDICTIVE BEHAVIOURS: RESEARCH FINDINGS

Personality Precursors of Addictive Behaviours

During the past three decades the search for personality precursors of addictive behaviours has been intense, particularly with regards to alcoholism and drug abuse. Although a distinctive addictive personality has not yet been identified, research findings suggest that there are certain premorbid personality characteristics which may accompany the later development of alcohol and drug abuse. These characteristics include independence, aggressiveness, rebelliousness, rejection of societal values, antisocial behaviour, impulsivity, psychopathology, low self-concept and hyperactivity.[16, 18-20] However, none of these characteristics have been found to specifically, inevitably, uniformly or exclusively predict the development of addictive behaviours, and it is therefore important that they are considered as pre-existing or predisposing factors rather than determining factors.

One of the first major longitudinal studies in the search for precursors and developmental factors in alcoholism was undertaken by McCord and McCord.[21, 22] Using data collected as part of a project to prevent delinquency, the behaviours of 225 lower-class boys aged nine to fourteen, were studied in 1935 and followed up by McCord and McCord in 1956. The investigators found that by the time the subjects had reached approximately 30 years of age, twenty-nine had developed problems relating to alcoholism. When comparisons were made between the child-hood personality characteristics of the alcoholic group and a control group of 158 boys who had no alcoholism or criminal record but who had been part of the original sample, the alcoholic group were found to be to be more self confident, somewhat sadistic, sexually anxious, had higher levels of unrestrained aggression, and were more disap-proving of their mothers.

In another study undertaken in the same year, Robins, Bates and O'Neal[23] followed up a group of 505 men and women who had at one time been patients in a children's mental health clinic. They found that as adults 84 had become alcoholic. Using information contained in the agency records, the researchers compared the childhood descriptions of the alcoholic group with those of other individuals who had also been patients at the hospital but had not developed any alcohol prob-lems. They found that the childhood descriptions of the alcoholics had a higher frequency of antisocial behaviour.

A further significant longitudinal study was carried out by Jones,[24] who assessed the personality characteristics of approximately 50 middle-class males at three different stages during their developments (junior high, high school and adulthood). As adults she classified all of the subjects as problem, heavy, moderate or light drinkers or abstainers using ratings of frequency and levels of alcohol consumption. Six males were classified as problem drinkers and at all three stages of their development they were reported to be more uncontrolled, hostile, ex-pressive, impulsive, indulgent and rebellious than their peers.

In spite of the differences in methodology and the economic status of the individuals who participated in the above studies, all three in-vestigations found that pre-alcoholics appeared to be non-conforming, aggressive and impulsive.

Further support for these findings has been obtained from a number of other studies in which comparative data have been gathered through the use of standardised personality questionnaires, particularly the Minnesota Multiphasic Personality Inventory (MMPI).[25–27] Between the late 1940s and 1962, as part of the admissions procedure, the MMPI was routinely administered to all new college students at the University of Minnesota. Eventually, of course, some of the students who at-tended the University developed problems with alcohol and sought treatment. A search of 12 000 files from two of the major alcoholic treatment services in Minnesota revealed that approximately 600 pa-tients diagnosed as suffering from alcoholism may have attended the university between 1947 and 1961. From these 600, proof of attendance was established for 38 men, and the MMPIs which they completed as college freshmen were found and scored. In the first of a series of studies, the pre-alcoholic personality characteristics of this group were compared with profiles obtained on admission to the two treatment centres.[25] It was found that a progression to overt alcoholism was accompanied by an increase in irritability, depression, hostility, anxiety, impulsivity and resentment, by a strong need to manipulate and use others and by difficulties with interpersonal relationships. In the second study, the personality characteristics of the alcoholics as college freshmen were compared with those of a randomly selected control group consisting of 148 of their classmates. Unfortunately no follow-up testing was conducted on the controls. Nevertheless, the results suggested that the college pre-alcoholics were more likely to be gregarious, impulsive and less conforming than their classmates, but were otherwise no more maladjusted compared to their peers.[26]

Later, in another related MMPI study, Hoffman *et al.*[27] examined the scores of pre-alcoholics and controls on two empirically derived scales from the MMPI, the Rosenberg (ARos)[28] and the MacAndrew (MAC),[29] both of which were designed to differentiate alcoholics from various control groups. Hoffman and his colleagues found that before the onset of problem drinking, pre-alcoholics scored significantly higher than controls on both of these scales. They also found that there was very little difference in the scores obtained prior to and after the onset of problem drinking. In fact, 72 per cent of subjects who participated in the study could be accurately classified as either control or pre-alcoholic on the basis of their personality profiles as college freshmen.

In a similar study, Goldstein and Sappington[30] compared the MMPI protocols of a group of college freshmen who later became heavy illicit drug users, with a group of control subjects. The researchers suggested that the pre-drug users were more adventurous, impulsive, less compliant and had greater social skills than the controls.

Building upon the possible MMPI differences between alcoholics and controls, several studies were undertaken during the 1980s to try and identify personality characteristics associated with a heightened risk of alcoholism, by virtue of family history. In one such study, Saunders and Schuckit[31] proposed that non-alcoholic young men with positive family histories of alcoholism might score differently on the various alcohol-related subscales of the MMPI compared with controls. They therefore administered the MMPI to 30 non-alcoholic men aged 20–25 who had a first-degree alcoholic family member and to a control group matched on demography and drinking behaviour but with no family history of alcoholism. Comparisons were made between the scores obtained by the two groups on various alcohol-related MMPI scales including the ARos and MAC. Initially, the subjects with the positive family histories of alcoholism were found to score significantly higher on the MAC scale than the control group, but no significant differences were found between the scores of the two groups on the ARos scale. However, further analysis of the data revealed that the scores of both groups fell within the normal range on the MAC scale, and that the averages between the two groups differed only slightly by just more than two points. In addition, it was also found that the two groups differed significantly on only one of the six MAC subfactors, *Interpersonal Competence*.

In another investigation, Schuckit[32] also found that there were no significant differences between the neuroticism or extraversion scores of sons of alcoholic fathers and sons of non-alcoholic fathers. In contrast, however, other evidence has been obtained which does suggest that adolescent sons with a positive family history of alcoholism present a more neurotic personality profile than sons with no family history of alcoholism[33] and that they tend to be more compulsive, insecure, fearful, subdued and detached.[34]

Within recent years, the work of Cloninger and his co-workers has attracted increasing attention. Cloninger has developed a theory of personality[35] and a typology of alcoholism[36] – both of which will be discussed in more detail in a later section of this chapter. In addition, he and his colleagues have also attempted to identify the personality characteristics which predict alcohol abuse in young adults by undertaking a prospective longitudinal study of a group of Swedish children. Using data collected as part of a project concerned with the development of adopted children, Cloninger *et al.*[37] studied the behaviours of 233 boys and 198 girls at the ages of 11 and 27 years. They found that by the age of 27, thirty boys and two girls had been registered for alcohol abuse. They also found deviations on three personality dimensions – novelty seeking, harm avoidance and reward dependence – were associated with an exponential increase in the risk of later alcohol abuse. High novelty seeking (for example, the tendency to be impulsive, exploratory, quick tempered and easily bored) and low harm avoidance (for example, the tendency to be confident, relaxed, optimistic, carefree and outgoing) were most strongly predictive of early-onset alcohol abuse.

Personality Characteristics of Addicts

Numerous studies have to date been undertaken to try and identify whether there are certain personality characteristics that can distinguish between addicts and non-addicts. However, from such studies it is difficult to draw any conclusions as to whether such characteristics are antecedents of addictive behaviours or whether they are the consequences of such behaviours. Only a brief review of some of the major research findings is included here, and readers wishing to obtain additional information are advised to refer to the more comprehensive reviews by Cox,[151] Nathan,[3] Lang[5] and Platt and Labate,[38] or to the later chapter in this book which focuses specifically on the relationship between addictive behaviours and the locus of control.

As mentioned earlier, much of the information about the personality characteristics of addicts has been gathered from individuals who have been clinically diagnosed as being alcoholic or drug-dependent and who are receiving treatment for their various addiction problems. One of the most commonly used approaches within this area of research is to administer standardised personality tests to such patients or clients, and then to report on their average group scores, or to compare their scores with a control group of non-addicts. Through this approach it has been shown that several of the pre-morbid personality characteristics which seem to accompany the development of addictive behaviours are also apparent after the onset of such behaviours. For example, it has been found that sensation seeking, which is defined as 'the need for varied and novel and complex sensations and experiences and the willingness to take physical and social risks for the sake of such experience' (Zuckerman[39], p. 10) is positively correlated with both non-dependent and dependent drug and alcohol use.[40, 41] It has also been found that both pre-drug abusers and drug abusers show antisocial behaviours[23, 22, 42] and from studies in which the MMPI has been employed, it has been repeatedly demonstrated that both alcoholics and pre-alcoholics have elevations of Scale 4, the *Psychopathic Deviate* scale.[26, 43, 44] Elevations of Scale 4 are generally interpreted as a disregard for social customs, impulsivity, a low tolerance for frustration, an inability to profit from punishing experiences and an emotional shallowness in relation to others.[45]

Elevations of the MMPI Scale 4 have also been found to be characteristic of cocaine abusers,[46, 47] heroin addicts,[48, 49] and heavy marijuana users,[50] and in a comparative study of the personality characteristics of cocaine abusers and alcohol abusers, Johnson *et al.*[46] found that there were no significant differences between the scores of the two groups of substance abusers on this scale. However, in an early study McLellan *et al.*[51] had reported that mixed stimulant abusers had greater levels of MMPI-associated psychopathy than opiate abusers.

According to Irwin *et al.*[52] research findings indicate that 75–80 per cent of individuals with psychopathy, otherwise referred to as antisocial personality disorder, will at sometime during the course of their disorder develop severe enough alcohol-related life problems to fulfil the criteria for secondary alcoholism. Irwin and his colleagues also cite evidence which suggests that between 10 and 20 per cent of alcoholic men being treated for alcoholism probably have a pre-existing antisocial personality disorder. However, in a recent study of 178 hospitalised alcoholics and 86 polydrug addicts, DeJong *et al.*[53] found that 48 per cent of the alcoholics and an even larger percentage of the drug addicts, met the criteria for the diagnosis of antisocial personality disorder.

In comparison with primary alcoholics or drug addicts, those with antisocial personality disorder have been found to be more likely to show an earlier age at onset, a more rapid progression from minor to major alcohol/drug-related problems, and to have more problems associated with their alcohol and other drug abuse.[54–58] It has therefore been suggested that individuals who develop alcohol or drug problems within the context of antisocial personality disorder should be distinguished from those who, as a result of alcohol or drug abuse, become involved in activities and behaviours (criminal activity, frequent fights, impulsivity) which could be labelled as psychopathic or antisocial.[52, 56]

In addition to meeting the diagnostic criteria for antisocial personality disorder, alcoholics and drug addicts also meet the criteria for the diagnosis of other psychiatric disorders – particularly affective disorders – with considerable frequency. Schuckit *et al.*[59] suggest that there are several lines of evidence which indicate that about one-third of all alcohol-abusing patients experience such severe depressive episodes as could qualify for a diagnosis of a major depressive disorder. Furthermore, from studies in which the MMPI has been administered to both alcoholics and drug addicts, it has been repeatedly shown that in addition to their elevations on Scale 4, many alcoholics and drug abusers typically show elevations on Scales 2 (*Depression*) and 7 (*Psychasthenia*).[43, 44, 46] Elevations on these latter two scales reflect pessimism and despair, lack of psychic energy, an inability to enjoy life, anxiety, worry, indecisiveness and irrational fears.[60] Heroin and cocaine addicts have also been found to score high on Scales 8 and 9 (the *Schizophrenia* and

Hypomania scales), reflecting overactivity, emotional excitement, sociability, confused thinking and unusual perceptions.[49, 61, 62]

Evidence which has linked both depression and anxiety with addictive behaviours has also been obtained from a number of studies which have utilised other psychometric tools besides the MMPI. For example, in comparison with controls, individuals diagnosed as suffering from alcoholism or drug abuse have been found to score significantly higher on the Neuroticism scale of Eysenck's Personality Questionnaire;[63-65] the Somatic Anxiety, Psychic Anxiety, Muscular Tension and Psychasthenia Scales of the Karolinska Scales of Personality;[64] the Hamilton Rating Scale and the Beck's Depression Inventory.[66-68] Furthermore, low self-esteem, a characteristic which may also be related to both depression and anxiety, has also been associated with various addictive behaviours. Alcoholic, bulimic, and drug-dependent patients have all been found to have deficiencies of self-esteem,[44, 69-72] and female addicts have been found to have more depressed levels of self-esteem than male addicts.[72] It has also been shown that whilst female cocaine addicts tend show a greater incidence of depression, male cocaine addicts tend to exhibit more antisocial personality disorder.[73]

Studies which have used one of Eysenck's personality questionnaires or inventories (EPI;[74] EPQ;[75] EPQ-R[76]) to compare the personality characteristics of alcoholics and non-alcoholics, have consistently found that alcoholics score significantly higher on both the neuroticism and psychoticism scales than non-alcoholics.[63, 77] Likewise, drug addicts have also been found to score significantly higher on both of these scales, as have gamblers and bulimics.[65, 78-81] However, data concerning the scores of alcoholics and drug addicts on the extraversion–introversion scale has been somewhat more inconsistent. Some studies have shown that drug addicts and alcoholics score significantly lower on the extraversion scale than non-addicts;[63, 64, 82-84] other studies have shown that there are no significant differences;[85, 86] and at least one study has reported finding higher levels of extraversion within an alcoholic population.[87]

Using Eysenck's personality scales evidence has also been obtained to show that different types of drug users may have different personality characteristics.[84, 88, 89] For example, Rosenthal *et al.*[84] used the EPQ to compare the personality characteristics of 202 male and 95 female substance users. Sixty-five subjects were classified as cocaine users, 34 as opiate users, and 75 as polydrug users. The remaining 46 comprised a residual mixed group. Rosenthal and his co-workers found that, in comparison with controls, all of the drug users were more introverted, impulsive and anxious. The cocaine users were found to be the most impulsive (the alcohol and opiate users were found to be the least so) and the least anxious of the different drug using groups. The polysubstance abusers and the mixed group were found to be the most extroverted whereas the opiate users were reported to be the most introverted.

Eysenck's personality dimensions, particularly his extraversion and neuroticism scales have also been linked with tobacco smoking.[90-92] Furthermore, a recent study by Breslau *et al.*[93] has suggested that even within the smoking population there may be certain personality characteristics which are related to different smoking behaviours. In a sample of 1007 21–30-year-old tobacco smokers, Breslau *et al.*[93] found that dependent smokers scored significantly higher on neuroticism than both non-dependent and non-smokers, whereas non-dependent smokers did not differ from non-smokers. Non-dependent smokers were also found to score higher on extroversion than both non-smokers and dependent smokers. No differences were found between the scores of the three groups on the psychoticism scale.

Personality Characteristics Associated with Subtypes of Alcoholism and Drug Abuse

Although the personality characteristics described above have all been found amongst people with addictive behaviours, it can not be assumed that they are necessarily common to all individuals, or that they are present to the same degree. For more than a century now researchers and clinicians have recognised that addictive behaviours are not homogenous disorders, but are composed of various subtypes for which causes, courses, clinical features and associated personality characteristics may differ.

Within the past sixty years or so numerous attempts have been made to identify different subtypes of alcoholism and drug addiction.[13, 14, 94-99] The early alcoholic typology proposed by Knight[13] included two types of alcoholism – 'essential' and 'reactive'. Knight described the essential alcoholic as having an early onset of abusive drinking that was typically insidious in nature, more severe and unrelated to identifiable environmental stressors. In contrast, the reactive alcoholic was described as having a later onset of problem drinking, more precipitating environmental stressors and a less severe course. According to Knight, essential alcoholism was theoretically and empirically linked to a positive family history of alcoholism whereas reactive alcoholism tended to be non-familial. To these two categories, Menninger[14] added 'neurotic characters' who drank heavily as a manifestation of their disturbance and 'psychotic personalities' for whom drinking was a symptom of a paranoid, schizoid or psychotic disorder.

A better known typology of alcoholism was proposed by Jellinek in the early 1960s. Jellinek differentiated between individuals who had persistent alcohol seeking-behaviours (or as he termed it an 'inability to abstain') and those who could abstain from alcohol for relatively long periods of time but were unable to terminate drinking binges once they had started (i.e those that showed a 'loss of control'). He identified and described five different types or 'species' of alcoholism: alpha, beta, gamma, delta and epsilion. Each so-called species was, according to Jellinek, associated with certain drinking behaviours, problems and varying degrees of psychological and physical dependency. Despite the popularity of this classification scheme, there has, according to Babor and Dolinsky,[100] been little empirical research to tests its validity and clinical utility, and very few researchers have attempted to investigate hypotheses derived from his theory. However, Babor and Dolinsky do give details of three studies in which the personality characteristics of gamma and delta alcoholics were compared. These studies showed that gamma alcoholics were more reticent, depressed, hostile and emotionally unstable than delta alcoholics, but had less self-esteem and were less conforming.[101-103]

Many of the studies which have been undertaken to identify alcoholic subtypes have used information obtained through the MMPI, and a sophisticated statistical procedure known as cluster analysis to group together alcoholics whose personality characteristics are similar. Using the cluster analysis technique, and data collected from 513 alcoholics, Goldstein and Linden[104] identified four distinct subgroups of alcoholics. Type I was characterised by an elevated MMPI Scale 4 (Psychopathic scale), and individuals within this type of alcoholism were described as having an emotionally unstable personality, with poorly controlled anger and/or psychopathy. Type I was characterised as having an elevated MMPI 2-8-7-4 (Depression, Schizophrenic, Psychasthenia, Psychopathic) profile, marked by the presence of either anxiety reaction or reactive depression, with somatic complaints and suicidal ideation. Type III was characterised by a 4-9-2 (Psychopathic, Hypomania, Depression) profile, and was seen as chronically alcoholic with sporadic attempts at abstinence. Denial of difficulties, uncooperative attitudes and poor prognosis were also associated with this type. Type IV was associated with a 4-9 (Psychopathic, Hypomania) profile, and secondary characteristics of drug addiction and paranoid features. Relatively lengthy periods of abstinence were characteristic of this group.

Several attempts have subsequently been made to try and replicate the MMPI alcoholic personality subtypes that were derived by Goldstein and Linden,[99, 105, 106] and the majority of these studies have shown some degree of comparatibility with the profile types.

Using a somewhat different methodological approach, Cloninger *et al.*[96] and Bohman *et al.*[95] have provided evidence for the existence of two subtypes of alcoholism. Utilising information obtained from national registers in Scandinavia and tracing adoptees into adulthood, Cloninger and his colleagues[96] have identified two distinct subgroups of alcoholics, Type I and Type II, which they claim are differentiable in terms of their alcohol-related symptoms, patterns of inheritance and personality characteristics. According to Cloninger *et al.*, Type I alcoholism is associated with loss of control, guilt and a fear about dependence on alcohol. It usually develops in late adulthood, after a period of heavy drinking which has been reinforced by external circumstances. It can occur in both males and females. In contrast, Type II alcoholism is thought to occur almost exclusively in males and is associated with an early onset of alcohol-seeking behaviour regardless of external circumstances, and frequent impulsive–aggressive behaviour, such as fighting or reckless driving after drinking (Table 7.1).

During the late 1980s, Cloninger[35, 107] also proposed a unified biosocial theory of personality in which he postulated that personality is comprised of three genetically homogenous and independent dimensions that activate, maintain and inhibit behaviour in response to specific types of environmental stimuli. He defines these dimensions as novelty seeking: 'a hereditable tendency toward intense exhilaration or excitement in response to novel stimuli or cues for potential rewards or potential relief of punishment, which leads to frequent exploratory activity in pursuit of potential rewards as well as active avoidance of monotony and potential punishment'; harm avoidance, 'a hereditable tendency to respond intensely to signals of aversive stimuli thereby learning to inhibit behaviour to avoid punishment, novelty and frustrative nonreward'; and reward dependence, 'a hereditable tendency to respond intensely to signals of reward (particularly verbal signals of social approval, sentiment and succour) and to maintain or resist extinction of behaviour that has previously been associated with rewards or relief from punishment' (1987a[107], p. 574).

Individuals with higher than average novelty seeking are described as being impulsive, exploratory, fickle, excitable, quick-tempered, extravagant and disorderly. They readily engage in new interests and activities, but tend to neglect detail and are easily bored and quickly distracted. They are also easily provoked to prepare for fight or flight.

TABLE 7.1 *Distinguishing characteristics of two types of alcoholism*

Characteristic features	Type I	Type II
Usual age of onset (years)	After 25	Before 25
Spontaneous alcohol-seeking (inability to abstain)	Infrequent	Frequent
Fighting and arrests when drinking	Infrequent	Frequent
Psychological dependence (loss of control)	Frequent	Infrequent
Guilt and fear about alcohol dependence	Frequent	Infrequent

In contrast, individuals who are lower than average in novelty seeking are reflective, rigid, loyal, stoic, slow-tempered, frugal, orderly and persistent. They are typically slower to engage in new activities, often become preoccupied with narrowly focused details and require considerable thought before making decisions. Individuals who are higher than average in harm avoidance are described as being cautious, tense, apprehensive, fearful, inhibited, shy, easily fatigable and apprehensive worriers, whereas those that are lower than average in harm avoidance are characterized as confident, relaxed, optimistic, carefree, uninhibited, outgoing and energetic. Individuals with high reward dependence are viewed as being eager to help others, emotionally dependent, warmly sympathetic, sentimental, sensitive to social cues and persistent, those with low reward dependence are considered to be socially detached, emotionally cool, practical, tough-minded and independently self-willed.

According to Cloninger's theory each of the three dimensions follows a normal distribution in the general population, with most people having intermediate values. Extreme variations have however been found to correspond closely with traditional subtypes of personality disorders.[107]

In addition to describing the behavioural characteristics associated with the three dimensions, Cloninger has hypothesised that individual differences along the behavioural dimensions are regulated neurochemically by specific monoamine brain systems.[35] Novelty seeking is considered to be associated with the behavioural activation system and the neurotransmitter dopamine, harm avoidance with the behavioural inhibition system and the neurotransmitter serotonin, and reward dependence with the behavioural maintenance system and the neurotransmitter noradrenalin (Table 7.2).

To measure the three personality dimensions of novelty seeking, harm

TABLE 7.2 *Cloninger's proposed personality dimensions and related brain systems*

Personality dimension	Brain system	Principal monoamine modulator
Novelty seeking	Behavioural activation	Dopamine
Harm avoidance	Behavioural inhibition	Serotonin
Reward dependence	Behavioural maintenance	Noradrenalin

TABLE 7.3 *Tridimensional Personality Questionnaire scales and subscales*

Novelty Seeking	NS1: exploratory excitability vs stoic rigidity
	NS2: impulsiveness vs reflection
	NS3: extravagance vs reserve
	NS4: disorderliness vs regimentation
Harm Avoidance	HA1: anticipatory worry vs uninhibited optimism
	HA2: fear of uncertainty vs confidence
	HA3: shyness with strangers vs gregariousness
	HA4: fatigability and asthenia vs vigour
Reward dependence	RD1: sentimentality vs insensitivess
	RD2: persistence vs irresoluteness
	RD3: attachment vs detachment
	RD4: dependence vs independence

avoidance and reward dependence, Cloninger has developed the Tridimensional Personality Questionnaire (TPQ) and more recently the Temperament and Character Inventory (TCI).[108–110] The TPQ consists of 100 self-report statements which people might use to describe their attitudes, opinions, interests and other personal feelings. The statements correspond to three domain scales designed to measure the three higher-order dimensions of novelty seeking, harm avoidance and reward dependence. Each scale is divided into four subscales (Table 7.3).

Relating his theory of personality with the onset of alcohol problems, Cloninger[36] proposes that the development of Type I alcoholism, i.e that which is associated with loss of control and guilt and fear about dependence, is also associated with the triad of traits characteristic of individuals with passive dependent or 'anxious' personalities, for example low novelty seeking, high harm avoidance and high reward dependence. In contrast, he suggests that the Type II alcoholism, which is typically associated with an inability to abstain and antisocial behaviour, is associated with the triad of traits characteristic of indi-

TABLE 7.4 *Distinguishing personality traits of two types of alcoholism*

Personality Trait	Type I alcoholism	Type II alcoholism
Novelty seeking	Low	High
Harm avoidance	High	Low
Reward dependence	High	Low

viduals with an antisocial personality, for example high novelty seeking, low harm avoidance, low reward dependence (Table 7.4).

Although several studies have to date been undertaken to evaluate Cloninger's theory of personality,[111-114] far fewer attempts have been made to validate his Type I/Type II theory of alcoholism and test the clinical utility of his two proposed subgroups. Penick *et al.*[115] attempted to categorise 360 hospitalised alcoholic men into Cloninger's two subtypes, but found that there was a marked overlap between the symptom-clusters used to define the two subtypes: 91 per cent of their sample group satisfied the symptom cluster criteria for both the Type I and Type II subgroups. In another study, Nixon and Parsons[116] administered the TPQ to 267 substance abusers, 172 of whom were alcoholic. However, their study also failed to support Cloninger's predictions and raised serious doubts about the reliability of the TPQ as a tool for classifying alcoholics into the expected frequencies for Type I and Type II. Similarly, Nagoshi *et al.*[117] administered the TPQ to a group of 173 male drug users but they also found that the TPQ failed to predict alcohol and drug abuse within the sample group. However, data obtained from their study did show that novelty seeking was significantly correlated with marijuana, barbiturate, amphetamine and cocaine abuse.

In a comparison study of the personality characteristics of sons of alcoholic and non-alcoholic fathers, Schuckit *et al.*[118] administered the TPQ to 33 males with a positive family history of alcoholism and 33 males with no family history of the disorder. Using information provided by the men, the father of each individual with a family history positive was assigned a score from 0 to 5 depending on the number of Type II alcohol-related symptoms reported. All 66 men were asked to complete the TPQ and were asked about their own drinking patterns and problems. It was hypothesised that among the 66 men the heaviest drinkers would be more likely to demonstrate higher levels of novelty seeking, and lower levels of harm avoidance and reward dependence. It was also hypothesised that individuals with family histories of alcoholism would have different TPQ scores than those with no family histories. Comparisons were also made between the alcoholic fathers' scores of 0–5 and the TPQ scores of their sons. The results of the study showed that there were no significant differences in the novelty seeking, harm avoidance or reward dependence scores of the heavier and lighter drinkers. There were also no significant differences between the two family history groups on any of the personality traits. Furthermore no significant correlations were found between the TPQ scores of the men with alcoholic fathers and their fathers' alcohol-related problem scores. Similar findings were also obtained by Zaninelli *et al.*[119] and Peterson *et al.*[120] Peterson *et al.* administered the TPQ to four groups of young men. The first group consisted of non-alcoholic sons of male alcoholics with extensive multigenerational family histories of male alcohol problems. The second was composed of non-alcoholic males with alcoholic fathers. The third group was made up of non-alcoholic males from the general population with no family histories of alcoholism and the fourth group consisted of male undergraduates with no family histories of alcoholism. Despite Cloninger's predictions, no significant differences were found between the mean TPQ scores obtained by the members of the four groups.

The TPQ has also been used to examine the personality traits of females with eating disorders;[121] females with bulimia nervosa;[114] and male and female smokers.[122] However, to date there is very little evidence on which to test Cloninger's theory concerning the neurobiological basis of personality, and its relevance to the Type I and Type II subgroups.

Using criteria which are somewhat different to Cloninger's, von Knorring *et al.*[92, 123] have also identified two subgroups of alcoholics. According to their typology, Type II alcoholism is associated with any early onset of subjective problems, early contact with treatment services, and more severe social complications including aggressiveness, difficulties at work, drink-driving and illegal drug abuse, whereas Type I alcoholism is associated with a later onset of alcohol-problems and for fewer social complications. von Knorring *et al.*[56] have also reported that the two subgroups of alcoholics have distinguishing personality characteristics. Type II alcoholics have significantly higher scores on sensation seeking, extraversion, somatic anxiety, and verbal aggression than Type I alcoholics, but lower scores on socialisation and inhibition of aggression.

Compared with the number of proposed typologies for alcoholism, considerably fewer attempts have been made to distinguish between different subgroups of drug addicts.[124–126] Using MMPI data collected from 1500 opiate addicts, and grouping together highly similar personality profiles, Berzins *et al.*[124] found two homogenous subgroups of heroin addicts. One group, labelled 'Type I' tended to have elevations on Scales 2 (Depression), 4 (Psychopathic) and 8 (Schizophrenic), reflecting high levels of subjective distress, nonconformity and confused thinking. It was thought that addicts within this group used drugs to 'control or attenuate feelings of anxiety, depression, distress and so on' (p. 72). In contrast, the other group, labelled Type II, tended to have a single elevation of Scale 4 (Psychopathic) and were believed to use drugs to 'enhance hedonistic pursuits or possibly reduce feelings of hostility'. It is interesting to note that less than half of the individuals who participated in this study could be classified as being either Type I (33 per cent) or Type II (7 per cent). As part of their study, Berzins and his co-workers also compared the characteristic features associated with their two types of drug addicts with Goldstein and Linden's[104] alcoholic subgroups. They concluded that their two drug addict groups bore a striking resemblance to two of Goldstein and Linden's alcoholic subgroups. Drug addict Type Is were found to have similarities with alcoholic Type IIs whereas Type II addicts had similarities with alcoholic Type Is.

The identification of alcoholic and drug-abuser subtypes has obvious practical implications for both treatment and prevention. If clinicians and researchers were able to identify whether certain subgroups of alcoholics or drug abusers responded more effectively to one form of treatment than another, appropriate matches could be made, resulting in better treatment outcomes. It is therefore important that further progress in made within this field of research.

Effects of Alcohol and Other Addictive Drugs on Personality

Since the 1960s, a growing number of clinical studies have been undertaken to assess objectively the effects of alcohol and other addictive drugs on human behaviour. It is now well established that the psychophysiological effects of such drugs are complex and diverse, and may be modulated by a whole range of non-pharmacological factors including the personality characteristics of the user, his/her emotional state, his/her previous experiences with the drug, his/her expectations and the social circumstances in which the substance is taken.[127, 128] Only the effects of alcohol and other addictive drugs on mood and aggression are reviewed in this section, and readers wishing to study this area in greater depth are advised to read the reviews by Mello,[128, 129] Mello and Mendelson,[127] and Cox.[44]

As mentioned earlier, depression and anxiety have frequently been linked with alcoholism and drug addiction. However, the question which has puzzled many researchers and clinicians is whether these negative feelings proceed or result from such behaviours. Many of the studies which have been undertaken to assess the psychological effects of alcohol and other addictive drugs have focused on changes in mood states which accompany the acute or chronic ingestion of such substances. Although it has been repeatedly demonstrated that alcoholics and drug addicts tend to have positive expectancies about their use of alcohol and other drugs,[130, 131] evidence from controlled clinical research studies, in which individuals have been observed during intoxication, has not substantiated these self-report findings. In fact, in her review of the literature, Mello[128] cites evidence from several studies which have consistently demonstrated that although low doses of alcohol tend to result in positive affective reactions, chronic alcohol consumption gives rise to increases in depression, anxiety and dysphoria in both alcoholics and social drinkers. Furthermore, there is also evidence which suggests that the effects of alcohol on mood are related to the personality characteristics of the individuals. Sher and Levenson[132] found that male college students who were characterised as outgoing, aggressive, impulsive and antisocial, had more intense affective reactions to alcohol, than other college males.

Mello[128] also cites evidence which indicates that chronic heroin use, like alcohol consumption, may give rise to increases in anxiety, depression, dysphoria, tension, irritability, feelings of hostility and somatic concerns. Only within the first day or two of heroin use, does the drug appear to produce the anticipated feelings of euphoria, elation and decreases in anxiety and depression. However, there is evidence which does suggest that even though the positive effects do not seem to be sustained during chronic use, heroin users do report experiencing a brief elevation in mood after acutely injecting heroin.[133] More recently, Dackis and Gold[134] have associated prolonged cocaine use with severe depression and anxiety, and in a study which was undertaken to assess the acute effects of tetrahydrocannabinols (THC – the most active ingredient in cannabis), Kamien et al.[135] showed that use of THC was also associated with increases in confusion, depression and general mood disturbance.

The severity of anxiety, depression and dysphoria in alcoholics and other drug users tends increase as heavy drinking and drug taking continues.[136, 137] In their study of 30 young women for example, Lex and his co-worker showed that heavy marijuana users consistently reported higher negative moods and lower positive moods than light users. Heavy caffeine consumers have also been found to be more depressed and anxious than light caffeine users.[138] Studies of the mood changes in hospitalised alcoholics and drug addicts have also clearly indicated that one of the long-term consequences of habitual alcohol or drugs abuse is to intensify in the users negative affect. Using the Beck's Depression Inventory, Strain *et al.*[139] assessed self-reported depressive symptoms of 58 opiate addicts at admission to a methadone treatment programme and weekly during the first four weeks of treatment. They found that depression declined after the first week of treatment and remained stable over subsequent weeks. In a study of benzodiazepine patients, Higgitt *et al.*[140] showed that both anxiety and depression improved with reduced benzodiazepine intake and, similarly, it has also been shown that when alcoholics and drinkers reduce their alcohol intake, they experience significant improvements in affect.[141, 142]

In addition to studying the effects of alcohol and other addictive drugs on mood, clinical laboratory studies have also investigated the effects that such substances can have on aggression. There is considerable evidence that aggressive patterns of behaviour are frequently associated with substance abuse, particularly with the excessive use of certain drugs such as alcohol, amphetamines and cocaine.[143-145] Many murders, armed robberies, incidents of domestic violence, incidents of child abuse and other violent behaviours have been found to be accompanied by excessive alcohol and drug abuse.[146] It has also been found that alcohol-dependent men tend to report more anger and aggression when drinking than when sober, especially those with a history of childhood aggression.[147, 148]

Studies of social drinkers support the impression that alcohol facilitates the expression of aggressive behaviours.[149, 150] In a study of 60 intoxicated and non-intoxicated male undergraduates with self-reported high, moderate and low aggressive tendencies, Bailey and Taylor[149] found that all three groups of subjects including those who reported themselves as non-aggressors became more aggressive when intoxicated. Comparable findings have also been obtained from experimental studies in which other psychoactive drugs besides alcohol have been systematically administered. In a recent study which was undertaken to study the effects of cocaine on human aggression, 30 male undergraduates were administered a placebo, or a low or high oral dose of cocaine. The subjects were then given the opportunity to administer electric shocks to an increasingly aggressive fictitious opponent. The results indicated that irrespective of the level of provocation the subjects who had been given the high dose of cocaine reacted more aggressively than those who had been given the placebo.[130]

CONCLUSION

This chapter has shown that despite a wealth of studies, no specific 'addictive personality' has been consistently identified. Nevertheless, certain personality characteristics have been associated with the development and expression of addictive behaviours, and it is has also been demonstrated the behaviours themselves can have a variety of effects on personality.

Gaining a greater understanding of the relationship between personality and addictive behaviours has serious implications for future prevention, education and treatment strategies. If individuals at risk of developing addictive behaviours can be identified by their personality characteristics, more effective primary prevention and education programmes could be designed and targeted to meet the needs of such individuals. Similarly, if it were possible to identify whether individuals with certain personality characteristics responded more favourably to one form of treatment than another, clinicians would be able to allocate their treatment resources more efficiently and effectively. It must, however, be recognised that determinants of addictive behaviours are unlikely to be found within the constraints of a single discipline. Perhaps, therefore, one of the most productive ways forward would be for future researchers to undertake more multidisciplinary research, integrating what is already known about the psychological, biological, and sociological correlates of addictive behaviours, and building upon this knowledge.

NOTES

1. L. Levy, *Concepts of Personality: Theories and Research* (New York: Random House, 1970).
2. R. L. Atkinson, R. C. Atkinson and E. R. Hilgard, *Introduction to Psychology*, 8th edn (New York: Harcourt Brace Jovanovich, 1983).
3. P. E. Nathan, 'The Addictive Personality is the Behaviour of the Addict', *Journal of Consulting and Clinical Psychology*, 56 (1988):183–8.
4. W. H. Sheldon, *Atlas of Men: A Guide for Somatotyping the Adult Male At All Ages* (New York: Harper & Row, 1954).
5. A. R. Lang, 'Addictive Personality: A Viable Construct?', in P. K. Levison, D. R. Gerstein and D. R. Maloff (eds), *Commonalities in Substance Abuse and Habitual Behaviour* (Lexington, MA: Lexington Books, 1983), pp. 157–235.

6. W. M. Cox, 'The Addictive Personality', in S. H. Snyder (ed.), *The Encyclopedia of Psychoactive Drugs* (New York: Chelsea House Publication, 1986).

7. B. Rush, 'An Inquiry into the Effects of Ardent Spirits upon the Human Body and Mind, with an Account of the Means of Preventing and of the Remedies for Curing Them', *Quarterly Journal of Studies on Alcohol*, 4 (1785):143–74.

8. T. Trotter, 'An Essay, Medical, Philosophical and Chemical on Drunkeness', *Quarterly Journal of Studies on Alcohol*, 2 (1804):321–41.

9. N. Heather and I. Robertson, *Problem Drinking*, 2nd edn (New York: Oxford University Press, 1989).

10. K. Abraham, 'The Psychological Relations Between Sexuality and Alcoholism', in *Selected Papers of Karl Abraham, M.D.* (New York: Brunner/Mazel, 1954).

11. W. M. Cox, 'Personality Theory', in D. A. Chaudron and D. A. Wilkinson (eds), *Theories on Alcoholism* (Canada: Alcoholism and Drug Addiction Research, 1988).

12. S. Freud, 'Mourning and Melancholia', in I. Starchey (ed.), *The Standard Edition of the Complete Psychological Works of Sigmund Freud* (London: Hogarth Press, 1917).

13. R. P. Knight, 'The Dynamics and Treatment of Chronic Alcohol Addiction', *Bulletin of the Menninger Clinic*, 1 (1937):233–50.

14. K. A. Menninger, *Man Against Himself* (New York: Harcourt, Brace, 1938).

15. E. M. Blum, 'Psychoanalytic Views of Alcoholism', *Quarterly Journal of Studies on Alcohol*, 27 (1966):259–99.

16. W. M. Cox, K. Lun and R. G. Loper, 'Identifying Pre-Alcoholic Personality Characteristics', in W. M. Cox (ed.), *Identifying and Measuring Alcoholic Personality Characteristics* (San Francisco: Jossey-Bass, 1983).

17. C. Johanson and M. Fischman, 'The Pharmacology of Cocaine Related to its Abuse', *Pharmacology Review*, 41 (1989):3–52.

18. R. Jessor and S. L. Jessor, *Problem Behaviour and Psychological Development* (New York: Academic Press, 1977).

19. J. A. Wingard, G. J. Huba and P. M. Bentler, 'A Longitudinal Analysis of Personality Structure and Adolescent Substance Use', *Personality and Individual Differences*, 1 (1980):250–72.

20. D. J. Samuels and M. Samuels, 'Low Self-Concept as a Cause of Drug Abuse', *Journal of Drug Education*, 4 (1974):421–38.

21. W. McCord and J. McCord, *Origins of Alcoholism* (Stanford, CA: Stanford University Press, 1960).

22. W. McCord and J. McCord, 'A Longitudinal Study of the Personality of Alcoholics', in D. J. Pittman and C. R. Snyder (eds), *Society, Culture and Drinking Patterns* (New York: Wiley, 1962).

23. L. N. Robins, W. M. Bates and P. O'Neal, 'Adult Drinking Patterns of Former Problem Children', in D. J. Pittman, and C. R. Snyder (eds), *Society, Culture and Drinking Patterns* (New York: Wiley, 1962).

24. M. C. Jones, 'Personality Correlates and Antecedents of Drinking Patterns in Adult Males', *Journal of Consulting and Clinical Psychology*, 32 (1968):2–12.

25. M. L. Kammeier, H. Hoffman and R. G. Loper, 'Personality Characteristics of Alcoholics as College Freshmen and at Time of Treatment', *Quarterly Journal of Studies on Alcohol*, 34 (1973):390–9.
26. R. G. Loper, M. L. Kammeier and H. Hoffman, 'MMPI Characteristics of College Freshmen Males who Later Became Alcoholics', *Journal of Abnormal Psychology*, 82 (1973):159–62.
27. H. Hoffman, R. G. Loper and M. L. Kammeier, 'Identifying Future Alcoholics with MMPI Alcoholism Scales', *Quarterly Journal of Studies on Alcohol*, 35 (1974):490–8.
28. N. Rosenberg, 'MMPI Alcoholism Scales', *Journal of Clinical Psychology*, 28 (1972):515–28.
29. C. MacAndrew, 'The Differentiation of Male Alcoholic Patients from NonAlcoholic Psychiatric Outpatients', *Quarterly Journal of Studies on Alcohol*, 26 (1965):238–46.
30. J. W. Goldstein, 'Personality Characteristics of Students Who Become Heavy Drug Users: An MMPI Study of Avantgarde', *American Journal of Drug and Alcohol Abuse*, 4 (1977):401–12.
31. G. R. Saunders, and M. A. Schuckit, 'MMPI Scores in Young Men with Alcoholic Relatives and Controls', *The Journal of Nervous and Mental Disease*, 169 (1981):456–8.
32. M. A. Schuckit, 'Extraversion and Neuroticism in Young Men at Higher and Lower Risk for Alcoholism', *American Journal of Psychiatry*, 140 (1983):1223–4.
33. R. E. Tarter *et al.*, 'Adolescent Sons of Alcoholics: Neuropsychological and Personality Characteristics', *Alcoholism: Clinical and Experimental Research*, 8 (1984):216–22.
34. S. C. Whipple and E. P. Noble, 'Personality Characteristics of Alcoholic Fathers and Their Sons', *Journal of Studies on Alcohol*, 52 (1991):331–7.
35. C.R. Cloninger, 'A Unified Biosocial Theory of Personality and Its Role in the Development of Anxiety States', *Psychiatric Developments*, 3 (1986):167–226.
36. C. R. Cloninger, 'Neurogenetic Adaptive Mechanisms in Alcoholism', *Science*, 236 (1987):410–6.
37. C. R. Cloninger, S. Sigvardsson and M. Bohman, 'Childhood Personality Predicts Alcohol Abuse in Young Adults', *Alcoholism*, 12 (1988):494–505.
38. J. J. Platt and C. Labate, *Heroin Addiction: Theory, Research and Treatment* (New York: Wiley, 1976).
39. M. Zuckerman, *Sensation Seeking: Beyond the Optimal Level of Arousal* (New York: Wiley, 1979).
40. M. Zuckerman, 'Sensation Seeking and Psychopathy', in R. D. Hare and D. Schalling (eds), *Psychopathic Behaviour: Approaches to Research* (New York: Wiley & Sons, 1978), pp. 165–85.
41. D. G. Kilpatrick, P. B. Sutker and A. D. Smith, 'Deviant Drug and Alcohol Use: The Role of Anxiety, Sensation Seeking and Other Personality Variables', in M. Zuckerman and C. D. Spielberger (eds), *Emotions and Anxiety: New Concepts, Methods and Applications* (Hillsdale, NJ: L. Erlbaum Associates, 1976).
42. R. B. Kandel, *Longitudinal Research on Drug Use* (New York: Wiley, 1978).
43. P. Owen and J. Butcher, 'Personality Factors in Problem Drinking: A

Review of the Evidence and Some Suggested Directions', in R. Pickens and L. Heston (eds), *Psychiatric Factors in Drug Abuse* (New York: Grune & Stratton, 1979).

44. W. M. Cox, 'The Alcoholic Personality: A Review of the Evidence', in B. A. Maher (ed.), *Progress in Experimental Personality Research* (New York: Academic Press, 1979) pp. 89–148.

45. W. G. Dahlstrom and G. S. Welsh, *An MMPI Handbook: A Guide to Use in Clinical Practice and Research* (Minneapolis: University of Minnesota Press, 1960).

46. R. S. Johnson, J. W. Tobin and T. Cellucci, 'Personality Characteristics of Cocaine and Alcohol Abusers: More Alike Than Different', *Addictive Behaviours*, 17 (1992):159–66.

47. S. Walfish, R. Massey and A. Krone, 'MMPI Profiles of Cocaine-addicted Individuals in Residential Treatment: Implications for Practical Treatment Planning', *Journal of Substance Abuse Treatment*, 7 (1990):151–4.

48. P. B. Sutker, 'Personality Differences and Sociopathy in Heroin Addicts and Nonaddict Prisoners', *Journal of Abnormal Pschology*, (1971):247–51.

49. J. E. Overall, 'MMPI Personality Patterns of Alcoholics and Narcotic Addicts', *Quarterly Journal of Studies on Alcohol*, 34 (1973):104–11.

50. N. Brill, 'Personality Factors in Marajuana Use', *Archives of General Psychiatry*, 24 (1971):163–5.

51. A. T. McLellan, A. R. Childress and E. G. Woody, 'Drug Abuse and Psychiatric Disorder: Role of Drug Choice', in A. I. Alterman (ed.), *Substance Abuse & Psychopathology* (New York: Plenum Press, 1985) pp. 137–72.

52. M. Irwin, M. A. Schuckit and T. L. Smith, 'Clinical Importance of Age at Onset in Type 1 and Type 2 Primary Alcoholics', *General Archives of Psychiatry*, 47 (1990):320–4.

53. C. A. de Jong et al., 'Personality Disorders in Alcoholics and Drug Addicts', *Comprehensive Psychiatry*, 34 (1993):87–94.

54. M. A. Schuckit, 'Alcoholism and Sociopathy – Diagnostic Confusion', *Quarterly Journal of Studies on Alcohol*, 34 (1973):157–64.

55. D. W. Goodwin, 'Alcoholism and Heredity: A Review and Hypothesis', *Archives of General Psychiatry*, 36 (1979):57–61.

56. L. von Knorring et al., 'Personality Traits in Subtypes of Alcoholics', *Journal of Studies on Alcohol*, 48 (1987):423–527.

57. M. J. Randolph and W. R. Yates, 'Antisocial Personality in Alcohol and Drug-Dependent Individuals: A Study of Gender Effects', *American Journal on Addictions*, 2 (1993):9–17.

58. M. N. Hesselbrock, V. M. Hesselbrock, T. F. Babor, J. R. Stabenau, R. E. Meyer, and M. Weidenman, 'Antisocial Behaviour, Psychopathology, and Problem Drinking in the Natural History of Alcoholism', in D. W. Goodwin, K. T. Van Dusen and S. A. Mednick (eds), *Longitudinal Research of Alcoholism* (Boston, Mass.: Kluwer-Nijhoff Publishing) pp. 197–214.

59. M. A. Schuckit, M. Irwin and T. L. Smith, 'One-Year Incidence Rate of Major Depression and Other Psychiatric Disorders in 239 Alcoholic Men', *Addiction*, 89 (1994):441–5.

60. W. G. Dahlstrom, G. S. Welsh and L. E. Dahlstrom, *An MMPI Handbook* (Minneapolis: University of Minnesota Press, 1972).
61. R. J. Dougherty and N. J. Lesswing, 'Inpatient Cocaine Abusers: An Analysis of Psychological and Demographic Variables', *Journal of Substance Abuse Treatment*, 6 (1989):45–7.
62. S. Walfish, R. Massey and A. Krone, 'Anxiety and Anger Among Abusers of Different Substances', *Drug and Alcohol Dependence*, 25 (1990):253–6.
63. H. Rankin, T. Stockwell and R. Hodgson, 'Personality and Alcohol Dependence', *Personality and Individual Differences*, 3 (1982):145–51.
64. J. Hallman *et al.*, 'Personality Traits and Platelet Monoamine Oxidase Activity in Alcoholic Women', *Addictive Behaviours*, 16 (1991):533–41.
65. P. H. Lodhi and S. Thakur, 'Personality of Drug Addicts: Eysenkian Analysis', *Personality and Individual Differences*, 15 (1993):121–8.
66. R. A. Steer, M. G. McElroy and A. T. Beck, 'Correlates of Self-Reported and Clinically Assessed Depression in Outpatient Alcoholics', *Journal of Clinical Psychology*, 39 (1983):144–9.
67. R. A. Steer, A. T. Beck and F. B. Shaw, 'Depressive Symptoms Differentiating between Heroin Addicts and Alcoholics', *Drug and Alcohol Dependence*, 15 (1985):145–50.
68. S. Darke, W. Swift and W. Hall, 'Prevalence, Severity and Correlates of Psychological Morbidity Among Methodone Maintainance Clients', *Addiction*, 89 (1994):211–7.
69. C. S. Rand, B. A. Lowlor and J. M. Kuldau, 'Patterns of Food and Alcohol Consumption in a Group of Bulimic Women', *Bulletin of the Society of Psychologists in Addictive Behaviours*, 5 (1986):95–104.
70. K. S. Kendler *et al.*, 'The Genetic Epidemiology of Bulimia Nervosa', *American Journal of Psychiatry*, 148 (1991):1627–37.
71. L. S. Fidell, 'Sex Differences in Psychotropic Drug Use', *Professional Psychology*, 12 (1981):156–62.
72. M. Gossop, 'Drug Dependence and Self-esteem', *International Journal of Addictions*, 11 (1976):741–53.
73. M. L. Griffin *et al.*, 'A Comparison of Male and Female Cocaine Abusers', *Archives of General Psychiatry* 46 (1989):122–6.
74. H. J. Eysenck and S. B. G. Eysenck, *Manual of the Eysenck Personality Inventory* (London: University of London Press, 1964).
75. H. J. Eysenck and S. B. G. Eysenck, *Manual of the Eysenck Personality Questionnaire* (London: Hodder & Stoughton, 1975).
76. H. J. Eysenck and S. B. G. Eysenck, *Manual of the Eysenck Personality Scales* (London: Hodder & Stoughton, 1991).
77. H. J. Eysenck and S. B. G. Eysenck, *Psychoticism as a Dimension of Personality* (London: Hodder & Stoughton, 1976).
78. M. R. Gossop and S. B. G. Eysenck, 'A Further Investigation into the Personality of Drug Addicts in Treatment', *British Journal of Addiction*, 75 (1980):305–11.
79. G. Sahasi *et al.*, 'Eysenck's Personality Questionnaire Scores in Heroin Addicts in India', *Indian Journal of Psychiatry*, 32 (1990):25–9.
80. J. Feldman and S. B. G. Eysenck, 'Addictive Personality Traits and Bulimic Patients', *Personality and Individual Differences*, 7 (1986):923–6.
81. A. P. Blaszczynski, N. Buhrich and N. McConaghy, 'Pathological Gam-

blers, Heroin Addicts and Controls Compared on the EPQ "Addiction Scale"', *British Journal of Addiction*, 80 (1985):315–19.
82. M. R. Gossop, 'A Comparative Study of Oral and Introvenous Drug-Dependent Patients on Three Dimensions of Personality', *International Journal of Addiction*, 13 (1978):135–42.
83. O. Doherty and G. Matthews, 'Personality Characteristics of Opiate Addicts', *Personality and Individual Differences*, 9 (1988):171–2.
84. T. L. Rosenthal *et al.*, 'Substance Abuse Patterns Reveal Contrasting Personality Traits', *Journal of Substance Abuse*, 2 (1990):255–63.
85. A. Kaldegg, 'Aspects of Personal Relationships in Heroin Dependent Young Men: An Experimental Study', *British Journal of Addiction*, 70 (1995):277–86.
86. H. Blumberg *et al.*, 'British Opiate Users: I. People Approaching London Treatment Centres', *International Journal of Addiction*, 9 (1974):1–23.
87. C. MacAndrew, 'Male Alcoholics, Secondary Psychopathy and Eysenck's Theory of Personality', *Personality and Individual Differences*, 1 (1980):151–60.
88. J. V. Spotts and F. C. Shontz, 'Correlates of Sensation Seeking by Heavy, Chronic Drug Users' *Perceptual and Motor Skills*, 58 (1984):427–35.
89. J. V. Spotts and F. C. Shontz, 'Drugs and Personality: Extraversion–Introversion', *Journal of Clinical Psychology*, 40 (1984):624–8.
90. H. J. Eysenck, 'Smoking, Personality and Psychosomatic Disorders', *Journal of Psychosomatic Research*, 7 (1963):107–30.
91. G. M. Smith, 'Personality Correlates of Cigarette Smoking in Students of College Age', *Annals of New York Academy of Sciences*, 142 (1967):308–21.
92. L. von Knorring, V. Palm and H. E. Andersson, 'Relationship Between Treatment Outcome and Subtype of Alcoholism in Men', *Journal of Studies on Alcohol*, 46 (1985):388–91.
93. N. Breslau, M. M. Kilby and P. Andreski, 'DSM-III-R Nicotine Dependence in Young Adults: Prevalence, Correlates and Associated Psychiatric Disorders', *Addiction*, 89 (1994):743–54.
94. E. M. Jellinek, *The Disease Concept of Alcoholism* (New Haven, CT: Hillhouse Press, 1960).
95. M. Bohman, S. Sigvardsson and C. R. Cloninger, 'Maternal Inheritance of Alcohol Abuse: Cross-Fostering Analysis of Adopted Women', *Archives of General Psychiatry*, 38 (1981):965–9.
96. C. R. Cloninger, M. Bohman and S. Sigvardsson, 'Inheritance of Alcohol Abuse: Cross-Fostering Analysis of Adopted Men', *Archives General Psychiatry*, 38 (1981):861–8.
97. T. F. Babar and J. Laverman, 'Classification and Forms of Inebriety: Historical Antecedents of Alcoholic Typologies', in M. Galanter (ed.), *Recent Developments in Alcoholism* (New York: Plenum Press, 1986).
98. H. A. Skinner, D. N. Jackson and H. Hoffman, 'Alcoholic Personality Types: Identification and Correlates', *Journal of Abnormal Psychology*, 83 (1995):658–66.
99. D. M. Donovan, E. F. Chaney and M. R. O'Leary, 'Alcoholic MMPI Subtypes: Relationship to Drinking Styles, Benefits and Consequences', *Journal of Nervous and Mental Disease*, 166 (1978):553–61.

118 *Addictive Behaviour*

100. T. F. Babor, and Z. S. Dolinsky, 'Alcoholic Typologies: Historical Evaluation and Empirical Evaluation of Some Common Classification Schemes', in R. M. Rose and J. Barrett (eds), *Alcoholism: Origins and Outcome* (New York: Raven Press, 1988), pp. 245–66.
101. H. J. Walton, 'Personality as a Determinant of the Form of Alcoholism', *British Journal of Psychiatry*, 114 (1968):761–6.
102. R. A. Brown, 'Conformity in Gamma and Delta Alcoholics', *Journal of Clinical Psychology*, 33 (1977): 895–6.
103. R. A. Brown, 'Personality Measure in Gamma and Delta Alcoholics: A Brief Note', *Journal of Clinical Psychology*, 36 (1980):345–6.
104. S. G. Goldstein and J. D. Linden, 'Multivariate Classification of Alcoholics by Means of the MMPI', *Journal of Abnormal Psychology*, 74 (1969):661–9.
105. P. R. Whitelock, J. E. Overall and J. H. Patrick, 'Personality Patterns and Alcohol Abuse in a State Hospital Population', *Journal of Abnormal Psychology*, 86 (1981):925–37.
106. V. J. Nerviano and W. F. Gross, 'Personality Types of Alcoholics on Objective Inventories', *Journal of Studies on Alcohol*, 44 (1983):837–51.
107. C. R. Cloninger, 'A Systematic Method for the Clinical Description and Classification of Personality Variants: A Proposal', *Archives of General Psychiatry*, 44 (1987):573–88.
108. C. R. Cloninger, *The Tridimensional Personality Questionnaire* (Washington, DC: Washington University School of Medicine, 1987).
109. C. R. Cloninger, T. R. Pryzybeck and D. M. Svrakic, 'The Tridimensional Personality Questionnaire: US Normative Data', *Psychological Reports*, 69 (1991):1047–57.
110. C. R. Cloninger et al., *The Temperament and Character Inventory (TCI): A Guide to Its Development and Use* (St Louis, MO: Centre for Psychobiology of Personality, Washington University, 1994).
111. M. Earlywine et al., 'Factor Structure and Correlates of the Tridimensional Personality Questionnaire', *Journal of Studies on Alcohol*, 53 (1992):233–8.
112. W. F. McCourt, R. J. Guerra and H. S. Cutter, 'Sensation Seeking and Novelty Seeking. Are They the Same?', *Journal of Nervous and Mental Disease*, 181 (1993):309–12.
113. R. D. Wetzel et al., 'Correlates of Tridimensional Personality Questionnaire Scales with Selected Minnesota Multiphasic Personality Inventory Scales', *Psychological Report*, 71 (1992):1027–38.
114. D. A. Waller et al., 'Tridimensional Personality Questionnaire and Serotonin in Bulimia Nervosa', *Psychiatry Research*, 48 (1993):9–15.
115. E. C. Penick et al., 'Examination of Cloninger's Type I and Type II Alcoholism with a Sample of Men Alcoholics in Treatment', *Alcoholism: Clinical and Experimental Research*, 14 (1990):623–9.
116. S. J. Nixon and O. A. Parsons, 'Application of the Tridimensional Personality Theory to a Population of Alcoholics and Other Substance Abusers', *Alcoholism: Clinical and Experimental Research*, 14 (1990):513–7.
117. C. T. Nagoshi et al., 'Validation of the Tridimensional Personality Questionnaire in a Sample of Male Drug Users', *Personality and Individual Differences*, 13 (1992):401–9.

118. M. A. Schuckit, M. Irwin and H. I. M. Mahler, 'Tridimensional Personality Questionnaire Scores of Sons of Alcoholic and Non-Alcoholic Fathers', *American Journal of Psychiatry*, 147 (1990):481–7.
119. R. M. Zaninelli, B. Porjesz and H. Begleiter, 'The Tridimensional Personality Questionnaire in Males at High and Low Risk for Alcoholism', *Alcoholism: Clinical and Experimental Research*, 16 (1992):68–70.
120. J. B. Peterson *et al.*, 'The Tridimensional Personality Questionnaire and the Inherited Risk for Alcoholism', *Addictive Behaviours*, 16 (1991):549–54.
121. T. D. Brewerton *et al.*, 'The Tridimensional Personality Questionnaire in Eating Disorder Patients', *International Journal of Eating Disorders*, 14 (1993):213–8.
122. C. S. Pomerleau *et al.*, 'Relationship of the Tridimensional Personality Questionnaire Scores and Smoking Variables in Female and Male Smokers', *Journal of Substance Abuse*, 4 (1992):143–54.
123. L. von Knorring and L. Oreland, 'Personality Traits and Monoamine Oxidase in Tobacco Smokers', *Psychological Medicine*, 15 (1985):327–34.
124. J. Berzins *et al.*, 'Subgroups Among Opiate Addicts: A Typological Investigation', *Journal of Abnormal Psychology*, 83 (1974):65–73.
125. R. J. Craig and R. Olson, 'MMPI Subtypes for Cocaine Abusers', *American Journal of Drug and Alcohol Abuse*, 18 (1992):197–205.
126. P. D. Moss and P. D. Weiner, 'An MMPI Typology of Cocaine Abusers', *Journal of Personality Assessment*, 58 (1992):269–76.
127. N. K. Mello and J. H. Mendelson, 'Alcohol and Human Behaviour', in L. L. Iversen, S. D. Iversen and S. H. Snyder (eds), *Handbook of Psychopharmacology, Drugs of Abuse* (New York: Plenum Press, 1978).
128. N. K. Mello, 'A Behavioural Analysis of the Reinforcing Properties of Alcohol and Other Drugs in Man', in B. Kissin and H. Begleitter (eds), *The Biology of Alcoholism*, vol. 7: *The Pathogenesis of Alcoholism: Biological Factors* (New York: Plenum Press, 1983).
129. N. K. Mello, 'Behavioural Studies of Alcoholism', in B. Kissin and H. Begleitter (eds), *The Biology of Alcoholism*, vol. 2: *Physiology and Behaviour* (New York: Plenum Press, 1972).
130. A. Licata *et al.*, 'Effects of Cocaine on Human Aggression', *Pharmacology, Biochemistry and Behaviour*, 45 (1993):549–52.
131. M. T. McGuire, J. H. Mendelson and S. Stein, 'Comparative Psychosocial Studies of Alcoholic and Non-Alcoholic Subjects Undergoing Experimentally Induced Ethanol Intoxication', *Psychosomatic Medicine*, 28 (1966):13–25.
132. K. J. Sher and R. W. Levenson, 'Risk for Alcoholism and Individual Differences in the Stress-Dampening Effect of Alcohol', *Journal of Abnormal Psychology*, 91 (1982):199–209.
133. S. M. Mirin *et al.*, 'Psychopathology, Craving and Mood During Heroin Acquisition: An Experimental Study', *International Journal of Addictions*, 11 (1976):525–44.
134. C. A. Dackis and M. S. Gold, 'New Concepts in Cocaine Addiction: The Dopamine Depletion Hypothesis', *Neuroscience Behavioural Review*, 9 (1985):469–77.
135. J. B. Kamien *et al.*, 'The Effects of D-Sup Tetrahydrocannabinol on Repeated Acquisition Performance of Response Sequences and Self-Reports

in Humans', *Behavioural Pharmacology*, 5 (1994):71–8.
136. A. I. Alterman, E. Gottheil and H. D. Crawford, 'Mood Changes in an Alcoholism Treatment Program Based on Drinking Decisions', *American Journal of Psychiatry*, 132 (1994):1032–7.
137. B. W. Lex *et al.*, 'Alcohol, Marijuana and Mood States in Young Women', *International Journal of Addiction*, 24 (1989):405–24.
138. J. E. James and D. P. Stirling, 'Caffeine: A Survey of Some of the Known and Suspected Deleterious Effects of Habitual Use', *British Journal of Addiction*, 78 (1983):251–8.
139. E. C. Strain, M. L. Stitzer and G. E. Bigelow, 'Early Treatment Time Course of Depressive Symptoms in Opiate Addicts', *Journal of Nervous and Mental Disease*, 179 (1991):215–21.
140. A. Higgitt *et al.*, 'Group Treatment of Benzodiazepine Dependence', *British Journal of Addiction*, 82 (1987):517–32.
141. S. A. Brown and M. A. Schuckit, 'Changes in Depression among Abstinent Alcoholics', *Journal of Studies on Alcohol*, 49 (1988):412–7.
142. I. M. Birnbaum *et al.*, 'Alcohol and Sober Mood State in Female Social Drinkers', *Alcoholism: Clinical and Experimental Research*, 7 (1983):362–8.
143. M. M. Miller and R. T. Pooter-Efron, 'Aggression and Violence Associated with Substance Abuse. Special Issue: Aggression, Family Violence and Chemical Dependency', *Journal of Chemical Dependency Treatment*, 3 (1989):1–36.
144. B. J. Bushman, 'Human Aggression while under the Influence of Alcohol and Other Drugs: An Integrative Research Review', *Current Directions in Psychological Science*, 2 (1993):148–52.
145. S. P. Taylor and S. T. Chermack, 'Alcohol, Drugs and Human Aggression', *Journal of Studies on Alcohol*, 11 (Suppl.) (1993): 78–88.
146. Royal College of Psychiatrists, *Alcohol Our Favourite Drug* (London: Tavistock, 1986).
147. J. H. Jaffee, T. F. Babor and D. H. Fishbein, 'Alcoholics, Aggression and Antisocial Personality', *Journal of Studies on Alcohol* 49 (1988):211–18.
148. D. H. Fishbein *et al.*, 'Drug Users' Self-Reports of Behaviours and Affective States under the Influence of Alcohol', *International Journal of Addiction*, 28 (1993):1565–85.
149. D. S. Bailey and S. P. Taylor, 'Effects of Alcohol on Aggressive Disposition on Human Physical Aggression', *Journal of Research on Personality*, 25 (1991):334–42.
150. A. Bond and M. Lader, 'The Relationship between Induced Behavioural Aggression and Mood after Consumption of two Doses of Alcohol', *British Journal of Addiction*, 81 (1986):65–75.
151. W. M. Cox, *Identifying and Measuring Alcoholic Personality Characteristics* (San Francisco: Jossey-Bass, 1983).

8 Locus of Control and Addictive Behaviour
Colin Martin and Catherine Otter

INTRODUCTION

The locus of control (LOC) construct[1] represents an enduring approach to the investigation of personality, it being a fundamental part of social learning theory.[2] It has also been used widely in the clinical field to investigate many examples of psychopathology including those purportedly involved in addictive behaviour.[3] In this chapter we shall address, amongst others, the following questions:

1. Where does the LOC construct come from?
2. How useful is the LOC construct in understanding the complexity of human behaviour?
3. In clinical terms, how useful is the LOC construct in predicting an individuals future behaviour?

Prior to examining the extensive use of the LOC construct in the clinical arena and in particular, addictions, let us consider the more rudimentary questions regarding this much used (and possibly abused) personality dimension.

ORIGINS AND ESSENTIAL PREAMBLE

The locus of control is an example of a single-trait theory of personality. Single-trait theories of personality, unlike multi-trait theories of personality, do not seek to explain the entire personality, rather, single-trait theories attempt to explain the *dominant* personality dimension that is *central* in mediating an individual's behaviour. The LOC construct describes a generalised expectancy regarding an individual's beliefs concerning his or her personal control over situations. The LOC scale is administered using a questionnaire that comprises twenty-nine pairs of statements. An example of a statement pair would be (a) 'Many times I feel that I have little influence over the things that happen to me', (b) 'It is impossible for me to believe that chance or luck plays an important part in my life'. The respondent chooses the one statement from each pair which he most strongly believes and from the subject's choice of responses a sum score is obtained representative of the subject's LOC orientation along the dimension. The unidimensional LOC continuum ranges from internal to external, therefore an individual who is nearer to the internal extreme of the dimension would be described as having an internal LOC and believe themselves to be more in control of situations. In contrast, an individual nearer to the external extreme of the dimension would be described as having an external locus of control and believe themselves to be less in control of situations. Relating this to the example above, statement (a) would be considered an 'external' choice, whereas choice (b) would be considered an 'internal' choice. To illustrate the concept of the internality/externality LOC continuum, consider the following scenarios.

Scenario One

Mike, a talented pianist, is sitting an exam the goal of which is to attain a not inconsiderable scholarship. It is unlikely that he will have an opportunity to sit this exam again should he fail. He has travelled to London to sit the exam from his home, a small industrial town in Northern England. Let us now examine control orientation on Mike's perception of events. If Mike had an *internal* LOC then if he passed the exam and were awarded the scholarship, he would believe this success as being down to his individual ability and effort. If Mike had failed the exam he would believe his failure to be due to lack of ability or lack of personal effort. Consider though the same situational outcomes (success or failure) if Mike had an *external* LOC. In both instances Mike would believe the outcome was due to chance factors that were beyond his control.

Scenario Two

Frank, an alcoholic, is currently an in-patient in a drug dependency unit (DDU) undergoing detoxification. This is Frank's seventh detoxification and it is unlikely that Frank will be admitted for detoxification as a priority if he were to relapse again. Frank's stated goal on discharge is to remain abstinent. Following discharge there are essentially two possible future outcomes (assuming that the goal of abstinence remains unchanged and, for the sake of argument, controlled drinking is not considered an option), Frank will either remain abstinent or he will relapse. Let us now examine control orientation on Frank's perception of events. If Frank has an *internal* LOC and remains abstinent he is likely to attribute this positive outcome to his own determination, ability and personal resources. If Frank were to relapse he would, again, be likely to attribute this to internal personal factors such as lack of personal ability or poor resolve. If Frank has an *external* LOC, however, he is likely to perceive these outcomes entirely differently. In the case of continued abstinence Frank would be likely to believe that chance factors were important such as not 'bumping into' previous drinking partners who would 'encourage him to drink'. In the case of Frank relapsing, he is likely to attribute this negative outcome to chance factors such as personal relationship difficulties which 'made him' drink or his relapse was due to a 'slip'.

These two quite different scenarios illustrate how the concepts of internality and externality are incorporated into the LOC construct. In both cases, however, locus of *perceived* causality is explicit and consistent across the two scenarios, i.e. external LOC associated with external factors such as 'chance'. This is an important point as any foundation for a theory of personality must incorporate features of *stability* over time and *consistency* across different situations. It should be noted that a critique of both single- and multi-trait theories of personality maintains that stability and consistency of this type has, in certain experimental manipulations, been found to be lacking.[4] It has also been found that many demographic variables can have a strong influence on control orientation[5] which can be both an advantage, i.e. inherent sensitivity to covariates, or a disadvantage, i.e. a source of extraneous variance and experimental confounding.

It is clear from the scenarios presented that the LOC construct is a broad personality concept and, as such, attempts have been made to enhance its specifity. Examples include the Health Locus of Control Scale, designed to measure control orientation in relation to health-related behaviour[6] and the Drinking Related Internal-External Locus of Control Scale (DRIE scale),[7] designed to measure control orientation in relation to substance misuse. Test-retest reliability of the LOC scale has been found in many studies to be high[8] thereby satisfying the consistency criteria for the dimension with regard to a wide variety of behaviours. The perennial problem with the LOC construct is, as with all single-trait theories of personality, a fundamental limitation in providing a complete explanation of behaviour.

LOCUS OF CONTROL AND ADDICTION

The LOC dimension has been used extensively in the study of addictive behaviour.[3] Most studies have, however, focused on LOC in relation to alcoholism rather than illicit drugs, although a significant number of studies have investigated this area. It is interesting to note that, in comparison to the United Kingdom, a large number of studies in the United States have explored LOC in relation to caffeine often as a covariable in an otherwise non-addiction centred design,[9] this probably being a reflection of the 'cultural dependence' on coffee in the US.

It would seem intuitive that individuals whose lives have been affected by the abuse of substances and who often report feeling out of control of their lives would be expected to have an *external* LOC orientation. This general expectation for substance misusers to have an external LOC has been investigated in many LOC studies in addiction. Since the majority of LOC studies have focused on alcoholism this section will, necessarily, address this area much more closely.

Alcoholism

Many studies have demonstrated that individuals with alcoholism have a more external LOC orientation than non-alcoholics.[10] These findings are supportive of the notion that individuals who feel they have little control over their drinking would also have an *external* LOC orientation. Other studies have found conflicting evidence against this prediction and have found alcoholics to be more *internal* in control orientation than non-alcoholics.[11] There is also some evidence from retrospective studies that pre-alcoholics are more likely to be external in control orientation compared to their peers, thus enhancing the LOC concept as an enduring personality dimension that has discriminatory power. Paradoxically, it has also been demonstrated that alcoholics during the course of treatment become more internal.[12] Though a shift toward internality would be desirable in terms of gaining control over one's drinking, this finding also rather usurps the concept of the LOC construct having inherent stability which is a prerequisite of a reliable measure of personality. This is more than merely a semantic point of definition because by using personality measures in the clinical field are we describing behaviour change, i.e. drinking cessation, or personality change, i.e. shift in control orientation, or an interaction between the two? Potentially then, there is at best some confusion, and at worst confounding, when observed behaviour and personal beliefs become circumscribed by a *single* LOC dimension. Since this issue is rarely raised in the clinical literature it is mentioned here to enlighten the reader to the wider issues that must be considered when attempting to equate personality dimensions to maladaptive or undesirable behaviour. The reader is therefore advised to be cautious when considering general personality theory and specific application, particularly in the light of the LOC studies in addiction which are replete with examples of the contradictions stated at the beginning of this section.

The apparent inconsistencies highlighted above may be explained by other factors that may covary with LOC orientation and drinking behaviour. Haack's[13] study of nursing students indicates some of the possible additional factors that need to be considered. Haack found that during a two-year affiliation, most student's frequency of alcohol use increased and that there was also a corresponding increase in burnout symptoms. Interestingly, these behaviours were related to a lack of social support and an external attribution style (conceptually related to external LOC). These findings would seem indicative of the role of stress, i.e. no support, as an important variable in increased drinking consumption. Social support may also be an important factor in the aetiology of problem drinking behaviour. Davis,[14] for example, found that children of alcoholics have lower self-esteem and have a more external LOC orientation than children of non-alcoholics. Since personality characteristics such as self-esteem and LOC are believed to be relatively stable from childhood to adulthood, researchers have explored the possibility of low self-esteem being a risk factor involved in alcoholism,[15] although the findings from self-esteem studies are by no means conclusive. Depression and anxiety should also be considered in any assessment of the clinical application of the LOC construct since depression and anxiety are often reported in cases of alcoholism[16] and depressed and anxious individuals demonstrate differences in LOC orientation compared to non-depressed and non-anxious controls.[17]

A practical measure of the validity of any personality dimension in the clinical field is its usefulness as a predictor of outcome and indicator of therapeutic change. Canton *et al.*[18] found that alcoholics entering treatment who were LOC internal had a better outcome in terms of drinking status at six-month follow up compared to those who were LOC external; however, it was also found that those alcoholics who experienced more independent life events of high negative impact were more likely to relapse. It would therefore seem that, for the LOC construct's value in predicting treatment outcome to be maximised, social context and personal circumstances need to be firmly considered as a co-determinate of outcome.

Using the drinking-related locus of control scale (DRIE Scale),[19] Annis and Peachey[12] explored the possibility that type of treatment was implicated in determining alcoholics' control orientation and their follow-up status. Subjects participated in a clinical trial and were prescribed calcium carbimide, a short-acting alcohol sensitising drug. Subjects received this medication in combination with either medical advice emphasising the medical management of their problem drinking or relapse-prevention counselling emphasising the development of more adaptive coping strategies for dealing effectively with high risk drinking situations. In the relapse-prevention condition, subjects were encouraged to gradually reduce their reliance on the medication in conjunction with graded exposure to high-risk drinking situations. Subjects receiving relapse-prevention counselling demonstrated a shift toward internality, whereas those in the medical advice condition showed no shift in control orientation. There was also some indication that treatment gains were more effectively maintained at 18 months post-treatment follow-up for those subjects who had received relapse-prevention counselling.

These studies provide support for the cognitive social learning model of behaviour change in the applied clinical setting. This also concords with the philosophy underpinning motivational interviewing, an approach that is now popular in the counselling treatment of addictive behaviour, which emphasises that personal control and responsibility are crucial to adaptive behaviour change. While there is evidence to suggest that high externality scores are a good indicator of active substance misuse behaviour[20] and that issues surrounding LOC orientation are important to address if the chances of a positive treatment outcome are to be maximised, it is important to add a note of methodological caution. Both Canton et al.[18] and Annis and Peachey[12] used LOC scales, and the results from both studies were supportive of a shift to internality as a desirable treatment outcome. In the former study, Rotter's LOC scale was used and in the latter the alcohol-specific DRIE LOC scale was used. Other studies have found using the DRIE LOC scale that drinking alcoholics were more externally orientated than recovering or abstinent alcoholics,[21] whereas there are contrary findings that alcoholics are internally controlled when measured on Rotter's LOC scale.[11] In view of this, the apparent, 'closeness of fit' between the findings and conclusions of Canton et al.[18] and Annis and Peachey[12] may be reduced or undermined by LOC scale differences. Contradictory findings between studies using the LOC construct seem to be the rule rather than the exception. Methodological inconsistencies between studies are likely to be an important contributing factor to this state of affairs, with the result that not only will any potential usefulness of the LOC dimension in clinical practice become diluted, but also the conceptual framework from which LOC dimension originated will become increasingly undermined. Effectively, a situation begins to emerge where we can determine that the LOC measures 'something', and does this reliably 'sometimes'! Clearly then, fundamental conceptual issues involving the LOC continuum need to be addressed; principal among these is the problem of applying a personality dimension derived from social learning theory to the clinical area on a 'let's try it and see basis'. At this conceptual level, the metaphor 'fitting a square peg into a round hole' comes increasingly to mind. It would seem appropriate then, that hypothesis generation based on social learning theory, and applied to a social learning model of substance misuse at more than a surface level, is an important consideration in formulating ways of *meaningfully* applying the LOC construct to clinical work.

The above paragraph serves to highlight potential limitations regarding the general usefulness of the LOC scale as a unidimensional measure of personality in addiction research. Attempts have been made to isolate salient personality characteristics pertinent to individual beliefs imbedded in the LOC continuum by developing multi-dimensional models of LOC orientation.[22] Walston and Walston's Multi-Dimensional Health Locus of Control Scale (HLC) has recently been applied to addictions research.[23] The HLC scale isolates three dimensions within the construct relating to individuals beliefs regarding their health. These are the degree to which people believe their health is under their own control (internal, IHLC), the degree to which they believe their health is influenced by others (powerful other, PHLC) and finally, the degree to which they believe their health is influenced by chance or luck factors (chance, CHLC). The HLC is administered using a questionnaire and the individual obtains a score on each of the three dimensions. Individual and group comparisons can then be made between these three dimensions. Dean[23] administered the HLC to forty-seven alcoholics entered into a treatment programme using the rationale that the subject populations health would be affected by chronic alcohol abuse. The results revealed that the subject population generally expressed a greater belief that health status was more under their own control than under the control of chance or 'powerful other' factors. Since the subjects were already in treatment, the finding of an internal

HLC is of no surprise (there was no control group in this study for comparison with non-drinkers or actively drinking alcoholics). A significant finding from this study was, however, that those alcoholics who expressed a greater 'powerful other' HLC would attempt treatment more frequently than those alcoholics with an internal HLC or chance/luck HLC. This group also maintained contact with Alcoholics Anonymous (AA) longer, sought help sooner, and began heavy drinking at a later age than alcoholics with an internal HLC or chance/luck HLC. Dean and Edwards point out that this finding contrasts with studies that have found that alcoholics with internal LOC have a greater involvement with AA.[24] It is clear from studies that use multidimensional LOC scales, such as the HLC scale, that new and meaningful interpretations can be introduced in the analysis of the data set that might otherwise be obscured if a general unidimensional LOC measure were used. Certainly, multidimensional LOC measures offer the opportunity to examine clinical evidence at a higher level of abstraction, thereby enhancing the possibility of relating more closely to advances in social learning and attribution approaches such as learned helplessness theory.[25]

APPLICATION OF LOCUS OF CONTROL TO OTHER ADDICTIVE DOMAINS

Many of the general comments made in the previous section regarding LOC and alcoholism apply to other addictive domains. This section will, therefore, primarily emphasise novel approaches to LOC areas of addiction other than alcoholism.

Opiates

Investigations that have used the LOC construct in studies of opiate addiction have found many inconsistencies similar to those of the alcoholism studies. Berzins and Ross[26] found opiate addicts to be LOC-internal compared to controls, while a study by Eiser and Gossop[27] demonstrated a correlation between external LOC and the individual addicts perception of being 'hooked' on drugs. Type of opiate administration technique may also be implicated in the opiate users subjective experience of control. des-Jarlais[28] interviewed intranasal heroin users regarding their reasons for not using needles and for entering treatment. The results demonstrated that these heroin users perceived using needles as being associated with loss of control and entering a treatment programme as a means of re-establishing control. This is of interest since many treatment regimes use methadone, itself a synthesised opiate, as a replacement of the illicit drug in systematic withdrawal programmes. It would therefore seem plausible to assume that control orientation and beliefs are important in treatment outcome. Recognising inconsistencies in previous LOC research, Bradley *et al.*[29] examined the beliefs of opiate users entering in-patient detoxification regarding responsibility for positive and negative outcomes, and their specific causal attributions regarding relapse. Addicts that attributed greater responsibility for negative outcomes to themselves, and attributed relapse episodes to personally controllable factors demonstrated better outcomes at six-month follow-up. Focusing on specific beliefs in this way may be a more sensitive method of predicting specific outcomes, Rotter's LOC scale has been found to correlate more significantly with responsibility for positive outcomes than negative outcomes.[30]

Using a subject population of 165 heroin users in the initial stage of withdrawal, Murphy and Bentall[31] used factor analysis to isolate three factors from an initial 30-item motivation scale that was administered to this cohort. Levensen's[32] LOC scale was also administered to the subject population. It was found that the first factor 'private affairs motivation' correlated significantly with the internal orientation subscale of Levensen's LOC scale. The items with a high loading on the private affairs motivation factor seemed to indicate that this factor was primarily concerned with positive personal reasons for withdrawing from heroin. Factor two 'external constraints motivation', appeared to be concerned with externally imposed constraints that make using heroin an uncomfortable option for the user. Factor two correlated significantly with the powerful others sub-scale of Levinsen's LOC scale. Since the factors were deduced from items measuring motivation and LOC sub-scales correlated significantly with factors one and two, it is conceivable that the LOC construct may also provide a useful measure of motivation. This is an important point since much addiction therapy, as mentioned previously, emphasises high levels of motivation for change as a prerequisite to achieving a good post-treatment outcome.

It would appear that with the development of important theoretical approaches to the problems of relapse,[33] more sophisticated attributional approaches may be required to account for both opiate and other substance abuse, to formulate treatment interventions, and to predict outcome.

It would also seem, however, from the evidence of factor analytic studies, that the LOC construct may provide a useful measure of motivation beyond its theoretical base as a measure of personality.

Obesity

Obesity may seem an unlikely candidate to be included in an evaluation of control orientation, but it is included here for a number of reasons. Firstly, when considering obesity, we are compelled to address our own conceptualisation of what constitutes addictive behaviour, i.e. can we really equate the 'withdrawal hunger' of the obese individual with the 'cold turkey' withdrawal experience of the chemically dependent heroin addict, or the sweats, shakes and occasional withdrawal fits and delirium tremens of the chemically dependent alcoholic? Secondly, by questioning and expanding upon our own implicit stereotypes of addictive behaviour we can begin to look at the wider issues of addiction, i.e. if we can be addicted to eating then can we be addicted to television, 'bad' personal relationships, sex, laxatives, gambling, crime, smoking, red shoes, etc.? The answers to the above questions are likely to be defined by degree and context in relation to the wider community, and such social sanctioning that may exist, rather than by 'yes' or 'no' statements. The point here is that 'addiction' in one guise or another is likely to affect us all at some point in our lives.

It has been found that successful reduction of weight and the maintainance of weight loss have been associated with an internal LOC.[34] Individuals entering treatment for obesity have been found to have an external LOC.[35] Mills,[36] contrary to expectation, found that adult females prior to entering an obesity treatment programme expressed an internal locus of control. Mills[3] then conducted a unique study comparing the LOC of male alcoholics entering residential treatment and male men seeking out-patient treatment for obesity within the same experimental design. The alcoholics demonstrated an external LOC orientation in contrast to the obese individuals who were LOC internal. Furthermore, Mills observed that both these groups had more extreme scores on the LOC continuum than had previously been reported. Mills concluded from these findings that though obese individuals may report little control over their eating behaviour, his obese subject population seemed in control of non-eating or weight-related behaviour.

Mills' study may have an important methodological legacy. Since both groups demonstrated extreme LOC scores in comparison with other studies, it is possible that inconsistencies in LOC results between studies may be strongly influenced by variations in experimental design. Since eating disorder has gained increasing clinical and research interest, studies utilising the LOC dimension may provide a valuable contribution to our understanding of eating disorder, as well as helping to identify the site of treatment focus, and development of predictive tests of treatment outcome. Such a contribution is likely to be enhanced by consistency in the experimental designs used in studies in this area.

LOCUS OF CONTROL AND PSYCHOPHYSIOLOGICAL PROCESSES

Blankstein[37] reported data from Cromwell *et al.*'s[38] investigation into the LOC orientation of 229 cardiac patients and 80 medical control patients. It was generally found that the cardiac patients were significantly more LOC external than the medical patient controls. However, it was further found that control orientation was a predictor of many of the physiological and biochemical measures taken while the patients were in hospital. It was found that those patients with an internal LOC had lower sedimentation rates, lower serum glutamic oxalacetic transaminase levels, lower lactate dehydrogenase levels and lower cholesterol. It was further found that internality predicted better prognosis. Cardiac patients with an internal LOC also spent less time in intensive care, and left hospital sooner, than cardiac patients with an external control orientation. These startling findings suggest strongly that social learning approaches to defining and qualifying personality may not be complete without examination of the interaction between biological and psychological processes. Blankstein's[37] excellent review of work in this area indicates that control orientation can differentiate individuals on a variety of physiological indices. Since addiction, particularly in the instance of chemical dependency, intrinsically implicates the importance of biological processes, and the variety and complexity of these biological processes have only recently started to become clear,[39] it would seem that the utility of the LOC construct's application to this clinical arena is further affirmed.

CONCLUSION

This chapter has shown that the LOC construct can be applied to the study of a range of addictive behaviours and may have potential as a predictor of treatment outcome. It has also been highlighted that, for the application of the LOC construct to the addictions domain to be in any way meaningful, important conceptual, methodological and clinical issues need to be addressed. The development of subscales and multidimensional LOC scales have, however, facilitated the productive study and application of control orientation to the clinical field of addiction. This adaptability in the context of both clinical application, and development of theory, would seem to assure a place for the LOC construct in future addictions research. Perhaps the limitation of the LOC construct to the study of addictive behaviour is one inherent in many approaches to psychopathology – essentially the heterogeneous nature of the groups of clinical interest. It is also clear that improvements in methodology, conceptual thinking and the formulation of hypotheses are crucial to the future development and application of the LOC construct to addiction research and clinical practice.

It should be noted, and no doubt be obvious at this stage, that attempts to understand addiction in terms of a small number of factors are inevitably reductionist, since addiction involves psychological and biological processes interacting within specific situational (social) contexts. It is concluded that the LOC construct has much potential in making a valuable contribution to the study of the psychology of addiction.

NOTES

1. J. B. Rotter, 'Generalised Expectancies for Internal versus External Control of Reinforcement', *Psychological Monographs*, 80 (1966):609.
2. J. B. Rotter, *Applications of a Social Learning Theory of Personality* (New York: Holt, Rinehart & Winston, 1972).
3. J. K. Mills, 'Differences in Locus of Control among Obese Adult and Adolescent Females undergoing Weight Reduction', *Journal of Psychology*, 125 (1991):195–7.
4. W. Mischel, *Personality and Assessment* (New York: Wiley, 1968).
5. R. W. Schmidt, H. Lamm and G. Tromsdorf, 'Social Class and Sex as Determinants of Future Orientation (Time Perspective) in Adults', *European Journal of Social Psychology*, 8 (1978):71–90.
6. K. A. Walston, B. S. Walston and R. Devellis, 'Development of the Multidimensional Health Locus of Control (MHLC) Scales', *Health Education Monographs*, 6 (1978):161–70.

7. D. M. Donovan and M. R. O'Leary, 'The Drinking Related Locus of Control Scale: Reliability, Factor Structure and Validity', *Journal of Studies on Alcohol*, 39 (1978):759–84.
8. E. J. Phares, *Locus of Control in Personality* (Morristown, N.J.: General Learning Press, 1976).
9. S. M. Labs, 'Fetal Health Locus of Control Scale: Development and Validation', *Journal of Consulting and Clinical Psychology*, 54 (1986):814–9.
10. D. J. Rohsenhow, *Identifying and Measuring Alcoholic Personality Characteristics* (San Francisco, CA: Jossey-Bass, 1983).
11. G. Hulbert, 'Sex and Race Factors on Locus of Control Scores with an Alcoholic Population', *Psychological Reports*, 52 (1983):517–8.
12. H. M. Annis, 'The Use of Calcium Carbimide in Relapse Prevention Counselling: Results of a Randomised Controlled Trial', *British Journal of Addiction*, 87 (1992):63–72.
13. M. R. Haacks, 'Stress and Impairment among Nursing Students', *Research in Nursing and Health*, 11 (1988):125–34.
14. R. B. Davis, 'Adolescents from Alcoholic Families: An Investigation in Self-esteem, Locus of Control, and Knowledge: Attitudes toward Alcohol', PhD dissertation, Boston College, US, 1983.
15. J. C. Churchill, J. P. Broida and N. L. Nicholson, 'Locus of Control and Self-esteem of Adult Children of Alcoholics', *Journal of Studies on Alcohol*, 51(4) (1990).
16. A. L. Errico, 'The Influence of Depressive Symptomology on Alcoholics Locus of Control: A Methodological Note and a Correction', *Journal of Clinical Psychology*, 47 (1991):600–4.
17. V. Molinari, 'Locus of Control and the Denial of Anxiety', *Psychological Reports*, 47 (1980):131–40.
18. G. Canton, 'Locus of Control, Life Events and Treatment Outcome in Alcohol-Dependent Patients', *Acta Psychiatrica Scandinavica*, 78 (1988):18–23.
19. D. M. Donovan, 'The Drinking Related Locus of Control Scale: Reliability, Factor Structure and Validity', *Journal of Studies on Alcohol*, 39 (1978):759–84.
20. P. Haynes, 'Locus of Control of Behaviour: Is High Externality Associated with Substance Misuse?', *British Journal of Addiction*, 86 (1991): 1111–7.
21. A. Huckstadt, 'Locus of Control among Alcoholics, Recovering Alcoholics, and Non-alcoholics', *Research in Nursing and Health*, 10 (1987): 23–8.
22. B. S. Walston, 'Development and Validation of the Health Locus of Control (HLC) Scale', *Journal of Consulting and Clinical Psychology*, 44 (1976): 580–5.
23. P. R. Dean, 'Health Locus of Control Beliefs and Alcohol Related Factors that may Influence Treatment Outcomes', *Journal of Substance Abuse Treatment*, 7 (1990):167–72.
24. C. D. Emrick, 'Alcoholics Anonymous: Affiliation Processes and Effectiveness of Treatment', *Clinical and Experimental Research*, 11 (1987):416–21.
25. M. E. P. Seligman, *Helplessness on Depression, Development and Death* (New York: W. H. Freeman, 1992).

26. J. L. Berzins and W. F. Ross, 'Locus of Control among Opiate Addicts', *Journal of Consulting and Clinical Psychology*, 40 (1973):84–91.
27. J. R. Eiser and M. R. Gossop, '"Hooked" or "sick": Addicts' Perceptions of their Addiction', *Addictive Behaviours*, 4 (1979):185–9.
28. D. C. des-Jarlais, 'Locus of Control and Need for Control among Heroin Users', *National Institute on Drug Abuse Research Monograph Series*, 74 (1986):37–44.
29. P. B. Bradley, 'Attributions and Relapse in Opiate Addicts', *Journal of Consulting and Clinical Psychology*, 60 (1992):470–2.
30. C. R. Brewin, 'Beyond Locus of Control: Attributions of Responsibility for Positive and Negative Outcomes', *British Journal of Psychology*, 75 (1984):43–9.
31. P. N. Murphy, 'Motivation to Withdraw from Heroin: A Factor-analytic Study', *British Journal of Addiction*, 87 (1992):245–50.
32. H. Levenson, 'Activism and Powerful Others: Distinctions within the Concept of Internal–External Control', *Journal of Personality Assessment*, 38 (1974):377–83.
33. *Relapse Prevention: Maintainance Strategies in the Treatment of Addictive Behaviours* (New York: Guilford Press, 1985).
34. E. B. Saltzer, 'The Weight Locus of Control (WLOC) Scale: A Specific Measure for Obesity Research', *Journal of Personality Assessment*, 46 (1982):620–8.
35. L. L. Tobias, 'Internal Locus of Control and Weight: An Insufficient Condition', *Journal of Consulting and Clinical Psychology*, 45 (1977): 647–53.
36. J. K. Mills, 'Control Orientation as a Personality Dimension among Alcoholic and Obese Adult Men undergoing Addictions Treatment', *The Journal of Psychology*, 125 (1991):537–42.
37. K. R. Blankstein, 'Psychophysiology and Perceived Locus of Control: Critical Review, Theoretical Speculation and Research Directions', in H. M. Lefcourt (ed.), *Research with the Locus of Control Construct* (Orlando, FL: Academic Press, 1984).
38. R. L. Cromwell, E. C. Butterfield, F. M. Brayfield *et al.*, *Acute Myocardial Infarction: Reaction and Recovery* (St Louis, MO: Mosby, 1977).
39. A. B. Bonner, 'Biological Mechanisms of Alcohol Dependence', *Current Opinion in Psychiatry*, 7 (1994):262–8.

9 Alcohol, Memory and Cognition
Colin Martin and Gwen Hewitt

INTRODUCTION

Memory can be influenced by alcohol to produce a wide variety of distinct recall phenomena, not only memory *impairment*, as one might, perhaps, intuitively expect, but also, under special conditions, *enhancement* of memory performance. There are many circumstances under which memory performance can be affected by alcohol and this is largely a function of the style of alcohol ingestion. The anterograde amnesia characteristic of the Korsakoff's syndrome patient is a result of the chronic abuse of large quantities of alcohol, resulting in a seemingly permanent, and irretrievable, loss of information. Acute ingestion of a large amount of alcohol (a binge) may cause amnesia only for events immediately before the binge; further, information apparently 'lost' may be retrieved following a second ingestion of a similar amount of alcohol. Interestingly, acute administration of small amounts of alcohol can produce either a deterioration, or an improvement in memory dependent on the type of memory being tested and the experimental conditions of testing. It is important, therefore, to differentiate between both style of drinking *and* type of memory, in order to understand the mechanisms by which alcohol can influence memory performance. Since distinct types of memory may be mapped onto specific physiological sites within the brain, and since there is a number of psychological models of memory, a truly integrative unitary model of memory encompassing neurobiological and cognitive processes seems an impossibly tall order. The result of this 'melting pot' of theory and divergent clinical and experimental philosophies is the application of models of memory that 'best fit' specified patterns of recall performance within a particular picture of consumption. It will become clear from the bulk of this chapter that memory processes are viewed as an intrinsic part of human cognitive function although they have, in the past, often been treated as totally separable entities. However, this is a result of the traditional delineation of the topics themselves within experimental psychology rather than memory and cognition actually being independent of each other. The relatively recent development of information-processing models of cognition implicate cognitive processes as being fundamental to memory function and vice versa. It is clear that to get a grasp of the important issues involved when contemplating the role of alcohol in memory and cognition, it is necessary to cast a broad net. Developments in social psychology too, implicate the role of social context in determining what is, and what is not, retrieved from memory.

To facilitate an understanding of the salient issues regarding alcohol and memory, while attempting to maintain clarity, the sections in this chapter have been organised in the following manner. Firstly, a brief description of a number of influential models of memory will be described, the purpose being that the reader will find these models applied where relevant in the sections that follow. Secondly, the effects of the chronic abuse of alcohol on memory will then be explored, followed by an examination of the psychophysiological effects of short-term exposure to alcohol on memory. Finally, following on from a section on the action of alcohol on social cognition, the last section will examine the implications of memory function for treatments for alcoholism.

MODELS OF MEMORY

Many theoretical models of memory have been postulated. Each model has been developed with the view to accounting for a variety of empirical observations of memory phenomena. Presented here are the central aspects of the more enduring models of memory. The models vary in complexity from the relatively simple to extremely complex and are not necessarily exclusive. It should be noted that a full account of these models is beyond the scope of this chapter. It is the intention that this section illustrates the complexity of the processes involved in memory function, without examining the models in great detail.

Duplex Model

The duplex model of memory (Waugh and Norman, 1965) postulates the existence of two memory stores, these being a short-term memory store (STM) and a long-term memory store (LTM). The short-term memory store has *limited* capacity, items being *temporarily* held in STM via a process of rehearsal. To attain permanence, information

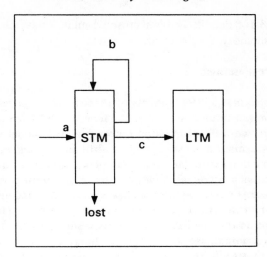

Figure 9.1   The duplex model of memory: information entering STM (a) is either rehearsed (b) or transferred (c) to LTM for permanent storage. Information that is not rehearsed or transferred is lost

must be *transferred* from this limited capacity short-term store to the long-term memory store for permanent consolidation. For information to be successfully retrieved from LTM it must first have been successfully *encoded*, then *transferred*, and finally *consolidated* within LTM. Fundamentally then, the duplex model consists of two separate memory stores (STM and LTM), acted on by the processes of encoding, transfer, consolidation and retrieval. These components must work interactively to promote successful recall function (see Figure 9.1).

Tulving's Model of Memory

The model of memory suggested by Tulving (1972) proposed that memories are organised according to three categories. *Procedural* memories include knowledge of which we are not explicitly conscious of the content. This includes memories of acts such as walking, talking and writing. *Episodic* memories, includes memories of specific events such as memories of holidays, past employment, personal friends, etc. Episodic memory is often referred to as our *autobiographical* memory. *Semantic* memory refers to meaning. Factual knowledge such as knowing that a chair is an object to be sat on is an example of semantic memory. These three components are largely independent, therefore, an individual may have deficits in their episodic memory system while their procedural memory system remains intact.

Levels of Processing

Craik and Lockhart's (1972) levels of processing model of memory is essentially a reformulation of the modular model of memory based within a framework of information processing. The model suggests that incoming information is subjected to different levels of processing dependent on the particular properties of the target information. The level of processing is crucial to the persistence of information in memory. According to this model, sensory analyses and pattern recognition would be subjected to a surface level of processing, stimulus identification would require an intermediate level of processing, and the deepest levels of processing would use knowledge to interpret the meaning of the stimuli and its significance. According to this model, the durability of a memory trace is largely a function of the depth of processing used to encode it; essentially, the deeper the level of processing, the more durable the memory trace, and the more likely the memory trace will be available for retrieval.

Working Memory

Working memory (Baddeley and Hitch, 1974) shares some of the properties of STM. Information in working memory is short-lived, however, within working memory information is actively manipulated and processed. Crucial to the concept of working memory is the notion of *competition* between information storage and information processing. A separate 'articulatory loop' which deals exclusively with the short-term storage of verbal information is also central to the working memory concept. Since the emphasis of this model is on competition between resources, it is possible that at full memory span, working memory, the articulatory loop, and to a lesser extent LTM, may all be utilised. It has also been speculated that there are several distinguishable working memories for different modalities, i.e. a working memory geared specifically for visual/spatial information, a working memory for verbal information, etc.

Summary

The brief descriptions of the models of memory presented above clearly imply that different processes act on incoming information and that the *accessibility* of the information for future *recall* depends on not only these processes, but also the properties of the information itself. Beyond separable processes, distinct memory stores are postulated. The main point regarding most of these models is that memories are not memories *per se*, rather, memory traces are essentially records of processes. Such records are the result of active manipulation of the information to interpret *meaning*. Essentially, there are no 'deep frozen' memories of specific events awaiting extraction which have not been 'adulterated' by processing. It should be noted that although attempts have been made to extrapolate these psychological models of memory function to specified anatomical sites within the brain, there is much disagreement as to whether it is possible, or even desirable, to localise aspects of higher order cognitive function.

CHRONIC EFFECTS OF ALCOHOL ON MEMORY

It has been widely reported in the literature that chronic abuse of alcohol can produce a decline in memory performance (Ryan and Lewis, 1988). It is also clear that such decrements in memory function are often accompanied by deficits within other areas of cognitive function such as intelligence ratings. It is not generally clear however, whether such deficits are permanent or improve with abstinence (Reed *et al.*, 1992). The exception to this case is the amnesia associated with the condition known as Korsakoff's psychosis which remains persistent with abstinence.

Korsakoff's Psychosis

Korsakoff's psychosis: an 'essential' neuropsychology?
Historically, the study of alcohol-related memory deficits has been dominated by investigations into the condition known as Korsakoff's psychosis. Though systematic investigation may reveal to us important information regarding a specific condition, in this case Korsakoff's psychosis, such investigations may also make accessible for scrutiny the motivation behind such investigations within a wider context, essentially the context of 'alcoholism'. Though alcohol use and abuse

may be viewed from a number of perspectives, for example social, psychological, etc., a dominant view in both research efforts, and treatment regimes, has been the conceptualisation of alcoholism as a 'disease' process. There are indeed, some social benefits to this 'disease' notion. By inferring a disease process we can legitimise the offering of 'treatment' and talk of 'cures'. The down side to this disease concept of alcoholism is the general absence of any supportive evidence for the notion itself (see Chapter 7), in essence no aetiology or pathology. Korsakoff's psychosis represents a consequence of 'alcoholism'. Though we cannot identify a *cause* of alcoholism we can identify that alcoholism *causes* Korsakoff's psychosis; more importantly, we can identify a cluster of symptoms, a prognosis and structural changes to the brain which we can integrate into a pathology, and that provides us with *real* patients. It would seem then, that Korsakoff's psychosis sits rather more comfortably in the realm of a disease than alcoholism. Therefore, for those motivated to believe in the disease concept, abstraction from the *disease* of Korsakoff's psychosis to (or back to) the *disease* of alcoholism would not be particularly effortful. Readers with a more liberal view will see the obvious problems of circularity with this issue in terms of *causality*; however, it is hoped that the reader is drawn to the wider issues involved when a particular area of a research field becomes focused, essentially, research and clinical interest influenced by ideological expediency.

Memory deficits associated with Korsakoff's psychosis

Individuals presenting with a diagnosis of Korsakoff's psychosis invariably demonstrate an anterograde amnesia, though whether there is a co-existing retrograde amnesia is uncertain. The defining feature of anterograde amnesia is the loss, or severe impairment of, the ability to learn new information. The Korsakoff's amnesic will typically, as an example, not be able to recall what he had just had for lunch or what he was doing yesterday evening. The hospitalised Korsakoff's amnesic may not recognise the nurse who has been looking after him for several months. This particular facet of the anterograde amnesia in relation to the Korsakoff's patient may not initially be obvious due to the common ability among Korsakoff's patients to *confabulate*. Confabulation is a description of the manner in which the Korsakoff's amnesic 'fills in' the gaps in memory by giving, on demand, a plausible, if fictional account of events not held in memory. To illustrate this, here is an example: When asked 'What did you have for lunch?' the Korsakoff's amnesic, even though he has no memory of what he did in fact have for lunch, may reply 'Cod and chips with peas, without tartare sauce for a change!'. The depth of the elaboration of the response ('without tartare sauce') adds plausibility to the statement, and if the enquirer had no knowledge regarding what was *actually* served for lunch, the account given could be taken as fact. Korsakoff's amnesics can often give the appearance of recognising certain staff members they may see frequently in a hospital environment, but whether they do in fact, learn over time to recognise, at some level, certain individuals or whether a strategy is invoked to give the appearance of recognition, i.e. a social desirability response, is unclear. Either way, it would seem that whether recognition does take place or a social strategy is invoked, some form of tacit learning would seem to have taken place.The amnesia associated with Korsakoff's syndrome is *episodic* in nature, therefore, the learning of simple *procedural* skills may be unaffected. In effect, the Korsakoff's syndrome patient may, for example, demonstrate improved performance with many trials on a mirror drawing task, but on presentation of the task for the twentieth trial he will experience the task as novel. It is impressed upon the reader to realise that the Korsakoff's syndrome patient does not present with an amnesia only. Other features of Korsakoff's syndrome, which may or may not present with the amnesic state, include confusion, mood lability and behavioural problems. Consequently, prognosis and treatment may be determined by the interaction of a number of distinguishable features of the syndrome.

Psychophysiology of Korsakoff's psychosis
It is emphasised that memory dysfunction associated with any amnesia is gauged by the amnesic patients' performance on memory tests; however, since a memory deficit may be due to a number of difficulties such as an encoding, a storage or a retrieval deficit, it seems increasingly implausible to localise an amnesic syndrome to any one structure. Conversely, it is entirely plausible that many different structures and pathways in the central nervous system are involved in the encoding, storage and retrieval of information (Morton, 1985). The scope of this section is, therefore, necessarily limited to a simple description designed to facilitate a basic understanding of what is, in effect, an extremely complex psychobiological phenomenon.

Korsakoff's psychosis (often referred to as Wernicke–Korsakoff's syndrome) occurs as a result of thiamine deficiency and is usually caused by chronic alcoholism. Excessive and prolonged consumption of alcohol causes disruption to the liver's metabolic pathways and leads to a failure to absorb thiamine in required quantities. This may also be exacerbated by the chronic alcoholics' inadequate diet; a bottle of spirits (40 per cent vol.) may provide up to half the normal daily calories requirement, but in the form of 'empty' calories, i.e. no vitamin content. Thiamine deficiency causes degeneration of neural tissue in, mainly, the diencephalic areas of the brain, particularly the mammilliary bodies and the thalamus. This neuronal degeneration eventually leads to an amnesic syndrome. Unlike other amnesias caused by brain damage, for example temporal lobe damage, which directly implicate damage to the hippocampus as a key feature of anterograde amnesia development, Korsakoff's psychosis need not necessarily directly involve the hippocampus; indeed, if the hippocampus is implicated at all in Korsakoff's syndrome, this would be indirect involvement, essentially secondary disruption to hippocampal function via degeneration of the mammilliary bodies, these being linked to the hippocampus via the fornix pathway. Though there is much dispute regarding the specific site of brain damage that is responsible for the amnesia associated with Korsakoff's syndrome, there is much evidence to support the notion of dorso-medial thalamus damage being implicated in not only Korsakoff's amnesia, but also in amnesias associated with tumour damage and accidental injury (McEntee *et al.*, 1976).

Psychological interpretation of the Korsakoff's amnesia
Identification of the psychological basis of an amnesia is important, not only from the point of view of giving insight into memory processes in the damaged brain, but also because such insights can be informative regarding memory processes in the normal brain. In effect, amnesics offer the opportunity to investigate psychological models of memory. A number of theories have been put forward to explain amnesia in psychological terms, and these can be largely differentiated on the basis of whether the deficit is seen as one of encoding or, alternatively, a deficit of retrieval of information.

Encoding deficit.   An encoding deficit explanation of anterograde amnesia posits that memory traces must be processed in some fashion in order to be stored. The problem from this perspective, lies in the transfer from an intact short-term memory (STM) to a long-term memory (LTM) store. This information processing model encapsulates memory and cognitive processes and, consequently, levels of representation become increasingly important. Cermak (1979, 1982) has conducted much work on the phenomena of amnesia and has consistently selected Korsakoff's amnesics' as the subjects of study. Cermak's view is that the amnesic deficit is generally a problem of encoding, specifically a problem of encoding *semantic* information.

The study by Cermak, Butters and Moreines (1974) is of particular interest in supporting the semantic deficit hypothesis. Essentially the study focused on the phenomena known as proactive inhibition. Proactive inhibition occurs on multiple trials of a memory task. The basic finding is that subjects recall performance deteriorates over successive trials *if* the material in successive trials is of the same semantic category. If the semantic category is changed at some point during a series of trials, recall performance drastically improves. This effect is known as release from proactive inhibition and has been accounted for by the process with which items are *encoded* in memory. Cermak *et al.* found that in normal controls, a change in category from letters to digits, and a shift from animals to vegetables *both* produced a release from proactive inhibition. The amnesic subjects, however, demonstrated release from proactive inhibition *only* when the category was changed from letters to digits. Hence it would appear that amnesics could encode at a superficial level (letters to digits), but not at the deeper semantic level (animals to vegetables). These findings have been interpreted as supportive of the semantic encoding hypothesis, though there are problems with such an interpretation, in particular, a semantic encoding deficit hypothesis does not explain why performance deteriorates across trials in a similar way to normal controls. If no encoding was taking place then there should be no proactive inhibition.

Retrieval deficit.   An alternative position to the encoding deficit hypothesis has been to speculate that the essential amnesic deficit is at the point of *retrieval*. A retrieval deficit hypothesis assumes that information has been encoded and stored but, the stored information cannot be accessed effectively. Warrington and Weiskrantz (1970) have proposed a possible mechanism whereby the retrieval process is degraded via interference at recall. According to Warrington and Weiskrantz, competing information in memory causes interference which reduces the efficiency of retrieval in the amnesic subject, whereas in non-amnesics, the competing information is either filtered out, or its influence actively suppressed. Interestingly, in this retrieval deficit hypothesis there thus exists a 'amnesic paradox': the amnesic cannot recall because he remembers too much. Warrington and Weiskrantz have conducted a number of elegant studies (1970, 1974, 1978) that have provided support for the notion of interference at retrieval being the salient feature of the amnesic syndrome; however, in many respects, an enduring feature of these studies has been to highlight the complexity of the mechanism of retrieval, and has questioned whether retrieval can be reduced to a single unitary process. Certainly, differences in the type of recall cue used, and their differential effect on recall performance, have strongly indicated that a number of different retrieval mechanisms may exist, the particular retrieval mechanism activated being dependent upon the particular characteristics of the memory task.

Summary. Though both the encoding, and retrieval deficit hypotheses are plausible explanations of the amnesic syndrome and have been important in providing insights into the function of normal memory, there exists a number of unanswered questions. Firstly, there exists the problem of mapping psychological models of the amnesic syndrome onto the particular physiological site/sites of damage, a not inconsiderable task given the complexity of the psychological mechanisms mooted and the difficulty of accurately identifying the sites of functional physiological localisation within the human brain. Secondly, there is a problem of whether the subjects used in amnesic studies demonstrate a heterogeneity in terms of type of damage. Cermak *et al.* (1974) have used exclusively Korsakoff's syndrome subjects for investigations, this, however, is not typical. Many investigators have used a 'mixed bag' of amnesic subjects that may comprise amnesics with Korsakoff's syndrome, temporal lobe damage, carbon monoxide poisoning or tumour invasion. It is, therefore, entirely possible that there may be several types of amnesia that can be differentiated at both the neuroanatomical and psychological level. It is very important that the salient features of such amnesic syndromes are classified so that techniques to aid recall can be devised that take into account specific underlying neuropsychological aspects, the point being that *if* mnemonic techniques can be devised to improve recall, the efficacy of such techniques is likely to be a function of the neuropsychological specicifity of the particular impairment, hence the obvious need to be able to classify the salient features of different amnesic syndromes. This particular aspect is especially important when it is considered that traditionally the individual with Korsakoff's syndrome has invariably followed a course of hospitalisation leading to eventual *institutionalisation*.

Korsakoff's psychosis: the wider issue

The government's current policy of 'Care in the Community' (Department of Health, 1989) has raised the issue of community placement of individuals with long-term mental health difficulties. Since the institutions that patients with Korsakoff's syndrome have been placed in are predominately psychiatric hospitals, it is of immediate concern that methods be investigated that maximise the residual memory function of Korsakoff's patients to facilitate function within the community with the appropriate support. More importantly, if mnemonic techniques could be developed that were effective with Korsakoff's syndrome patients, the consequent opportunity would present itself for the quality of life of these individuals to become much improved.

SHORT-TERM ACUTE EFFECTS OF ALCOHOL ON MEMORY

Impairment of Memory

Moderate alcohol intake of doses as low as 0.67 ml/kg body weight is known to impair the ability to acquire new information (anterograde amnesia) when tested in a laboratory setting. Such impairment is responsible for the inability of the reveller to recall the details of events which took place during a 'boozy night before'. Higher doses (3 ml/kg body weight) can result in a complete blackout for events experienced during the drinking episode. Neither level of alcohol consumption disrupts the capacity to retrieve old memories (retrograde amnesia) and therefore alcohol is widely thought to depress the mechanisms by which memory traces are consolidated rather than affecting the way information is recovered.

However, not surprisingly, there is little agreement about the precise mechanisms which are disrupted by alcohol, although it is assumed that alcohol must act as a depressant, but unravelling how this occurs is not an easy task. Memory is a complex, higher order function with many contributory components. Alcohol could produce a generalised slowing of the central nervous system (CNS) and of cognition as suggested by Maylor and Rabbitt (1993). On the other hand, alcohol could affect memory by modifying aspects of motivation or attention as reviewed by Lister *et al.* (1987), perhaps via the systems which modulate or regulate memory processes described by McGaugh (1989). Alternatively, alcohol could interfere directly with the neural substrates of memory, for example by modifying neuronal plasticity and by depressing the development of long-term potentiation (LTP) as reviewed by Bonner (1994).

Generalised Slowing of the CNS

Maylor and Rabbitt (1993) investigated the simple model of cognitive slowing caused by alcohol doses of 0.8–1.0 ml/kg body weight through a meta-analysis of eight of their own studies on the effects of alcohol on reaction times and a further four of their studies on the effects of alcohol on recognition memory. In both cases a regression analysis indicated that alcohol appeared to have a strongly linear depressant effect on information processing. For example, in the analysis of recognition memory studies the plot of accuracy with alcohol as a function of accuracy without alcohol resulted in linear fits explaining 96.2 per cent of the variance. The equivalent figure was even higher for reaction time performance (99.7 per cent). The authors consider that this general linear effect indicates that the cognitive consequence of alcohol is likely to be a general rather than a specific one. Alcohol might limit a few (unspecified) general processing resources and therefore cognitive impairment should increase as task complexity increases.

Alcohol and Attention

The above explanation does not fit comfortably with the ideas of others. For example, Lister *et al.* (1987) reviewed the acute sedative effects of alcohol on cognitive performance and suggested that drug-induced changes in factors such as arousal, attention and mood which they described as 'traditionally non-cognitive' have generally been ignored in discussions of the amnesic affects of alcohol. One area that has been studied experimentally is the effect of alcohol on attention. Some evidence for a depressant effect comes from electro-encephalogram (EEG) studies of event-related averaged potentials where low to moderate doses of alcohol have been shown to impair performance at detecting stimuli and to reduce the amplitude of peaks (such as the P300) generally associated with attentional and other relatively complex cognitive processes. This depressant effect is particularly marked in conditions where the task itself is relatively easy and not intrinsically interesting or attention 'grabbing'. These studies do not provide any evidence that alcohol impairs perceptions because the early peaks generally described as reflecting perceptual processes are unaffected by doses of alcohol which both impair performance and reduce the amplitude of the P300 peak. Clearly, in this case, the effect of alcohol seems to be a specific one affecting the later stages of information processing. There does not seem to be any evidence for a generalised effect because the earlier, perceptual stages of processing were not altered. The effect of alcohol on averaged event-related responses is also not what might be expected if alcohol was producing a generalised slowing effect which should result in a marked increasing of latencies rather than a depression in amplitude of the major peaks.

However, the effects of alcohol on attention are not straightforward, because some studies have shown impaired performance without a depression of the P300 amplitude in a task where the targets were difficult to detect. However, it is interesting that studies on alcoholics and their non-alcoholic relatives also indicate a possible attentional deficit in that the amplitude of the P300 is depressed under similar conditions. Therefore some evidence exists to support the idea that alcohol might impair trace consolidation by reducing attention in some way.

Arousal and Mood

Alcohol affects arousal levels and mood and such changes in arousal and mood could affect memory via state-dependent mechanisms. That is, subjects recall information best when they are in the same state of arousal or when their mood is identical to that when the information is learned. Therefore, alcohol should not impair memory if subjects are tested and then retested when drunk. Some studies have shown that information was recalled better when subjects were drunk than when they were sober. However, others such as that of Parker *et al.* (1980) reported that acute anterograde amnesia occurred even when subjects were retested with alcohol. Further evidence in the same direction comes from an unpublished study by Hewitt and Popoff (1993) who showed that alcohol increased arousal levels (measured by skin conductivity levels) but arousal levels were not related to performance on a kinaesthetic memory task.

Alcohol, Neuronal Plasticity and Long-term Potentiation

A specific effect of alcohol on receptors thought to be involved in long term potentiation (LTP) in the hippocampus, and perhaps in other areas of the brain indicate that alcohol (even at low doses) has a marked inhibitory effect on the NMDA receptor complex. (These effects are reviewed in more detail by Bonner in Chapter 13).

Facilitation of Memory

The picture is made more complex because the acute effects of alcohol are dose-dependent and are also influenced by whether blood alcohol levels are rising (the ascending limb of the blood alcohol curve (BAC) or falling (the descending limb of the BAC). For example, Parker *et al.* (1981) and Lewis and June (1994) have described a biphasic effect with low doses of alcohol and a rising BAC resulting in stimulant rather than depressant consequences. This could account for the phenomenon described earlier where low doses of alcohol on a rising BAC which are insufficient to produce anterograde amnesia enhance memory if the alcohol is drunk immediately after learning information (retrograde facilitation).

Facilitation of Memory by Alcohol Drunk after Initial Learning

Such a situation was first reported by Parker *et al.* in 1980. They showed that moderate doses of alcohol drunk immediately after learning new information enhanced recall of word lists and the recognition of slides of scenic views. Others have since confirmed these findings (Mueller *et al.*, 1983; Mann *et al.*, 1984). In addition, Lamberty *et al.* (1990) showed a similar facilitatory effect on recall of narrative prose and Hewitt *et al.* (1995) showed that both kinaesthetic and visual memory were enhanced in a similar fashion. All these studies reported enhancing effects of alcohol at doses which were too low to produce anterograde amnesia and therefore it seems likely that alcohol was acting as a stimulant rather that a depressant.

However, two main groups of theories have been proposed to explain this retrograde enhancement and the first assumes that alcohol acts by disrupting the consolidation of traces related to information perceived after the first task has been learned, presumably by acting as a depressant. Protection of recently acquired memory traces from interference by competing aspects of memory processing (or retroactive interference) has been shown in other drugs, such as valium, which presumably acts as a depressant.

The second group of theories suggest that the stimulant properties of low doses of alcohol on a rising BAC might enhance the formation and consolidation of memory traces directly or via the reward systems (particularly the dopaminergic–enkephalinergic pathways) in the brain. Evidence for the effect via the reward systems in humans is slight but alcohol has been reported to increase the rate at which rats will stimu-

late their own brains by pushing levers and delivering a stream of
electrical impulses to such areas and stimulation of these pathways is
thought to consolidate memory (Esposito *et al.*, 1984). However direct
testing of the second theory in human subjects by Hewitt *et al.* (1995)
showed that alcohol failed to protect against moderate interference.

Alcohol, Neuromodulatory Systems and Memory

An alternative explanation for retrograde enhancement is suggested by
the finding of Manning and colleagues (1992) that glucose could also
retroactively enhance the recall of prose in elderly humans. A number
of studies have reported that hormones such as adrenaline and other
neuromodulators can regulate memory storage. Indeed, it has been
suggested that the modulation of new memory by endogenous systems
could provide a mechanism by which the final strength of a memory
trace might relate to the importance of the experience (see, for example,
Esposito *et al.*, 1984; McGaugh, 1989). Information salient to survival
might be stored at the expense of less important information. For example,
such modulation could be important in 'flight–fight' situations where
it might be highly adaptive for threatening stimuli to be recorded accurately, speedily and permanently. Typically, such situations result in
raised levels of adrenaline and of blood glucose levels, the latter of
which have been shown to enhance memory retroactively in elderly
humans. Could alcohol-induced increases in adrenaline and blood glucose levels be the most likely mechanism for retrograde enhancement?
Interestingly such a mode of action could possibly provide some explanation for the strongly addictive effects. Social situations and alcohol
consumption might become linked via such mechanisms. Also individual differences in the degree that alcohol modulates learning might
provide reasons why some are more strongly affected. Although, as
Esposito *et al.* (1984) pointed out, more research is still needed here.

ALCOHOL AND SOCIAL COGNITION

Cognition is a term that has been used to refer to activities such as
reasoning, thinking, problem solving, etc. Cognitive psychologists use
the term to describe mental activity that is generally *abstract* in nature, and often involving complex manipulation of elements from which
higher-order concepts such as insight, belief, heuristics and intentionality

are accrued. Memory processes are an *intrinsic* part of human cognitive function and, within the social environment, memory-mediated cognitive processes interact with context via the process of *interpretation*. This section necessarily departs from the traditional boundaries of alcohol and memory research, to examine the role of memory in the wider social context, in terms of understanding the ways in which individuals seek to *explain* their problematical drinking behaviour, in a *functionally* productive manner (from the problem drinkers point of view). This stage of the chapter therefore represents the transition from a psychophysiological approach to memory, to a psychosocial cognitive perspective, and examines, in effect, the role of the intellect in problem drinking behaviour.

Memory as Interpretation: A Social Cognitive Catalysis

We have seen from the evidence of models of memory, and from the evidence of short-term and long-term alcohol mediated memory deficits, that memories are essentially the records of *processes*. This is an important point because information recalled will be instrumental in influencing decision-making processes and, therefore, guiding the behaviour of the individual. Since the cognitive processes that influence memory are interpretive, it makes sense to assume that retrieval processes will influence recall in relation to the social context. This need not be a difficult point to grasp, in fact, it is implicit to many models of social cognition including social identity theory (Tajfel, 1982) and attribution theory (Weiner, 1974). A dominant tenet in both social identity theory and attribution theory, albeit by arguably different processes, is the concept of the individual, in the presence of an overwhelming amount of incoming sensory information, attempting to make sense of the world by using cognitive rules of thumb such as *stereotyping*, in the case of social identity theory, and implying *causality* in the case of attribution theory. Though these processes seem to be primarily hard-wired in the brain, presumably for primitive species-specific reasons that were important to human survival, their role in modern humans, and in the dominant social context, would appear to be to maintain high *self-esteem* and to enhance *self-presentation*.

The application of these concepts to memory is that self-esteem and self-presentation issues will be factors that shape the retrieval process and hence the content of the retrieved memory. The upshoot of all this is that when such concepts are applied to behaviour which, by general concensus, is judged by society as being 'bad', such as alcoholism, it would be predicted that individuals indulging in such 'bad' behaviour are likely to use retrieval strategies that provide recalled information that can be used to *explain* their behaviour in the best possible light. In essence then, in terms of social explanation, memories are *constructed*. It is thus implied that *functionality* rather than any objective 'truth' is the criteria for recall within this model of attribution. Consider this in relation to the development of 'alcoholism'. Our society tends to offer punishment to people who do 'bad' things voluntarily; however, if individuals do 'bad' things but cannot help it, they are deemed to need treatment and are evaluated more sympathetically. It is no surprise then that 'alcoholism' is often viewed as a disease particularly by those who *suffer* from it since there are obvious *functional* benefits to this position – fundamentally having an illness of alcoholism removes culpability. A fundamental process in decision theory is that individuals will specify a *criterion* for responding. Taking an attributional perspective in regard to alcoholism, it is likely that factors such as social desirability, abdication of culpability for behaviour, the perceived costs and benefits of the response, etc., will be influential in setting the particular criteria for responding, i.e the criteria for memory search and memory *selection*. Chick and Duffy (1979) found in a study in which problem drinkers were asked to describe their symptoms, and the order in which they occurred, from a symptom list, that there was a significant concordance of order of occurrence of symptoms. Obviously, this finding was 'good news' from a 'disease' perspective, since it directly implicated a developmental process involved in alcoholism. Anderson, Aitken and Davies (1981) replicated this study and found similar results; however, in addition they also used a control group, screened to eliminate individuals with a current or past problem drinking history. The control group were asked to complete the same task *as if* they were problem drinkers. It was found that the control group produced a similar pattern of results as the problem drinkers. It would seem that in this study, both the problem drinkers and the control subjects adopted a common strategy in performing the task which basically amounted to arranging the list of symptoms in order of perceived seriousness. It would seem that what would, without the control group, be taken for a memory task is essentially, when a control group is added, simply representative of the demand characteristics of the situation. Extrapolating this to social cognition, where explanation is required, and on the basis of the response judgements made, recall is likely, as stated earlier, to be strongly influenced by the demand characteristics of the social context. It becomes increasingly clear that memories cannot be taken at surface value, indeed, in light of the Anderson *et al.* study, it is possible to take a more extreme position that, under certain circumstances, 'memories' need not be representative of recall at all.

Summary

The role of cognition and memory in mediating problem drinkers' *explanatory style* has been vastly overshadowed in alcohol research by the more traditional and, largely predictable, mnemonic pursuits such as giving alcoholic and control subjects a list of (for the most part) meaningless words, and looking for differences between alcoholic subjects and normal controls on recall performance. Though most memory studies involving problem drinkers are much more complicated at the experimental and conceptual level than this example, they invariably share a kind of 'looking through the goldfish bowl' quality. That is, they tend to view phenomena in isolation from *context*. It is our belief that, via the medium of causal attribution, a new fertile ground exists for researching memory and cognitive function in an altogether more meaningful way, that usefully combines process *and* context to create a gestalt of social explanation relevant to problem drinking behaviour.

MEMORY AND THERAPY

The application of the global term *therapy* to the treatment of alcoholism embraces a wide variety of interventions that broadly cover both *pharmacological* and *talking* approaches to the problem. This section is essentially interested in the talking approaches since these primarily invoke the processes of memory and cognition into promoting adaptive behaviour change in a dynamic manner.

The scope of what a talking approach represents is, of course, vast, typically ranging from giving advice about 'safe' drinking levels through to specialised alcohol counselling, cognitive behaviour therapy, group therapy and even psychoanalysis. Interestingly, within such diversity of approaches, it is possible to allude to some common factors involving memory and cognitive processes to achieve a therapeutic milieu. Specialised alcohol counselling may utilise the same basic philosophy of general client centred therapy (Rogers, 1951) which, by default, implicates retrieval processes. Essentially, by changing future behaviour it is necessary to understand our past behaviour.

The uncovering of the past is also a principle tenet of the psychoanalytic tradition, hence we have, at a definable level, a congruence between this approach and that of counselling. This would also be true of some, but not all, group therapy settings. Certainly, Alcoholics Anonymous (AA) would distance themselves from the notion that they were fundamentally a group therapy but, consider the AA individual who finds himself in the weekly *chair*, the role of which is to share with the group his *life story*. Again, memory function is implicated here as being essential to the *healing* process, even if the setting is not explicitly stated as being one of *therapy*. Finally, a conspicuous feature of cognitive behaviour therapy is the notion of *cognitive schemata*. Cognitive schemata refers to packets of information that have been learned. These cognitive schemata may guide beliefs and behaviour. The salient point here is that not only are these cognitive schemata learned, but also they were at some point in the past, assumed to be adaptive.

The role of cognitive behaviour therapy would, therefore, be to facilitate the problem drinker's adoption of new adaptive cognitive schemata, and abandonment of those schemata which are no longer positively functional. Paul Davies (Chapter 10), provides an in-depth examination of this particular therapy, but for our purposes it provides a further example of the requirement of intact memory and cognitive function to assimilate knowledge in order to change problem drinking behaviour. In view of this, it would seem relatively safe to assume that there is an onus on *retrospective* recall to promote psychological growth, irrespective of the exact nature of the therapy employed.

There are, however, problems with the content of retrospective accounts that are given in therapy. Some of these problems can be considered in relation to the issues raised in the previous section regarding attribution, basically, self-presentation factors will be important in shaping the clients account of their drinking behaviour. Implicitly, within any therapeutic setting is the issue of *demand characteristics*. Demand characteristics refers to those features of a particular environment/situation which influence performance. In terms of treatment for alcoholism we might be interested in the particular *setting*, i.e. community substance misuse team, psychiatric out-patients, domiciliary visit, AA group, etc. Attributionally speaking, however, we are likely to be interested in also, and to a greater degree, the attributional beliefs of the 'therapist'. The process of causal attribution does not preclude any individual groups such as 'therapists', the concept of attribution being a global one. In terms of a causal model, a therapist with a belief system of 'alcoholism as a disease' is likely to influence the client's search through memory for causal factors involved in their drinking, i.e. an emphasis for a family history of 'alcoholism'. A therapist with a belief structure of 'family systems' is likely to influence memory search for accounts of early family dysfunction that would explain the development of a *coping style* of problem drinking. This is not a process of manipulation, merely that aspect of attribution that is imbued within language. The important point is that memories, by being *reconstructions*, are necessarily influenced by the dominant causal belief structures of *both* the clients and the therapists. The notion of 'objective truth' cannot exist within the realm of attribution theory and evidence from cognitive science seems increasingly to support this view as well (Schank and Abelson, 1977). The problem here is that the 'pursuit of truth' is a fundamental feature of many therapies in identifying a *cause* of a problem; however, since there can be no objective truth, then the 'truth factor' assumption in therapies is seriously undermined. The current debate over false memory syndrome (FMS) highlights these issues perfectly. We would suggest that, in order to understand a problem drinkers difficulties, it is crucial to examine the discourse between client and therapist in the context of the therapeutic environment. A perfectly acceptable way of achieving this is to adopt an attributional style of therapy. It is suggested that when 'pursuit of truth' therapies are replaced by approaches that seek to *understand explanations in context*, it will be possible to make sense of seemingly illogical behaviour such as self-destructive drinking. To the mnemonic psychologist the idea of uncovering a 'truth' in order to facilitate desired behaviour change is no longer tenable. To the *pure* mnemonic psychologist, the clinical picture is even more controversial, since there are some doubts as to what actually constitute 'cognitive schemata', and as to whether the *mental models* which frame cognitive schematic processes actually operate in the manner originally theoretically conceived (Johnson-Laird, 1983). The choice between a counselling therapy or a cognitive behaviour therapy becomes, therefore, one of 'the lesser of two evils', and therapy *fashion*. We use these approaches *not* because of their arguable efficacy, but because we have *nothing else*.

CONCLUSION

This chapter has taken a broad perspective in exploring the ways in which alcohol may affect memory and cognition. The sections on the chronic and acute effects of alcohol on memory covered the role alcohol plays in affecting certain neurophysiological substrates and the consequential results on psychological function. Using the concept of psychological models of memory as a pivot, the role of memory as part of an integrated cognitive system was then investigated in relation to explanations for problem drinking within a social context. Finally, cognitive function, defined within a template of functional attribution, was used to focus upon the role of higher order cognitive processes within the therapeutic environment. It is hoped that the scope of topics covered in this chapter alert the reader to the complexity of memory and cognitive processes in relation to the study of problem drinking behaviour. It is ventured that to gain an understanding of the role of memory and cognition in problem drinking behaviour, it is necessary to adopt a multidisciplinary approach that encompasses an integrated psychological, biological and sociological perspective.

REFERENCES

Anderson, I., Aitken, P. P. and Davies, J. B. (1981) 'Recall of the Ordering of the Symptoms of Alcoholism', *British Journal of Clinical Psychology*, 20:pp. 137–8.

Baddeley, A. D. and Hitch, G. (1974) 'Working Memory', in G. H. Bower (ed.), *The Psychology of Learning and Motivation*, vol. 8 (New York: Academic Press).

Bonner, A. (1994) 'Biological Mechanisms of Alcohol Dependence', *Current Opinions in Psychiatry*, 7:pp. 262–268.

Cermak, L. S. (1979) 'Amnesia Patients' Level of Processing', in L. S. Cermak and F. I. M. Craik (eds), *Levels of Processing in Human Memory* (Hillsdale, New Jersey: Lawrence Erlbaum Associates).

Cermak, L. S. (1982) 'The Long and Short of it in Amnesia', in L. S. Cermak and F. I. M. Craik (eds), *Levels of Processing in Human Memory* (Hillsdale, New Jersey: Lawrence Erlbaum Associates).

Cermak, L. S., Butters, N. and Moreines, J. (1974) 'Some Analyses of the Verbal Encoding Deficit of Alcoholic Korsakoff's Patients', *Brain and Language*, 1:pp. 141–50.

Chick, J. and Duffy, J. (1979) 'Application to the Alcohol Dependence Syndrome of a Method of Determining the Sequential Development of Symptoms', *Psychological Medicine*, 9:pp. 313–9.

Craik, F. I. M. and Lockhart, R. S. (1972) 'Levels of Processing: A Framework for Memory Research', *Journal of Verbal Learning and Verbal Behaviour*, 12:pp. 599–607.

Department of Health (1989) *Caring for People: Community Care in the Next Decade and Beyond*, Cm. 849 (London: HMSO).

Esposito, R. U., Parker, E. S. and Weingartner, H. (1984) 'Encephalinergic–Dopaminergic "Reward" Pathways: A Critical Substrate for Stimulatory, Euphoric and Memory Enhancing Actions of Alcohol – A Hypothesis', *Substance and Alcohol Actions*, 5:pp. 111–119.

Hewitt, G. and Popoff, I. (1993), unpublished study.

Hewitt, G., Holder, M. and Larid, J. (1995) 'Retrograde Enhancement of Human Kinaesthetic Memory by Alcohol: Consolidation or Protection Against Interference?', in preparation.

Johnson-Laird, P. N. (1983) *Mental Models* (Cambridge: Cambridge University Press).

Lamberty, G. J., Beckwith, B. E., Petros, T. V. and Ross, A. R. (1990) 'Post-trial Treatment with Ethanol Enhances Recall of Prose Narratives', *Physiology and Behaviour*, 48:pp. 653–6.

Lewis, M. J. and June, H.L. (1990) 'Studies of Ethanol Reward and Activation', *Alcohol*, 7(3):pp. 213–9.

Lewis, M. J. and June, H. L. (1994) 'Synergistic Effects of Ethanol and Cocaine on Brain Stimulation Reward', *Journal of Experimental Analysis and Behaviour*, 61:pp. 223–9.

Lister, R. G., Eckardt, M. J. and Weingartner, H. (1987) 'Ethanol Intoxication and Memory: Recent Developments and New Directions', *Recent Developments in Alcohol*, 5:pp. 111–26.

Mann, R. E., Cho-Young, J. and Vogel-Sprott, M. (1984) 'Retrograde Enhancement by Alcohol of Delayed Free Recall Performance', *Pharmacology, Biochemistry and Behaviour*, 20:pp. 639–42.

Manning, C. A., Parsons, M. W. and Gold, P. E. (1992) 'Anterograde and Retrograde Enhancement of 24-hour Memory by Glucose in Elderly Humans', *Behavioural and Neural Biology*, 58:pp. 125–30.

Maylor, E. A. and Rabbitt, P. M. A. (1993) 'Alcohol, Reaction Time and Memory: A Meta-analysis', *British Journal of Psychology*, 84:pp. 301–17.

McEntee, W. J., Biber, M. P., Perl, D. P. and Benson, D. F. (1976) 'Diencephalic Amnesia: A Reappraisal', *Journal of Neurology, Neurosurgery, and Psychiatry*, 39:pp. 436–41.

McGaugh, J. L. (1989) 'Involvement of Hormonal and Neuromodulatory Systems in the Regulation of Memory Storage', *Annual Review of Neuroscience*, 12:pp. 255–87.

Morton, J. (1985) 'The Problem with Amnesia: The Problem with Human Memory', *Cognitive Neuropsychology*, 2:pp. 281–90.

Mueller, C. W., Lisman, S. A. and Spear, N. E. (1983) 'Alcohol Enhancement of Human Memory: Tests of Consolidation and Interference Hypotheses', *Psychopharmacology*, 80:pp. 226–30.

Parker, E. S., Birnbaum, I. M., Weingartner, H., Hartley, J. T., Stillman, R. C. and Lyatt, R. J. (1980) 'Retrograde Enhancement of Human Memory', *Psychopharmacology*, 69:pp. 219–22.

Parker, E. S., Morihisa, J. M., Wyatt, R. J., Schwartz, R. L. and Weingartner (1981) 'Alcohol Facilitation Effect on Memory: A Dose–Response Study', *Psychopharmacology*, 74:pp. 88–92.

Reed, R. J., Grant, I. and Rourke, S. B. (1992) 'Long-term Abstinent Alcoholics have Normal Memory', *Alcoholism: Clinical and Experimental Research*, 16(4):pp. 677–83.

Rogers, C. R. (1951) *Client-centred Therapy* (Boston: Houghton Mifflin).

Ryan, J. J. and Lewis, C. V. (1988) 'Comparison of Normal Controls and Recently Detoxified Alcoholics on the Weschler Memory Scale', *Clinical Neuropsychologist*, 2(2):pp. 173–80.

Schank, R. and Abelson, R. (1977) *Scripts, Plans, Goals and Understanding: An Enquiry into Human Knowledge Structures* (Hillsdale, New Jersey: Erlbaum).

Tajfel, H. (ed.) (1982) *Social Identity and Intergroup Relations* (Cambridge: Cambridge University Press).

Tulving, E. (1972) 'Episodic and Semantic Memory', in E. Tulving and W. Donaldson (eds), *Organisation of Memory* (New York: Academic Press).

Warrington, E. K. and Weiskrantz, L. (1970) 'Amnesic Syndrome: Consolidation or Retrieval?', *Nature*, 228:pp. 628–30.

Warrington, E. K. and Weiskrantz, L. (1974) 'The Effect of Prior Learning on Subsequent Retention in Amnesic Patients', *Neuropsychologia*, 12:pp. 419–28.

Warrington, E. K. and Weiskrantz, L. (1978) 'Further Analyses of the Prior Learning Effect in Amnesic Patients', *Neuropsychologia*, 16:pp. 169–77.

Waugh, N. C. and Norman, D. A. (1965) 'Primary Memory', *Psychological Review*, 72:pp. 89–104.

Weiner, B. (1974) *Achievement Motivation and Attribution Theory* (New Jersey: General Learning Press).

10 Cognitive and Behavioural Approaches to Changing Addictive Behaviours

Paul E. Davis

INTRODUCTION

It is arguably the case that changing an addictive behaviour is all about changing beliefs and behaviours; and that whilst many different approaches and interventions may be helpful in different ways for different people, it seems reasonable to assume that cognitive and behavioural techniques will play a significant role in this process of change. This is regardless of whether a person is changing a behaviour entirely by themselves and without outside help, whether the intervention appears wholly physical (such as with pharmacotherapy or acupuncture), or whether the person is receiving a structured programme of cognitive–behavioural interventions. In the former case, for example when a cigarette smoker stops without outside help, the person may simply be using what to that individual is simply common sense (e.g. replacing smoking with an alternative behaviour in risky situations associated with smoking, or rewarding oneself for abstaining); in the case of pharmacotherapy, contingent positive (or negative) reinforcement for treatment compliance, or exposure to craving, for example, will inevitably also be present, albeit accidental and not planned as part of therapy. When analysing how people change attitudes and behaviours, it is often the case that behavioural, social learning and cognitive theories of psychology provide the scientifically most acceptable explanations. There are numerous psychological approaches to treating addictive behaviour, for example, motivational interviewing, supportive expressive psychotherapy, group work and behaviour therapy, etc. This chapter will focus on the use of cognitive and behavioural approaches.

COGNITIVE AND BEHAVIOURAL MODELS

The empirical origins of cognitive–behavioural approaches to psychological problems go back to two principles of animal learning. The first is classical conditioning, based on the work of Pavlov and other Russian physiologists with dogs. They conducted experiments where a bell was first rung, followed by food. After repeating this sequence of events several times the dogs salivated to the bell, before the food was given. This became known as classical conditioning. The food produces salivation before learning (conditioning) takes place and is thus known as the unconditioned stimulus. The salivation response to the food is called the unconditioned response. After several pairings of the bell and the food, the bell (which has become the conditioned stimulus) itself elicits salivation (the conditioned response). If the bell continues to be presented without food, the conditioned response is eventually extinguished. In humans, it has been found that many responses, including emotional and cognitive ones, are subject to the same laws of classical conditioning. This is particularly relevant to addictive behaviours where stimuli are conditioned to a powerful unconditioned response (the immediate consequence of the addictive behaviour) and become important in mediating the experience of craving, amongst other things.

The second principle is known as operant conditioning and is most associated with the work of an American psychologist, B. F. Skinner. Put simply, the 'Law of Effect' in operant conditioning states that the frequency and/or the strength of a behaviour is a function of the consequences of that behaviour. Figure 10.1 describes how the behaviour is affected by different types of reinforcer being presented or omitted.

These two principles were combined by Mowrer (see, for example, Mowrer, 1960) into a 'two factor' theory in which a response (such as drug taking) is acquired through classical conditioning and maintained through operant conditioning (such as avoiding unpleasant withdrawal symptoms by further drug taking, i.e. negative reinforcement).

The next major principle to be added came largely from the work of A. T. Beck (see, for example Beck, 1976). He described a model in which behaviours and feelings are mediated by the thoughts and belief systems that an individual has. Between the stimulus (e.g. the opportunity to use drugs) and the response (e.g. drug use) there is a cognitive mediation, made up of cognitive schemata, cognitive processes, and thoughts.

Childhood and/or adult life events influence the 'cognitive schemata'

Reinforcer

	Added	*Omitted*
Positive Reinforcer (something good, e.g. effects of an (addictive behaviour)	**behaviour is strengthened** positive reinforcement)	**behaviour is weakened** (extinction or frustative non reward)
Negative Reinforcer (something bad, e.g. withdrawal symptoms)	**behaviour is weakened** (punishment)	**behaviour is strengthened** (negative reinforcement)

Figure 10.1 Summary of operant conditioning, showing the additive and subtractive effects of positive and negative reinforcers

or underlying assumptions that we have. Cognitive schemata can be thought of as stable knowledge structures which represent all of an individual's knowledge about themselves in their world; they are beliefs and theories we hold about other people, ourselves, and the world about us. They influence for example our attitude to experimentation with drugs, our self esteem and vulnerability to mood disorders, our 'locus of control' and proneness to sensation seeking.

Cognitive schemata are mediated by cognitive processes (the 'computer software'). The end result (or cognitive product) of the process is the conscious series of thought and beliefs. Errors, biases or distortions can occur in any of these structures or processes, and affect our emotional responses, behaviours and indeed our 'personality'.

The treatments described in this chapter are an integration of cognitive and behavioural approaches, but draw on other models as well, such as Rogerian style psychotherapy, and Ellis' Rational Emotive Therapy (see, for example, Ellis, 1962). It is not possible to introduce these in any detail here. Within cognitive and behavioural approaches, the client is helped to recognise patterns of distorted or unhelpful thinking and dysfunctional behaviour. Systematic discussion and structured behavioural assignments are used to help the clients evaluate and modify their unhelpful thoughts and behaviours. Some aspects of treatment have greater emphasis on cognitive, others on behavioural factors.

HOW DO WE START TO HELP SOMEONE REDUCE AN APPETITIVE BEHAVIOUR?

Before embarking on any intervention, it is vital to understand the person's motivational stage of change; once this is understood, a suitable intervention package can be offered which matches where the person is in their motivational stage to where they would like to be. A person's level of motivation for change is an important factor in determining the likely success of any intervention (and measurement of this will form part of the assessment interview). Of course not every person presenting with an addictive behaviour problem will be fully motivated to benefit from treatment, and a person's motivation for change will fluctuate depending on many factors. Most people have a degree of ambivalence, a number of reasons for and against giving up or changing a habit, and the salience given to each of these can fluctuate even in a short time period. A useful way of thinking of motivation for change is as a circle which the drug user may go round many times before achieving a long lasting change. Prochaska and DiClemente (described in Miller and Rollnick, 1991) identify five stages of change around this circle. The circle of motivation starts with the person not contemplating a change in their behaviour, either because of denial that a problem exists or a belief that the problem is unchangeable ('precontemplative' stage). The next stage is an awareness of the need and ability to change ('contemplative' stage) whilst nevertheless continuing with the behaviour. In the 'preparation' stage, the person wishes to make actual changes and therefore desires help with their problems, but feels at a loss as to how to do what is necessary to alter the habit. This is followed by a stage of 'active change' where the person's determination and commitment to change produces change directed behaviour. The next part of the motivational circle is a 'maintenance of change' stage. One person may remain for several years at each stage whilst someone else might experience all five on a daily basis! The important thing is that motivation is not viewed as static or dichotomous (motivated versus unmotivated). Most people do not progress smoothly around the circle, but rather 'get stuck' at certain points or alternatively jump around the circle in an apparently illogical manner.

The interventions offered will to some extent depend on the assessment of motivation for change, and we should not assume that everyone is at the active change stage nor that everyone will necessarily benefit from help directed at changing their behaviour. Therapy with someone with an addictive behaviour may be viewed as a process of

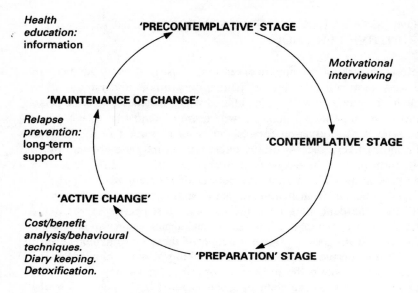

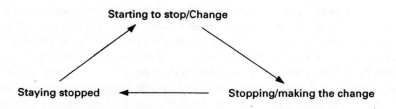

Figure 10.2   Adaptation of the motivational model presented by Prochaska
and DiClemente (described in Miller and Rollnick, 1991): some
suggestions as to the types of responses which might be appropriate
(in italics) and indicated

Figure 10.3   Levels of help provided by statutory and non-statutory services

'nudging' the client around the circle towards the 'maintenance of change'
stage, and this is helped most if both the client and the therapist are
focusing on the same stage of change. Figure 10.2 is an adaptation of
the model presented by Prochaska and DiClemente, with some suggestions as to the types of responses which might be appropriate. For
most clients the categories of help offered fall into one of three levels
(see Figure 10.3).

Some form of intervention will be considered appropriate at some time for most clients presenting for treatment, and a variety of treatment options are available; in virtually every case, for the treatment to be of any value it has to be on a voluntary basis and it is important that the client takes part in the choice of a treatment option. Negotiating with the client on a treatment package is alien to some treatment models, but is crucial to the cognitive–behavioural approach where the client has to be in the 'driving seat', and has to develop a sense of self efficacy. Sometimes this is thought of as a 'self-service cafeteria' approach, with the client deciding which components he or she will consume from the menu on offer.

Some treatments are directed at the underlying causes which may have initiated the addictive behaviour and/or are contributing to its continuation. Some help to resolve the problems associated with or consequences of the problem behaviour and some deal more directly with the addictive behaviour itself, aiming to reduce or stop the behaviour regardless of other problems or circumstances.

Other treatments are directed at helping the client's motivation for change rather than directly changing the behaviour, while others are aimed at helping to prevent relapse in those who have achieved change. The setting for these treatment options is likewise varied, from a residential programme through to self-help groups in the community. In recent years there have been considerable improvements in the provision of community treatments, often given by a multidisciplinary team seeing the client at home or in another community venue. Not all interventions are suitable for every person, nor are they mutually exclusive, but for all clients the important point is that treatment plans must be drawn up thoughtfully, according to the needs of the individual utilising, as appropriate, a single intervention or a 'mix' of interventions, or components of different interventions. It is always important to remember that there is no one approach that is 'right' or 'best'.

Motivational Interviewing

'Motivational interviewing' (described in detail in Miller and Rollnick, 1991) is a generic term encompassing numerous approaches and techniques, some of which will be described in detail here. Firstly it should be understood why there is a need for motivational interviewing. Perhaps the most compelling point is that treatment can only be successful when the client stays in treatment and participates in an active way. General practitioners and other doctors and therapists working in the field of addictive behaviour know from experience that people with addictive behaviours often do not recognise these problems and that their motivation to do something about it is sometimes very low. This is especially so in the early stages of motivation to change, usually at the beginning of the treatment process. The early contacts between a treatment agency and the problem drinker or drug user are therefore of crucial importance. In this first phase of the help-seeking process drop-out rates are highest. Motivational interviewing is a therapy approach which helps the client to 'nudge' himself/herself towards commitment for change. In addition, even with a determined 'active changer' or someone in the maintenance stage, a degree of ambivalence will always threaten to impede progress or contribute to a lapse, and so helping someone to maintain their motivation is important throughout the circle of change.

The fact that clients are often not highly motivated to change, and once started on a treatment programme clients often drop out, means that the aims of motivational interviewing are particularly pertinent to these client groups. Motivational interviewing is an approach that:

1. raises the client's self-esteem, self-efficacy and awareness of problems;
2. elicits self-motivational statements and pinpoints motivated behaviour;
3. attributes responsibility to the client.

Motivating the client is a crucial part of the therapy process. Three phases are involved:

1. *eliciting phase* – get the client to say why there is a problem ('lecturing' to the client may simply harden their denial attitude);
2. *information phase* – client receives from the therapist objective information about his medical, psychological and social situation; based on this, the client draws his/her own conclusions;
3. *negotiation phase* – therapist and client start negotiation about a possible treatment goal and plan.

Miller *et al.* (1988) describe the general characteristics of motivational interventions as consisting of giving clear advice to change (e.g. providing realistic and practical information on consequences of the person's continued level of addictive behaviour); removing practical barriers to change (offering a service that is easily accessible, available at times convenient to the client, and free or at least affordable to the client); and providing choice for the client. The phases described above are then added to these three characteristics. Much of motivational interviewing relies as much on the attitudes and approaches adopted by the therapist as on the individual techniques used.

STOPPING AND STAYING STOPPED

Much of the above is directed at engaging the client and helping the person to move around the motivational circle towards 'maintenance of change'. Although there is a place for motivational interviewing at all stages, someone in the active change or maintenance stage will be appropriate for many other interventions. It is only possible here to give a brief description of some of the cognitive behavioural therapies used, and the interested reader is referred to Gossop (1989), Miller (1980), Beck *et al.* (1993), Orford (1985) and Marlatt and Gordan (1985) for more detailed accounts.

Cognitive Behavioural Psychotherapy

This approach assumes that beliefs and assumptions that the person holds may be distorted (during childhood and learning experiences as an adult) and as a result the person may have negative interpretations of themselves, their future or the world around them which predisposes them, for example, towards low self-esteem, depression or anxiety, or the continued use of substances. Patients can learn, with the help of a trained therapist, to correct negatively biased attitudes and beliefs based on faulty assumptions, and as a result learn to cope better with life without drugs.

Cognitive therapy with, for example, a problem drug user, aims to address drug-related beliefs and automatic thoughts that contribute to continued use, urges and craving. Although many of the techniques used in cognitive therapy with addictive behaviours are adapted for specific use with these client groups, most are applicable to people across the full range of disorders and problems. As with motivational interviewing, the efficacy is dependent to a large degree on the therapeutic relationship in which the therapist is required to have warmth, accurate empathy and genuineness. The therapist in general uses what Beck (e.g. Beck *et al.*, 1993) describes as the Socratic method of interviewing, the goal of which is for the client to think autonomously and rationally (it is not to 'brainwash' the client into thinking in a misguided or over-optimistic way). In this method, the client is guided through a process of discovering their distorted pattern of thinking and behaving, rather than being told or lectured at. The cognitive therapist uses the interviewing techniques described earlier such as reflections, summarising, implying and probing questions, in order to examine and test the client's basic beliefs and automatic thoughts. This helps the client to become more aware of important information and to 're-think' some of this information. Examples of errors of thinking and unhelpful beliefs might be 'I've made a mess of my life so far therefore I will always be a worthless person') or 'the only time I can ever enjoy myself is when I am drunk'; or 'if I stop smoking I'll become overweight'; or 'how can I have a drink problem when I am so successful in my career'. The therapist's goal is to help the client recognise these as errors or unhelpful thoughts, and to challenge beliefs and restructure them using a number of techniques.

A common technique is for the client to perform a cost–benefit analysis or pay-off matrix on the effects of continuing to use:

	Benefits	**Costs**
Short-term	e.g. feel good, fun, part of the crowd	e.g. costs a lot, threat of arrest, overdose or infection
Long-term	e.g. overcomes problems such as low self confidence, gives a role identity	e.g. relationship problems, long-term health and social problems

A person with an addictive behaviour often maintains beliefs that minimise the disadvantages and maximise the advantages of their behaviour. In completing a pay-off matrix, the client is encouraged to list and evaluate the advantages and disadvantages of their addictive behaviour, with the aim of gaining a more accurate, objective and balanced view than previously held.

An important aspect of cognitive therapy is the client understanding, perhaps through examples and 'vignettes' as well as through literature supplied by the therapist, the cognitive model as applied to addictive behaviour. This is important in obtaining compliance with other exercises such as recording basic beliefs, automatic thoughts, feelings and behaviours which are of relevance to the addictive behaviour. When clients systematically monitor their basic drug-related beliefs and automatic thoughts, and when these cognitive processes are shown to be related to their subsequent addictive behaviour, clients tend to report an increased understanding of their addictive behaviour and how to change.

A common theme in cognitive therapy (see Chapter 8) is helping the client to reattribute responsibility for their addictive behaviour away from external factors (such as 'I drank because I was at a party where you were expected to drink') to internal responsibility ('I took the decision to say yes'). By doing this the 'locus of control' is internalised which places the client in a position where they can do something about their behaviour rather than being at the mercy of others (or their addictive behaviour). Reattribution of responsibility requires the skilful application of the Socratic method so that the client does not feel that the therapist is being accusatorial.

Other Strategies

Keeping a 'daily thought record' (DTR)

This is a fundamental strategy in cognitive therapy (e.g. Beck *et al.*, 1993). This usually consists of a five-column form with headings to record the situation (e.g. what was happening before and during the urge to drink); the automatic negative thoughts (with a rating of belief or salience of the thought); emotions and feelings which occurred; a description of a rational response to the thoughts with a rating of belief or salience of this response; a column to describe the outcome, what happened and what rating is now given to the automatic thoughts.

Techniques such as 'distancing' (asking the client to imagine he is advising a friend, 'what helpful advice would I give my best friend in this situation', or that he is observing himself in the situation) are sometimes used in order to help the client formulate a rational response. An example of the use of a DTR might be someone trying to avoid entering a betting shop on the way home from work, who recognises a risky thought such as 'nobody will know, and I need some pleasure in life'. By writing down on the DTR what he is thinking, the client is able to examine the belief and consider its validity in a more systematic and objective fashion. In addition, the DTR introduces a delay between the initial urge and the choice point, during which time he may choose not to gamble, etc. because of a natural diminution of the desire.

Another useful method for teaching clients using a DTR to generate objective rational responses, is to write down on the DTR a series of open ended questions, such as 'what evidence supports this thought', 'are there other ways I could view this situation', 'what is the worst thing that could happen – and what would happen then', 'what is the best thing', and 'what is the most likely realistically to happen'; 'what are pros and cons of changing the way I view this situation, and what constructive action can I take to deal with it'.

Completion of the DTR and practise of these questions is often set by clients as a 'homework assignment', so that the client is more likely to be able to use the techniques in situations where there is no opportunity to complete a DTR.

Imagery
This is another technique used both in cognitive and behavioural therapy (see, for example, Sharpe and Tarrier, 1992, who use this with a problem gambler). As an adjunct to cognitive therapy the technique involves the client visualising 'self control' as well as scenes where they are carrying out their addictive behaviour. Imagery can be a useful technique for focusing clients on addictive behaviour beliefs and automatic thoughts, or distracting them from their cravings and urges. When used as a method for changing (as opposed to eliciting) addiction-related beliefs, the client may be guided by the therapist to imagine coping scenes such as being assertive, engaging in positive enjoyable activities as alternatives to the addictive behaviour, or imagining a productive and healthy life as a result of changing their behaviour. Imaginal exposure to addictive behaviour situations can also act to sensitise the person to cues associated with the addictive behaviour and to get the client to associate addictive behaviour cognitions with self-management skills such as cognitive challenging, relaxation or turning away without carrying out the addictive behaviour.

Stimulus Control and Cue Exposure

Ideally an effective treatment would be the total elimination of all cues, triggers or stimuli associated with the addictive behaviour. While this is partially possible, for example, with drug injectors (needles and syringes are relatively easy to avoid, although other drug-taking paraphernalia such as spoons, sugar and silver paper are not), for most types of addictive behaviours avoidance is not an option. Walking past the tobacconist shop, turning down a drink at a party, or declining an office sweepstakes on the Grand National, are common occurrences for many people attempting to stay stopped. An alternative to avoidance is to help the client reduce the aroused cravings (see Beck *et al.*, 1993).

Techniques include various methods for distraction; the goal of distraction techniques is to get the clients to change their focus of attention from internal responses (such as automatic thoughts, 'positive outcome expectancies' where pleasurable memories are aroused, and physical sensations) to external stimuli and responses which are incompatible with the addictive behaviour. Distraction techniques might be cognitive (e.g. reciting a favourite poem or story; mental arithmetic or visualising complex shapes and movements practised in therapy, or describing the surroundings to oneself in detail); or behavioural (e.g. removing oneself from the cue-laden environment, talk to a friend, perform a household activity, or start a challenging activity which demands focused attention). When cravings are strong, distraction is unlikely to be sufficient alone. The ability to reason objectively may also be lost, in which case flashcards with coping statements are useful. The client writes out in advance relevant coping statements such as 'I don't want to blow all my hard work so far' or 'I know that just one cigarette will not be enough'. Another technique, already mentioned earlier, is the use of imagery to help control craving. The client may be taught to use a 'thought stopping' procedure such as shouting 'stop' and imagining the word in front of him. This might be followed by images of a negative consequence to the addictive behaviour, such as imagining oneself being operated on for lung cancer, followed by a positive image (e.g. playing sport, keeping custody of your children) for not engaging in the addictive behaviour. Imagery rehearsal is used to prepare clients when it is known they are going to be in cue-laden situations. Rehearsal might include as well mastery of the situation, getting the client to see themselves in the scene as strong and successful at coping with these urges.

Graded exposure to cues has also been used in behavioural programmes to reduce craving (see, for example, Miller, 1980). The client is asked to produce a list of situations, feelings, objects or anything else which has become associated with the addictive behaviour (including, in the case of alcohol, small amounts or primer doses of alcohol). The goal is to extinguish the conditioned response, by presenting the cue without the opportunity to engage in the addictive behaviour. This technique has been shown to be helpful with some clients, although there is a considerable risk of precipitating relapse in some clients, and in the absence of positive outcome evaluation in controlled studies, it is not a procedure which can be recommended for use by anyone not fully trained in the technique.

Rational responding (as described earlier for recording thoughts), can also be helpful in controlling craving. Clients are told to keep a notepad to record any urges and to then challenge their thoughts and feelings using the kinds of questions listed earlier. Detailed descriptions of the craving, broken down into cognitive, behavioural, affective and physiological components, help the client to be more objective about the experience and to approach the phenomenon in a constructive way.

Activity Monitoring and Scheduling

It is part of the definition of an addictive behaviour (see Chapter 1) that the person tends to focus their behaviours on activities that support their addiction, and give increased salience to their drug- or addiction-seeking behaviours over other behaviours. In many cases the person loses activities which formerly may have been rewarding, such as work, hobbies, relationships, etc. Activity monitoring and scheduling are relatively simple techniques which help the person to re-engage in non-addictive behaviours and to modify their addictive behaviours. The techniques (described in greater detail in Beck *et al.*, 1993), typically consist of the client recording on a chart divided into one-hour blocks each day what activities they have done in the last hour. This activity is rated both for how pleasurable the activity was and the extent to which the client felt 'mastery' at performing the task , thus giving measures of the level of the reward and satisfaction experienced. This chart is used retrospectively to analyse the client's activities and how they relate to drug use, and prospectively as a guide for planning future activities. Initially activity scheduling will seem artificial to the client, but with time the client sees that they can be successful at planning and completing non-addiction related behaviours, which in turn gives them positive reinforcement and builds self-efficacy.

Activity scheduling is also another helpful behavioural technique for controlling craving. Once someone has changed an addictive behaviour, it leaves gaps in their day and clients often report having time on their hands. The resulting boredom can often contribute to craving and relapse unless new activities are substituted. An activity schedule is used to obtain a baseline measure of how the client is spending his/her time, and what are the enjoyable activities. Often the client has to be helped to remember what they used to enjoy and how they spent their time before their behaviour became an addiction. The scheduling of activities can revive some of these old habits and pastimes which will help in coping with craving.

Behavioural rehearsal is another technique much used by behavioural therapists. The most common use is probably in relation to anger control, social skills and assertiveness training, relationships and other interpersonal skills training. Whatever the situation, the normal procedure is to set up the role play after firstly discussing the various options for how it might be handled in order to achieve the outcome desired by the client. The important principle is that the client is adding to their inter personal skills by firstly practising in a relatively safe environment before trying out it out in real life.

Negative moods (and often positive ones as well) are risk factors for many clients attempting to stay stopped. Clients are taught in therapy management strategies such as anger control, how to manage depression and anxiety, problem solving skills training, and how to celebrate. Coping with excitement or happiness may form part of the behavioural programme to help cope with urges and craving. Relaxation training is often used to help control craving. There are numerous types of relaxation exercises to try, including autogenic relaxation, autosuggestion, biofeedback, yoga and breathing exercises, but the easiest to apply in everyday situations is probably progressive muscle relaxation, learned as part of a course going from tensing and relaxing each of the muscle groups, to being able to relax muscles without the need to tense them firstly (see Bernstein and Borkovec, 1973).

Contingency Management

This is a procedure based on the principles of behaviour modification, or 'operant conditioning' described earlier. Translated into helping a person with an addictive behaviour, it is possible to have specified rewards which are made contingent upon continuation or initiation of an agreed behaviour. Such a programme is probably best suited to residential settings or more formal clinics which treat people who perhaps might benefit from the structure and clear boundaries of this approach. The desired (target) behaviour is defined and explained first, along with the contingent reward, before the procedure is initiated, rather than the individual learning by trial and error what is expected and what the price of failure/success is going to be. More importantly, the goals and methods are agreed with the client in advance as being what they want. Another important feature is that the procedures are based on scientific theory which allows for clear predictions to be made, again as opposed to trial and error.

In practice contingency management utilises positive reinforcers which are both ethically acceptable and under the control of the therapist. Punishment and negative reinforcement are never used as part of a therapeutic programme, nor is it ethical to use positive reinforcers to which the patient does not have a right of access. So, the therapist is restricted but nevertheless with, for example, an opiate-dependent individual who is attending a clinic regularly and frequently for a prescription for methadone (or heroin), a variety of reinforcers might be utilised for contingency management. For example, methadone take-home privileges (rather than having to take the methadone under supervision at the clinic), frequency of clinic attendance, time of appointment, and advantageous holiday arrangements can all be made contingent upon certain behaviours. In practice, similar systems may already exist but in an informal and unrecognised way, which makes consistency of approach unlikely. Thus if patients ask for special arrangements to be made for opiate prescription while they are on holiday, their request is more likely to be granted if they have been 'doing well' – i.e. attending regularly with no evidence of illicit drug abuse, etc. Planned contingency management, however, means that drug abusers learn much more directly and therefore more easily and more quickly, exactly what is expected of them. It is important to understand, however, that among the most potent reinforcers available to staff, particularly in a residential setting, are staff attention and time, which tend to be contingent on problematic or undesirable behaviour and thus unwittingly may increase these behaviours. An awareness of this and their use in a structured behavioural programme has obvious benefits for overcoming these problems.

Relapse Prevention as a Cognitive Behavioural Approach

Finally, no overview of addictive behaviour treatments would be complete without discussion of the 'relapse prevention' model (see Marlatt and Gordan,[10] 1985). A relapse is defined as a return to previous levels of activity following an attempt to stop or reduce that activity. So, any change, be it unsafe to safer injecting practices, controlled drinking or total abstinence, can be considered in this model. Relapse prevention equips the person with a plan of action (rather like a fire drill, which you hope will never be needed but is well rehearsed 'just in case') for how to cope with a 'slip' or the risk of this. The maxim for relapse prevention programmes is 'forewarned is forearmed'.

In the relapse prevention model, Marlatt and Gordan (1985) view the person who, for whatever reason, is at risk of lapse, as having a number of choice points. If the person has coping skills which are used and are effective, then drinking, etc. is avoided, the person's self-esteem and feeling of self-efficacy is enhanced, and their internal, global and stable attributions are positive and are reinforced. If, on the other hand, the person has ineffective or absent coping strategies, coupled with raised positive outcome expectancies, then a lapse is more likely to occur. There is another choice at this point; if the person has effective strategies for coping with a lapse then the abstinence violation effect will be avoided which will lead to relapse prevention and again a feeling of raised self-efficacy and self-esteem, with enhancement of the internal, global and stable attributions described earlier. If these are absent, then the abstinence violation effect will be present and this is more likely to lead to a risk of a full blown relapse. The programme uses cognitive–behavioural techniques, designed to teach individuals who are trying to maintain a behavioural change how to anticipate and cope with the problem of relapse. The various techniques used include most of those described already above, and may be classified into three groups:

1. Those that teach the client to recognise and deal effectively with high risk situations (using self-monitoring, inventories, autobiography, descriptions of past relapses, relapse fantasies, etc.). Once the client recognises the chain of events or thoughts leading to relapse, skills training and the other behavioural techniques described above are used for dealing with these, as well as learning how to change the environment to modify this chain.
2. Life-style modification.
3. Management of lapses (a lapse is defined as any discrete violation of a self-imposed rule over the level of an addictive behaviour).

Relapse prevention encompasses numerous techniques and may operate at any of the levels and choice points described by Marlatt and Gordan. These interventions are often best offered in groups although where specific cognitive therapy approaches are used these are probably difficult to manage other than on a one to one basis.

CONCLUSION

The present chapter has ignored social/milieu therapies, and family and couples interventions, not because these are not relevant within cognitive–behavioural therapies – they definitely are relevant – but because of personal interests of the author taking over all of the allocated space. In conclusion, cognitive – behavioural approaches have much to offer in the treatment and management of addictive behaviours. This chapter has attempted to describe some of these approaches. It has not been possible here to review the literature on the effectiveness of cognitive–behavioural therapies (for recent reviews, see Bien *et al.*, 1993; and Hodgson, 1994). The challenge for the future is to develop further these approaches, and to attempt to match the most appropriate techniques to the individual client's needs. We know that they are effective for some people some of the time. The question of what kinds of person, with what kinds and severities of addictive behaviour, will respond best to what kinds of treatments delivered in what kinds of ways, is a long way from being answered, but is, nevertheless, the correct question in need of addressing.

REFERENCES

Beck, A. T. (1976) *Cognitive Therapy and the Emotional Disorders* (New York: International Universities Press).

Beck, A. T., Wright, F. D., Newman, C. F., and Liese, B. S. (1993) *Cognitive Therapy of Substance Abuse* (New York: Guilford Press).

Bien, T. H., Miller, W. R. and Tonigan, J. S. (1993) 'Brief Interventions for Alcohol Problems: A Review', *Addiction*, 88:pp. 315–36.

Bernstein, D. A. and Borkovec, T. D. (1973) *Progressive Relaxation Training* (Champaign, IL: Research Press).

Ellis, A. (1962) *Reason and Emotion in Psychotherapy* (New York: Lyle Stuart).

Festinger, L. (1957) *A Theory of Cognitive Dissonance* (New York: Harper & Row).

Gossop, M. (1989) *Relapse and Addictive Behaviour* (London: Tavistock/Routledge).

Hodgson, R. (1994) 'Treatment of Alcohol Problems', *Addiction*, 89:pp. 1529–34.

Marlatt, G. A. and Gordan, J. R. (1985) *Relapse Prevention: Maintenance Strategies in the Treatment of Addictive Behaviours* (New York: Guilford Press).

Miller, W. R. (1980) *The Addictive Behaviors: Treatment of Alcoholism, Drug Abuse, Smoking, and Obesity* (Oxford: Pergamon Press).

Miller, W. R. (1983) 'Motivational Interviewing with Problem Drinkers', *Behavioural Psychotherapy*, 11:pp. 147–82.

Miller, W. R., Sovereign, R. G. and Krege, B. (1988) 'Motivational Interviewing with Problem Drinkers: II. The Drinker's Check up as a Preventative Intervention', *Behavioural Psychotherapy*, 16:pp. 251–68.

Miller, W. R., and Rollnick, S. (1991) *Motivational Interviewing: Preparing People to Change Addictive Behaviours* (New York: Guilford Press).

Mowrer, O. H. (1960) *Learning Theory and Behaviour* (New York: Wiley).

Orford, J. (1985) *Excessive Appetites: A Psychological View of Addictions* (Chichester: Wiley).

Sharpe, L. and Tarrier, N. (1992) 'A Cognitive–Behavioural Treatment Programme for Problem Gamblers', *Journal of Cognitive Psychotherapy*, 6: pp. 193–203.

Part IV
Molecules, Mood and Addictive Behaviour

11 Craving: Fancies, Fact and Folklore

David Peers

THE NATURE OF CRAVINGS

Craving is a concept which everyone vaguely thinks that they understand, and is usually thought of as an intense desire or longing. The use of the term in scientific studies is hardly more precise. The term is used to refer to different phenomena by different investigators. Opinions range from those who believe that craving is the dominant factor in drug addiction to the suggestion that it is a hypothetical construct, an 'epiphenomenon', which is more obscure than helpful – it is neither observable directly nor measurable. Despite such imprecision, the term has been widely used in a range of scientific investigations, particularly in studies of addiction, alcoholism and eating disorders. Such practice was criticised many years ago by the World Health Organisation.[1] The use of the term is still widespread, presumably because everyone thinks that they know what it means. An attempt was made in 1991 to reach consensus at a meeting of experts from several disciplines, sponsored by the Addiction Research Centre of the US National Institute on Drug Abuse.[2] The participants agreed that craving is a subjective state in humans that is associated with drug dependence but that little further could be certain. Unsurprisingly, it was suggested that, in order to advance knowledge, a substantial research programme is required.

The idea that craving is a distinct state is reinforced by Kilgus and Pumatiega.[3] They reported experimental manipulation of cocaine craving by showing videotaped environmental cues to subjects in a rehabilitation programme. The subjects self-rated their perceived degree of craving, mood, energy and wellness. Only craving showed a statistically significant change from pre-test to post-test.

The importance of a precise definition is more than of academic interest. Confusion has more serious implications for those working in the areas of prevention and education. Kozlowski *et al.*[4] found that whilst around half of smokers understood the term *craving* to mean a strong urge, another third of their sample interpreted it as any urge, even a weak one. One in six (15.2 per cent) stated that craving was neither of the above. Sithathian and McGraph[5] extending a similar approach to the attitudes of alcoholics found further confusion and disturbing difference in definition between health professionals and their clients. The communication issues resulting from inadequate definition of the concept of craving suggest a potential for problems for intervention strategies. Endeavours to define and measure craving broadly represent two approaches: descriptive or physiological.

The descriptive approach suffers from the usual problems in quantifying self-report. Typically, subjects are asked to estimate, on some arbitary rating scale, how much they crave or desire some substance. Whether ratings of 1 or 2 out of 10 should even be considered to be craving is rarely considered. With measures such as these it is difficult to generalise reported results. Attempts have been made to tighten quantitative rigour by measurement of consumption of the postulated craved substance. The more one consumes, the more one is presumed to have craved it. The circularity of this logic has been noted.[6] The weakness of this argument is illustrated by two opposites. Someone giving up smoking does not consume, but still craves. Similarly, from the opposite viewpoint, it is possible to engorge oneself with large amounts of food, for example at Christmas, without necessarily craving it. Psychophysiological parameters such as measures of arousal using skin conductance or salivation have been used in order to assess levels of craving. These measures have been reported to correlate with self-reports of craving for alcohol.[7] However, these may simply reflect anxiety or expectation.

A second approach focuses on a possible physiological basis for the phenomenon of craving. This is usually suggested to be neurological. The craved substance is presumed to affect the action of a neurochemical, such as a synaptic transmitter, used in signalling between neurons. This could suggest a variety of sub-classes of craving, depending on the specific transmitter involved, for example 'opiate' dependency as distinct from 'barbituate' dependancy. The **psychomotor stimulant theory** for the neurobiology of craving[8] posits separate mechanisms for positive or negative reinforcement. It is suggested that a wide range of addictive drugs share a common brain mechanism, probably mediated via dopaminergic fibres. In contrast, different addictive drugs are thought to have different mechanisms of negative reinforcement. In some cases, the drug may activate mechanisms which suppress pain and distress signals, including those associated with the drug's own withdrawal symptoms.

Another view of the possible integration of the various aspects of craving and addiction is summarised by Robinson and Berridge.[9] They suggest a combined biological and psychological mechanism, the '**Incentive-Sensitisation Theory**'. The suggestion here is that a psychological process is responsible for transforming the perception of stimuli, imbueing them with 'salience', making them attractive. Again, it is suggested that addictive drugs enhance dopamine transmission. In some individuals, the repeated use of addictive drugs produces adaptation in this neural system, making it increasingly sensitive to drugs and drug-induced stimuli. Such sensitisation is gated by associative learning, transforming ordinary *wanting* into excessive *craving*. Once again, different mechanisms are suggested for positive or negative reinforcement. Thus, sensitisation of incentive salience can produce addictive behaviour even if the expectation of drug pleasure or the aversive properties of withdrawal are diminished. This could apply even in the face of strong disincentives, such as legal consequences or loss of job, home or family.

EXPLANATIONS OF THE MECHANISMS OF CRAVING

Explanations for craving have two extremes; based on positive or negative affect, the reality probably comes somewhere in between. The craved substance may produce some desired state, 'euphoria' or 'pleasure', concepts which are hardly better defined than craving. Expectation models suggest that cravings are triggered by exposure to stimuli associated with the desired substance. It is a commonplace observation that the sight or smell of palatable food produces desire for it, or indeed any, food. Cornell *et al.*[10] demonstrate experimentally another truism, 'Stimulus-induced eating when satiated' as demonstrated by the lure of the sweet trolley. As well as negating simplistic explanations of hunger based on stomach distension or blood sugar levels, this indicates that expectation can override physiological reality. Engle and Williams[11] asked alcoholics to indicate their desire for alcohol after a drink. The taste of alcohol in the drink was disguised and only one-half of the subjects were informed that it was present. Only these subjects who were aware of the presence of alcohol reported significant cravings to drink more. Subjects who consumed the equivalent amount of alcohol, but who were unaware, reported no cravings.

Expectation may be for the sensory events accompanying the intake of particular substances. It is controversial whether provision of nicotine via gum or dermal patches is effective in relieving withdrawal distress or cravings for cigarettes[12] when this is the only intervention in attempts to stop smoking. The sensory correlates of smoking, especially the sensation of smoke in the throat, appear to have an important role in cigarette smoking. Mimicking such sensations or anaesthetisation of the sensory endings in the oropharynx have been reported to reduce craving.[13]

The opposite pole of explanations of cravings is that they are triggered after a period of abstinence from the highly desired or addicted substance. An early model involving alcohol was given by Jellinek *et al.*[14] Studies have been published supporting the view that cravings are most intense when the withdrawal state is most severe; for example, cravings for cigarettes are predicted by pre-abstinence levels of nicotine. Once again, this is an almost tautologous statement. Within this model, some have tried to identify possible mechanisms for abstinence-induced cravings. For example, Dakis *et al.*[15] suggest that chronic cocaine use depletes brain dopamine, resulting in dysphoria and, consequently, the triggering of cocaine craving in withdrawal. Several workers have suggested similar mechanisms based on serotonin, which is generally sedative, in relation to carbohydrate 'self-medication to avoid dysphoria'. This has been reviewed by Wurtman and Wurtman,[16] and Noach.[17] Gossop *et al.*,[18] investigating opiate addicts and cigarette smokers, found general agreement that craving was a dysphoric state, especially amongst the former. The authors do recognise that this may be reflective of context, as all subjects were in the early stages of abstinence.

FOOD CRAVINGS

There is a general folkloric assumption that food cravings serve body needs, the 'wisdom of the body'.[19] This is reinforced by vague references to animals, which are not supported by scientific agricultural studies (reviewed, Underwood[20]). Extreme cases may provide support. Adrenalectomised rats consume salt solutions in concentrations which are rejected by normal rats (reviewed Denton).[21] A parallel case in humans was a boy suffering from adrenal insufficiency who was prepared to break open cupboards in order to obtain salt.[22] Following his death when hospitalised, it appeared that his behaviour was directed at maintaining physiological homeostasis.

There are several suggestions linking food cravings with altered affect. These commonly involve carbohydrate, overlapping with sweetness. The underlaying assumption seems to be that animals, and particularly primates, evolved preference for sweet tastes as an indicator of ripeness in fruits. The best worked out version is that of the Wurtmans, (for review see Wurtman *et al.*[23]), based on a homeostatic balance between separate appetites for carbohydrate and protein, mediated by tryptophan, the precursor for the neurotransmitter, serotonin. As the rate limiting step in its synthesis is not saturated in normal physiological conditions, its availability can be affected by the quality and quantity foods in the diet (see Chapter 8). Serotonin, amongst its other, generally inhibitory, effects is sedative. Individuals are suggested to learn to self-medicate anxiety or depression with carbohydrates. This hypothesis is extended to the obese, where such behaviour could act as a contributive factor. The same explanation has been applied to pre-menstrual syndrome and seasonal affective disorder. The topic of 'precursor-control of neurotransmitter synthesis' is reviewed by Wurtman *et al* [23]. Opinions for and against are reviewed by a variety of authors.[24]

Many foods contain pharmacologically active substances, possibly evolved as defence mechanisms. These include the alkaloids, some of which are deliberately exploited by various methods of ingestion. Many foods contain biogenic amines, sometimes due to the processes of fermentation. The most studied physiologically active bioamine is probably histamine, a compound also involved in the mediation of allergic reactions. Another amine, tyramine, has been implicated in the initiation of migraine attacks, although there is growing controversy surrounding this proposal.[25] Ingestion of such substances can become critical in people taking monoamine oxidase inhibitors. The 'phenomenology of food cravings' is reviewed by Weingarten and Elston.[26]

An alternative aspect of cravings and food relates to 'eating disorders'. These are suggested to be widespread, bulimia nervosa may affect between 3 and 7 per cent of adolescent and young adult women. Mitchell *et al.*[27] reported 70 per cent of bulimic women ascribing the onset of binging to craving for specific, sweet foods. Many authors assume that disordered eating and, in particular, calorific restriction, can trigger cravings for carbohydrate (see Garner and Garfinkel).[28] Similar ideas can be extended to those with a history of dieting. It is known that carbohydrate cravings are more frequent in obese populations.[29] This could be interpreted as either cause or effect.

A number of authors have drawn attention to similarities between eating disorders and chemical dependency. Beresford and Hall[30] compare similarities and differences between alcoholism and eating disorders. They suggest that diagnostic, psychodynamic and therapeutic similarities are strong and may relate to a common breakdown in behavioural inhibition once abnormal patterns of consumption have been adopted. They compare the conditions against four criteria; tolerance, withdrawal, loss of control and social decline. Cooper [31] uses four rather different criteria to argue that chemical dependency and eating disorders are comparable. He suggests that in both cases, the person experiences uncontrollable self-destructive behaviour, both personally and socially, together with denial of the extent of involvement. There is progressive deterioration. Fourthly, there is a considerable familial involvement, in both aetiology and consequences. An attempt at integration of these various aspects is presented as a 'biopsychosocial perspective'.

EFFECTS OF FEMALE ENDOCRINE CHANGES

Reports of effects of changes in female hormone physiology on food cravings have a long tradition. The first reported scientific study [32] found that about one-third of pregnant women experienced *longings*. Dickens and Trethowan [33] reported that around a half of women in their study had such experience. Results, consistent over many studies, suggest that folklore contains a core of truth, pregnant women do have food cravings, especially in the first trimester, the time of most endocrine instability. However, the detail is less precise. The apochryphal pickles and salty foods are rarely craved in scientific observations. The most frequently reported longings are for fruit and fruit juice, followed by milk and dairy products. Suitably flavoured ice cream can score on both accounts. In contrast, in a population of pregnant adolescents, [34] cravings, which were reported by 86 per cent of subjects, often included available 'fast foods' This is perhaps influenced by American teenage culture. In this case, pickles did score higher than ice cream! These subjects also reported development of aversions during their pregnancy, commonly to meat, eggs and pizza. In contrast, Rodin [35] questions the ubiquity of intensity of cravings during pregnancy.

Endocrine fluctuation is cyclical in human females. This may give rise to fluctuation in a variety of physical and physiological signs. The luteal phase of menstrual cycles is dominated by progesterone, comparable to the first trimester of pregnancy. Most studies of the 'pre-menstrual syndrome' assume the inclusion of food cravings (reviewed Bancroft and Backstrom [36]). Various attempts have been made to group putative pre-menstrual signs into clusters. An example is provided by Reinken *et al.*,[37] who found food cravings reported by women in all their suggested sub-sets. There is generally an increase in energy intake. However, this is not simply due to heightened appetite. In self reports from 289 nurses, Smith and Saunder[38] found that foods with sweet tastes were desired in preference to spicy. Some reports suggest a specific appetite for chocolate, rather than generally sweet or carbohydrate, immediately preceding and during menstrual flow.[39] It must be remarked that the concept of 'PMS' has become so diffuse that attempts have been made to restrict the diagnostic criteria. It may be that in some cases it has become a self-fulfilling prophesy.

CASE STUDY

'Cravings' may be very specific. Chocolate is a topical example. The concept of the 'chocoholic' receives widespread coverage in the popular media.[40] Chocolate consumption in the UK in 1994 was 510 000 tonnes, with a market turnover of £3.1 billion. This represents 169 g/head/week, costing £1.03.[41]

It could be suggested that chocolate could satisfy several appetites: for carbohydrate, for sweetness and for fat . In addition, it may provoke a special 'craving'. This could be due to taste and/or other sensory criteria, such as texture (known in the industry as 'mouth feel').[42] It is widely suggested that chocolate has some special pharmacological appeal, possibly influenced by female hormonal shifts. Various explanations have been proposed. The already suggested appetites are non-specific. One example of a suggested specific demand is for magnesium. Some reports have suggested that premenstrual syndrome involves increased glucose tolerance and low plasma magnesium (e.g. Abraham).[43] Oral magnesium supplementation has been claimed to relieve pre-menstrual mood changes.[44] Chocolate could be postulated to redress both of these.

Alternatively, chocolate, has been suggested as providing some positive pharmacological imput. It contains significant levels of methylxanthines, especially caffeine. These have a number of physiological and psychotropic effects, notably arousal (reviewed Clementz and Dailey.[45] It has been suggested that people might self-medicate with caffeine either to obtain stimulation or in order to avoid dysphoria. However, the greater amounts available from, say, coffee, would seem to be more easily accessible. Rozin *et al.*[46] found little evidence for a relationship between 'addiction' to chocolate or the pharmacological (e.g. xanthine-based) effects of chocolate and any 'liking' for it. In addition, in the present context, caffeine has ambiguous impacts, it is recognised to aggravate pre-menstrual symptoms.[47]

Another constituent, phenylethylamine, has excited a good deal of interest. A whole sub-group of psychological disorders, 'hysteroid dysphoria,' was sugested to be linked with shortage of phenylethylamine.[48] Individuals, usually women, are suggested to have repeated episodes of abruptly depressed mood in response to feeling rejected. Leibowitz and Klein remarked that 'when depressed, hysteroid dysphorics often binge on chocolate, which is loaded with phenylethylamine'. The phenylethylamine hypothesis as explanation for various affective disorders has been criticised[49] and in the scientific literature has faded due to lack of further supportive evidence. It persists in folklore, with the appeal of the substance, and therefore of chocolate, ascribed to its production of momentary sensation mimicking, variously, 'love' or 'orgasm'.

Michever and Rozin[50] used chocolate in order to carry out what seems to be the first experimental study directed at differentiating between physiological or sensory accounts of satiation of non-drug cravings. Subjects, at the start of 'craving' consumed a range of chocolate related items. 'White chocolate' produced partial abatement, unchanged by addition of all of the purported pharmacological factors in cocoa. They further suggested a role for aroma, independent of sweetness, texture and calories.

A study[51] was carried out in order to test the hypothesis that there is a menstrual influence on food cravings in young women. The study combined prospective and retrospective methods of investigation. The methodology was developed from that used in a previously published report . The subjects ($n = 52$) were students with an informed interest in healthcare. They completed weekly questionaires recording their immediate 'fancies' for a range of food items, representing a number of categories, including a distinction between 'chocolate' and 'sweet'. Subjects similarly reported on a range of physical signs which could be menstrually influenced. The weekly sheets were completed under the same conditions for five subsequent weeks, encompassing a complete menstrual period. Additional questions solicited a range of further information, including one which enabled phase of menstrual cycle to be determined. The purpose of the enquiry was disguised.

At the end of the investigation, subjects completed a retrospective menstrual questionnaire for comparison. A general questionnaire provided information about a range of possibly confounding factors, such as habits of dietary restraint, use of oral contraceptives, previous pregnancy and self-perceptions.

A smaller number of subjects ($n = 10$) filled in daily sheets, indicating intensity of positive or negative mood and any perceived cravings at that time.

Few significant correlations were found, except for trivial ones, such as that subjects who had missed breakfast reported 'fancies' for foods in all categories. Few data were found to support the suggestion that cyclical changes in female physiology influence 'cravings' for particular foods. However, the concept of craving in relation to food items, in particular to chocolate, continues to attract media attention.

It is suggested that some women, and possibly some men, perceive themselves as feeling strong urges towards certain foods. These urges may be influenced by sensory expectations. Self-awareness may lead such women selectively to be aware during the pre-menstrual phase. This could contribute to an interpretation of their feelings as 'pre-menstrual chocolate craving', as an aspect of pre-menstrual syndrome. It may be that chocolate's image as 'naughty but nice' adds a sense of self-indulgence. Reporting of such perception is diluted in surveys of the general population.

Substantially similar conclusions were drawn by Hetherington and MacDiarmid[52] using different methodology. They recruited self-styled 'chocolate addicts'. Most (76 per cent) of their respondents considered the 'addictive' factor in chocolate to be orosensory (i.e. taste, smell, texture.)

SUMMARY

The phenomena of craving, no matter how contentious is its definition, is very real and a quite unique human sensation. Despite extensive work and attempts at unified theories, the concept of craving eludes rigorous definition. It is in a similar position to other apparently intuitively understood abstractions such as 'drive' or 'motivation'. Progress has been made in identifying possible neural pathways but the link between neural substrates and behavioural state is far from clear.

NOTES

1. Expert Committee on Mental Health and Alcohol, First Report (Geneva: World Health Organisation, 1954).
2. W. P. Pickens and C. E. Johanson, 'Craving: Consensus of Status and Agenda for Future Research', *Drug and Alcohol Dependence*, 30 (1992):127–31.
3. M. D. Kilgus and A. J. Pumariega, 'Experimental Manipulation of Cocaine Craving by Videotaped Environment Cues', *Southern Medical Journal*, 87 (11):1138–40.
4. L. Koslowski, D. Wilkinson, W. Skinner, C. Kent, T. Ranklin and M. Pope, 'Comments on Koslowski and Wilkinson's "Use & Abuse of the concept of craving": A Reply from the Authors', *British Journal of Addiction*, 82 (1989):489.
5. T. Sitharthan and D. McGraph, 'Meaning of Craving in Research on Addiction', *Psychology Report*, 71 (3 Pt 1) (1992):823–6.
6. L. T. Koslowski and M. A. Wilkinson, 'Use and Misuse of the Concept of Cravings by Alcohol, Tobacco and Drug Researchers', *British Journal of Addiction*, 82 (1987):31–6.
7. L. C. Laberg and B. Ellertson, 'Psychophysiological Indictors of Cravings in Alcoholics; Effects of Cue Exposure', *British Journal of Addiction*, 82 (1987):1341–8.
8. R. A. Wise, 'The Neurobiology of Craving: Implications for the Understanding and Treatment of Addiction', *Journal of Abnormal Psychology*, 97(2) (1988):118–32.
9. T. E. Robinson and K. C. Berridge, 'The Neural Basis of Drug Craving: An Incentive-Sensitisation Theory of Addiction', *Brain Research Review*, 18 (1993):247–91.
10. C. E. Cornell, J. Rodin and H. P. Weingarten, 'Stimulus Induced Eating when Satisfied', *Physiology and Behaviour*, 45 (1989):695–704.
11. K. B. Engle and T. K. Williams, 'Effect of an Ounce of Vodka on Alcoholics' Desire for Alcohol', *Quarterly Journal of Studies on Alcohol*, 33 (1972):1099–1105.
12. R. West, P. Hajek and M. Belcher, 'Time Course of Cigarette Withdrawal Symptoms While Using Nicotine Gum', *Psychopharmacology*, 99 (1989):143–5.
13. J. E. Rose, D. P. Tashkin, A. Ertle, M. C. Zinser and R. Lafer, 'Sensory Blockade of Smoking Sensation', *Pharmacology Biochemistry and Behaviour*, 23 (1985):289–93.
14. E. M. Jellinek, H. Isbell, G. Lundquist, H. M. Tiedbout, H. Duchene, J. Mardones, and L. D. Macleod, 'The "Craving" for Alcohol', *Quarterly Journal of Studies on Alcohol*, 16 (1955):33–66.
15. A. D. Dackis and M. S. Gold, 'New Concepts in Cocaine Addiction: The Dopamine Depletion Hypothesis', *International Journal of Psychiatry in Medicine*, 15 (1985):469–77.
16. R. J. Wurtman and J. J. Wurtman. 'Do Carbohydrates Affect Food Intake via Neurotransmitter Activity?', *Appetite*, 11 (Suppl.) (1988):42–7.
17. E. L. Noach, 'Appetite Regulation by Serotonergic Mechanisms and Effects of d-fenfluramine', *Netherlands Journal of Medicine*, 45(3) (1994):123–33.

18. M. Gossop, J. Powell, S. Grey and P. Hajek, 'What do Opiate Addicts and Cigarette Smokers Mean by "Craving"? A Pilot Study', *Drug & Alcohol Dependency*, 26 (1990):85–7.
19. C. P. Richter, 'Total Self-regulatory Functions in Animals and Human Beings. A Review', *Journal of Milk and Food Technology*, 39 (1942):353–403.
20. E. J. Underwood, 'The Mineral Nutrition of Livestock (Commonwealth Agricultural Bureaus, Australia)', cited in H. P. Weingarten and D. Elston, 'The Phenomenology of Food Cravings', *Appetite*, 15 (1990):231–460.
21. D. Denton, *The Hunger for Salt* (New York: Springer).
22. S. C. Wilkins and C. P. Richter, 'A Great Craving for Salt by a Child with Cortico-adrenal Insufficiency', *Journal of the American Medical Association*, 114 (1940):866–8.
23. R. J. Wurtman, F. Heftl, and E. Melamed, 'Precursor Control of Neurotransmittor Synthesis', *Pharmacology Review*, 32(4) (1981):315–415.
24. *Appetite*, Special Issue 8(3) (1987).
25. J. N. Blau, 'What Some Patients can Eat During Migraine Attacks', *Cephalalgia*, 13(4) (1993):293–5.
26. H. P. Weigarten and D. Elston, 'The Phenomenology of Food Cravings', *Appetite*, 15 (1990):231–46.
27. J. E. Mitchell, D. Hatsukami, E. D. Eckert and R. L. Pyle, 'Characteristics of 275 Patients with Bulimia', *American Journal of Psychiatry*, 142 (1985):482–5.
28. D. N. Garner and P. E. Garfinkel, *Handbook of Psychotherapy for Anorexia Nervosa and Bulimia* (New York: Guilford Press, 1985).
29. H. Bjorvell, S. Ronnberg and S. Rossner, 'Eating Patterns Described by a Group of Treatment-seeking Overweight Women and Normal Weight Women', *Scandinavian Journal of Behavioural Therapy*, 14 (1985):147–56.
30. T. P. Beresford and R. C. W. Hall, 'Food and Drug Abuse: The Contrasts and Comparisons of Eating Disorders and Alcoholism', *Psychiatric Medicine*, 7(3) (1989):37–46.
31. S. E. Cooper, 'Chemical Dependency and Eating Disorders: Are they really so Different?', *Journal of Counselling and Development*, 68 (1989):102–5.
32. A. Giles, 'The Longings of Pregnant Women', *Obstetrical Society of London Transactions*, 35 (1893):242–9.
33. G. Dickens and W. H. Trethowan, 'Cravings and Aversions during Pregnancy', *Journal of Psychosomatic Research*, 15 (1971):259–68.
34. J. E. Pope, J. D. Skinner and B. R. Carruth, 'Cravings and Aversions of Pregnant Adolescents', *Journal of the American Dietetics Association*, 92 (1992):1479–482.
35. J. Rodin, 'Cravings and Aversions during Pregnancy', *Appetite*, 12 (1989):76–7.
36. J. Bancroft and T. Backstrom, 'Premenstrual Syndrome', *Clinical Endocrinology*, 22 (1985):313–14.
37. J. A. Reinken, S. R. N. Pullon and M. J. Sparrow, 'Premenstrual Syndrome Defined by Symptom Sets', *Family Practice*, 7(3) (1990):201–4.
38. S. L. Smith and C. Sauder, 'Food Cravings, Depression and Premenstrual Problems', *Psychosomatic Medicine*, (1969) 312–88.

39. R. Tomelleri and K. K. Grunewald, 'Menstrual Cycle and Cravings in Young College Women', *Journal of the American Dietetics Association*, 87 (1987):311–16.
40. 'Chocs and the Single Girl', *Guardian*, 12 February 1993.
41. *Cadbury Market Review* (1995).
42. J. Morgan, 'Chocolate; A Flavour and Texture Unlike Any Other', *American Journal of Clinical Nutrition*, 60 (Suppl.) (1994):1060s–4s.
43. G. E. Abraham, 'Nutrition and the Premenstrual Syndrome', *Journal of Applied Nutrition*, 40 (1984):103–7.
44. F. Facchinetti, P. Borella, G. Sances, L. Fioroni, R. Nappi and A. R. Genazzani, 'Oral Magnesium Successfully Relieves Premenstrual Mood Changes', *Obstetrics and Gynecology*, 78(2) (1991):177–81.
45. G. L. Clementz and J. W. Dailey, 'Psychotropic Effects of Caffeine', *American Family Physicians*, 37 (1988):169.
46. P. Rozin, E. Levine and C. Stoess, 'Chocolate Craving and Liking', *Appetite*, 17 (1991):199–212.
47. A. M. Rossignol and H. Bonnlander, 'Prevalence and Severity of the Premenstrual Syndrome', *Journal of Reproduction Medicine*, 36(2) (1991):131–6.
48. M. R. Leibowitz, and D. F. Klein, 'Hysteroid Dysphoria', *Psychiatric Clinical Studies in North American*, 2(3) (1979):555.
49. A. D. Mosnaim and M. W. Wolf (eds), *Noncatecholic Phenylethylamines*, Part 1: *Biological Mechanisms and Clinical Aspects* (New York: Marcel Dekker).
50. A. D. Michever and P. Rozin, 'Pharmacological versus Sensory Factors in the Satiation of Chocolate Craving', *Physiology Behaviour* 56(3) (1994):419–22.
51. D. R. Peers, 'Perimenstrual Chocolate Craving in Healthy Young Women' thesis, University of Surrey.
52. M. M. Hetherington and J. I. Macdiarmid, '"Chocolate Addiction": A Preliminary Study of its Description and its Relationship to Problem Eating', *Appetite*, 21 (1993):233–46.

12 The Biological Basis of Bulimia Nervosa
Sarah Brien

INTRODUCTION

Bulimia nervosa is a distressing disorder. This chapter attempts to address some of the research findings from studies performed since 1979 when bulimia was first diagnosed as a psychiatric illness by Russell.[1] The increasing prevalence of bulimia in our society highlights the continuing need for research to aid our understanding as to why certain individuals will become bulimic and continue to maintain their behaviour in spite of the obvious physical and emotional detriment to themselves. A myriad of factors contribute to its initiation and maintenance and an eclectic view becomes both necessary and appropriate. Although the following chapter will concentrate specifically on the role of the neurotransmitter serotonin in its pathogenesis and maintenance, the disorder bulimia involves a range of other factors. A thorough discussion of the psychological and social aspects of this disorder is not feasible here, but where appropriate reference to pertinent aspects of these approaches will be made.

THE CLINICAL FEATURES AND THE PREVALENCE OF BULIMIA NERVOSA

Bulimia was first described by Russell in 1979 who described it as 'an ominant variant of anorexia nervosa'. It was in 1980 that bulimia was first classified as a distinct clinical entity by the American Psychiatric Association (APA)[2] and the current criteria (revised by the APA, 1987)[3] used for diagnosis of bulimia are shown in Table 12.1.

From a clinical view, bulimia nervosa normally commences with the individual starting a weight reducing diet which continues, triggering of a cycle of binging, purging (to get rid of the excess calories) and then starvation (as indicated in Figure 12.1). A binge has been defined as 'an episode or episodes of uncontrolled eating in which a

TABLE 12.1   *Diagnostic criteria for bulimia nervosa*

1. Recurrent episodes of binge eating (i.e. the rapid consumption of a large amount of food in a discrete period of time).

2. A feeling of lack of control over eating behaviour during the eating binges.

3. The person engages in either self-induced vomiting, use of laxatives or diuretics, strict dieting or fasting, or vigorous exercise in order to prevent weight gain.

4. A minimum average of two binge eating episodes a week, for at least three months.

5. Persistent overconcern with body shape and weight.

SOURCE: From *Diagnostic and Statistical Manual of Mental Disorders*, 3rd edn, revised (Washington, DC: American Psychiatric Association, 1987), pp. 68–9.

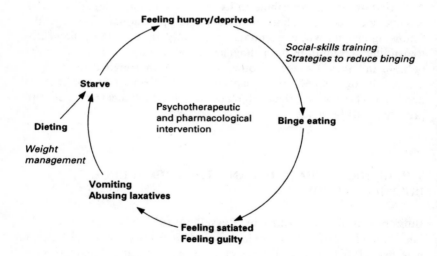

Figure 12.1   Phases of eating behaviour leading to bulimia, showing personal and professional interventions (*in italics*).
Source: Modified from L. K. Hsu and D. Holder, 'Bulimia Nervosa: Treatment and Short-term Outcome', *Psychological Medicine*, 16 (1986): 65–70.

TABLE 12.2   *Clinical features of bulimia nervosa and normal weight*
bulimic sufferers

Feature	Bulimia nervosa	Normal weight bulimia
Weight loss	Severe	Minimal to moderate
Body weight	Low	Normal
Amenorrhea	Present	Variable
Bulimia	Present	Present
Vomiting/purging	Present	Present
Fear of fatness	Present	Present

SOURCE: *European Diagnostic and Statistical Manual* (International Classification of Disease, 1993)

huge amount of food is consumed, often rapidly and in secret. These episodes often end because of stomach pains, interruptions by others, running out of food supplies or vomiting. Although the actual eating may be enjoyable, afterwards the individual invariably feels disgusted, guilty and depressed.'[4] The clinical features of the disorder have been described in detail[5] and they include a significant degree of psychological morbidity with a high degree of depressive symptoms including anxiety, irritability, insomnia and social withdrawal. In addition, alcohol or substance abuse and menstrual disturbances are common. Bulimic sufferers are clinically differentiated into two types as identified in Table 12.2, dependent on body weight; that is bulimia nervosa sufferers (i.e. who have previously experienced anorexia nervosa before) and normal weight bulimics (i.e. those whose weight is in the normal range but wish to be lighter).

Bulimia is often seen as a modern disease of Western society. However, the first detailed description of the disorder (although anecdotal) was published by Pierre Janet in 1903 who described a patient in the nineteenth century with the now-recognised classic symptoms. In his discussion, Janet suggested a possible association between the major affective disorders and the condition now referred to as bulimia. Since his observation, there has subsequently been numerous discussions by others concerning this putative link (for example, Pope *et al.*).[6] Since these early observations, the increase in the prevalence of the disorder in Western countries[5, 7] could be attributed, in part, to the growing cultural pressure on women to maintain thier body weight at (probably) unrealistically low levels. In the last three decades, slimness has been associated as a product of Western society, and related in the media with 'attractiveness' and 'success'. Indeed studies indicate that there has been an increase in binge eating and dieting amongst young 'healthy' women.[8] It is unlikely that sociocultural phenomena alone could explain the aetiology of the growing incidence of bulimia but it should be considered as one of the major modern influences amongst women today.

Although there are inherent difficulties in obtaining information regarding the prevalence of bulimia within the UK, the Eating Disorder Association estimates that three out of 100 women in the UK suffer from bulimia.[9] However, in 'at risk' populations such as female adolescents and college students, the prevalence is thought to be much higher. Bulimia is not, as commonly thought, a solely female disorder. Predominantly it is more common in females but male sufferers are known.[10] The ratio of female: male sufferers is thought to be in the region of about 10 : 1. However, this ratio may be misleading as the association of bulimia as a female disorder would result in more women than men seeking the help, thereby masking the real prevalence of male sufferers.

Over recent years, the prevalence of bulimia has increased. This could be a result of several factors. It could be of course solely due to an increase in the actual number of sufferers. However, other factors may be indirectly contributing to the rise. For example, the media has recently highlighted this disorder and has resulted in increased general awareness and understanding about this disorder. Bulimia is usually very much a secretive behaviour but increasing public awareness (aided by 'Royal patronage') is making it more common for personal exposés. Additionally since bulimic behaviour now has a 'label' it is therefore easier for sufferers to seek both professional and non-professional help.[11] This has been aided by the way that bulimia has been promoted (to the general public) as an illness or an addiction, since it conveys less responsibility for the individual and implicitly less self blame.

BULIMIA AS AN ADDICTION

In recent years it has been suggested that bulimia could be classified as an addiction, since it could be seen to conform to certain criteria indicative of an addictive style behaviour. For example, bulimic sufferers display the following:

- repeated episodes of excessive consumption;
- repeated unsuccessful attempts to stop the excessive consumption;
- changing lifestyle to provide the time and money for the behaviour;
- increase in severity of the symptoms over time;
- decreased social adjustment;
- increased urge to binge after consuming a small amount of food.

Russell[1] first noted that bulimic behaviour can occur in conjunction with other forms of addictive behaviours, such as alcoholism and drug abuse. Subsequently, there has been an increasing number of reports in the literature of coprevalence of substance use/abuse in eating disordered individuals. This appears to be more so in those with a bulimic component to their disorder (i.e. normal weight bulimia, bulimia nervosa and bulimic anorexia sufferers) rather than food restricting (i.e. anorexic) behaviour (reviewed by Holdensen *et al.*).[12] Bulimia can therefore be seen as an addiction, i.e. that the sufferer is addicted to the binging and purging behaviour.

Studies have indicated that bulimic sufferers do have increased frequency of other altered behaviours such as suicidal tendencies, self injury, substance misuse/abuse, and stealing.[13] These types of behaviours can all be distinguished by their core pathology of impulsivity. In 1993, Lacey[14] proposed that a distinct subgroup of individuals with bulimia existed, which he referred to as multi-impulsive bulimics. This was based on the findings of Lacey and Evans[15] who identified individuals who suffered from multi-impulsive personality disorder, abusing a range of substances. They suggested that these individuals failed to control their impulses resulting in abnormal control which is expressed, for example, as repetitive self-harm or overdosing, alcohol or substance abuse or dependence, shoplifting or sexual disinhibitions. The study by Lacey[14] was based on an assessment of 112 consecutive patients seeking treatment for bulimia, and showed that self-damaging and addictive behaviour are common in bulimic women. Forty per cent of the group reported self-damaging and other addictive behaviours. Alcohol abuse was significantly associated with drug abuse and repeated overdosing; and repeated self-mutilation was associated with alcohol and drug abuse. The study identified that bulimics did not restrict themselves to only one damaging or addictive behaviour, 80 per cent reporting at least three self-damaging behaviours. The subjects reported that each behaviour was associated with a 'similar sense of being out of control', and that they had a 'similar function', i.e. of reducing or blocking unpleasant or distressing feelings.

The link between eating disorders and substance abuse has been investigated from different perspectives than that of the 'poor impulse controller' defined by Lacey. For example, Brisman and Siegal[16] suggested that the existence of an 'addictive personality' would predispose an individual to become addicted to one or more substances. From a psychoanalytic construct, it is suggested that these individuals have regressed psychological to the oral phase of development.[17] However, subsequent research on personality characteristics commonly found in both food and substance misusers has not yielded any conclusive findings, with the exception of impulsive behaviours. Alternatively, it has been suggested that the consumption of food or substances is a coping mechanism which alleviates dysphoric feelings. Filstaed *et al.*[18] looked at individual responses in those situations that precipitate binges on food or other substances, to try to identify if it is the actual behaviour that is addictive and not the substance. No conclusions though were drawn from this study.

It has also been suggested that the physiological and behavioural patterns associated with an addiction could leave the individual vulnerable to other addictions. Evidence for this has been sought by Hudson *et al.*[19] and Mitchell *et al.*[20] Again, no specific conclusions were reached from these studies. Genetic factors have been implicated in comorbidity, indeed the role of inheritance in the development of eating disorders[21] and substance abuse (e.g. alcoholism)[22] indicate that this might be the case. Studies along similar lines suggest that the link between several addictions could be a result of genetic changes in neurochemical or neuropeptide physiology that may regulate the neural basis of those behaviours associated with addictions.

Therefore it can be seen that there could potentially be many complex factors which result in this comorbodity that yet to remain answered. Population data points to there being a higher co-prevalence with other addictions than would be expected by chance, but the reasons still remain open to speculation.

BIOLOGICAL FACTORS IN EATING DISORDERS

Historically, early attention focused on the hormonal changes seen in bulimia: initially bulimia was considered to be a manifestation of underlying pathological processes within the pituitary gland (Simmonds, 1914 as cited in Kaplan and Woodside[23]. This theory was dismissed in the

1940s and attempts to define a psychoanalytical construct were made. The therapies that derived from these psychological approaches, although providing valuable insight into the disorder, proved ineffective in treating the psychopathological disturbances and in normalising eating behaviour. Therefore in recent years attention focused once more on the biological aspects of this disorder.

During the 1980s and 1990s, there has been a large expansion in research into the biological basis of bulimia. Indirect clinical evidence suggests that biological factors may contribute to the development and/ or the persistence of this eating disorder. Many of the hormonal and neuroendocrinological abnormalities are now *thought* to be secondary to the disorder, i.e. as a result of the binge–purge cycle. A number of studies are presently addressing this issue. Four main areas of research have been reviewed[23] as follows.

Hypothalamic Pituitary Axis (HPA)

The hypothalamus, in response to neural and hormonal inputs, in association with the pituitary gland, is responsible for the regulation of most of the body's hormonal activities; those which are affected in normal weight bulimics are:

(a) reproductive functions: menstrual abnormalities are frequent;
(b) cortisol secretion: between 20 and 60 per cent of bulimics have an abnormal dexamethasone suppression test (DST), the neuroendocrine test used as a functional test of the HPA.

Central Nervous System Peptides

The *endorphins and enkephalins* play a role in the regulation of the pituitary gland. They are structurally similar to opiates and may act as neurotransmitters. Endorphins have been implicated both addictive behaviours and in the control of eating. The evidence linking opiates to eating behaviour is summarised below:

- that levels are elevated in genetically obese rats;
- that when injected into the ventromedial hypothalamus of satiated rats, food intake is stimulated;
- that the opioid antagonist, naloxone, reduces food intake in deprived rats, abolishes overeating in genetically obese mice and causes loss of weight and appetite when administered to humans, causing a decrease in binge frequency in bulimic patients.

Gastrointestinal Hormones

The gastrointestinal tract is active in hormone secretion. The function of many of these hormones in eating disorders remain unclear. However, the hormone cholecystokinin (CCK), which is located in both the gut and the brain, is involved in satiety regulation[24] and has been implicated in bulimia. In healthy individuals CCK is secreted after the ingestion of food, when the food passes from the stomach to the duodenum. Once the released CCK reaches a specific level, individuals become satiated and stop eating. However, in bulimia the levels of CCK secreted are generally low (perhaps because the food leaves their stomach slowly or not at all if it is vomited) so as a result bulimics will not reach the point of satiation so they remain hungry. The persistent hunger could therefore cause them to gorge repeatedly.[25]

Central Nervous System Amines

Several amines that act as neurotransmitters in the central nervous system (e.g. serotonin, noradrenaline and dopamine) are believed to be involved in the control of food intake. The actual mechanisms are still not clear but are thought to act via the hypothalamus. Serotonin (5-hydroxytryptamine, 5-HT), within the lateral hypothalamus, inhibits the process of food intake. Dopamine on the other hand stimulates the intake of food.[26] Noradrenaline has a dual action, dependant on its location. Within the lateral hypothalamus it acts to inhibit food intake; but in the medial hypothalamus it stimulated food intake.

THE ROLE OF SEROTONIN IN BULIMIA

The neurotransmitter serotonin is synthesised from the dietary essential amino acid tryptophan and was first identified in nerve cells in 1962[27] and then later distinguished in specific neurones using fluorescence microscopy.[28] The majority of serotonin (approximately 90 per cent) is found in the gastric mucosa enterochromaffin cells and blood platelets. However, serotonin is also synthesised within the CNS (where it acts as a neurotransmitter) from its dietary precursor by the action of the rate-limiting enzyme tryptophan hydroxylase (discussed in more detail in Chapter 4). The synthesis of central serotonin production is regulated and affected by several factors which are listed below.

1. **Ratio of bound to unbound tryptophan.** Tryptophan, normally bound to albumin, needs to be in an unbound state to cross the blood brain barrier to be converted centrally to serotonin.[29]
2. **Activity of the tryptophan pyrrolase enzyme.** Increased activity of this liver enzyme results in reduced tryptophan availability for 5HT synthesis (Chapter 4).
3. **Blood–brain barrier transport system competition.** The ratio of tryptophan to large neutral amino acids (as indicated by T/LNAA) determines the entry of tryptophan into the central nervous system (CNS); an increased T/LNAA ratio results in increased tryptophan entry into the CNS.[30] Kynurenine pathway metabolites also, to a limited extent compete with tryptophan for entry into the CNS.[31, 32]
4. **Immune system activation – the activity of the indoleamine 2,3 dioxygenase.** This enzyme also catalyses tryptophan to kynurenine but is only activated when the immune system is stimulated.
5. **Diet.** A high carbohydrate diet elevates the ratio of T/LNAA via the release of insulin,[33] resulting in the elevation of brain tryptophan and brain serotonin levels;[34] conversely a high protein diet leads to a reduction, reducing brain serotonin synthesis.[30]
6. **Gonadal hormones.** Findings (mainly from animal studies) have indicated that gonadal hormones can exert an effect, be it direct or indirect, on the metabolism of tryptophan.[32, 35–40]

It is becoming increasingly clear that particular aspects of feeding behaviour are mediated via specific receptors in the CNS. To date, four families of serotonin receptors have been identified within the CNS and the periphery[41] – see Table 12.3.

HOW COULD ALTERED SEROTONIN FUNCTION BE IMPLICATED IN BULIMIA NERVOSA?

Neurochemical alterations may have a pathological role in bulimia.[42] Several neurotransmitters and neuromodulators are known to be involved in the regulation of eating behaviour in animals and have also been implicated in symptoms such as depression and anxiety which are frequently observed in bulimics.

TABLE 12.3 *The distribution of serotonin receptors in the brain*

Receptor type	Localisation	Behaviour effected
5HT1a	Dorsal raphe Hippocampus Cortex	Antihypertensive Feeding Sexual behaviour
5HT1b	Substantia nigra Basal ganglia	Motor behaviour Emotional?
5HT1c	Choroid plexus Globus pallidus Substantia nigra	CSF regulation Motor behaviour
5HT1d	Substantia nigra Basal ganglia Subiculum	Motor behaviour Feeding behaviour Anxiety
5HT2	Claustrum Olfactory tubercle Cortex	Emotional Sleep
5HT3	Dorsal vagal nerve Solitary tract nerve Trigemminal nerve Area postrema Spinal cord Limbic system	Anti-emetic Learning Deficit Addiction Anxiety
5HT4	Colliculus Hippocampus	Feeding Emotional

Serotonin in the Control of Eating Behaviour

In support of the argument of a putative role for serotonin in bulimia is the fact that the serotonergic systems occupy a strategic anatomical location known to be pivotal in the control of feeding behaviour. [Serotonergic neurones arise from a series of nuclei in the middle of the brainstem (the raphe nuclei) which descend to the spinal cord to innervate peripheral organs. The terminals of the serotonergic neurones are diffusely distributed, specifically to the hypothalamus and the amygloid nucleus.] Additionally, serotonergic neurones are also widely distributed in the gut and this again points to serotonin having a potential role in the control of eating. Lesioning the paraventricular nuclei, ventromedial nuclei and the suprachiasmatic nuclei of the hypothalamus in the rat has been demonstrated to result in dysregulation of feeding. However, lesions of the midbrain raphe nuclei does not alter feeding[43] suggesting that feeding behaviour is mediated specifically via the hypothalamus. Recent advances in molecular biological techniques have identified specific serotonergic receptors which are involved in the control of eating. These include 5HT1a, 5HT1c, 5HT1d and possibly the 5HT4 family (refer to Table 12.3 for a summary of the serotonergic receptor subtypes identified to date).

Serotonin could be implicated in either the initiation or maintenance of bulimia for three reasons. Firstly, bulimia nervosa is characterised by frequent uncontrollable urges to binge, i.e. the process of satiety does not function in a normal manner. Secondly, bulimia is characterised by psychological disturbances, e.g. depression, anxiety and impulsivity, all of which have a neurobiological element. Thirdly, eating disorders are frequently preceded by a period of dieting which physiologically increase an individuals neurobiological vulnerability, leading the individual to develop bulimic behaviour . However, what is still unknown is whether serotonin plays a causal role in triggering bulimia; certainly altered serotonergic function can be seen to be a consequence of the behaviour.

There is increasing evidence, therefore, that serotonin plays an important role in the inhibition of feeding and could have a very important role in the pathogenesis and continuation of bulimic behaviour. If central serotonin function is decreased in bulimia, as various studies suggest, then this would alter the satiety cascade that brings a period of eating to a halt, resulting in an excessive quantity of food intake, i.e. a binge. It has been suggested that the post-absorptive phase involved in the termination of feeding would be lost in a bulimic episode, as a result of the accompanying vomiting, and as such would destroy the satiety cascade. Serotonin has been shown to play a very important stage in this inhibitory stage.

The Role of Serotonin in Mediating Mood States: Possible Evidence to Implicate Altered Serotonergic Activity in Bulimics

The behavioural disturbances of bulimia are accompanied by a wide range of mood disturbance in particular depression and anxiety.[1, 5] Indeed it has been demonstrated that one of the precipitating antecedents of a binging episodes is a negative mood state. Schlundt *et al.*[44] showed that negative moods were predictive of binging whereas positive moods were associated with a reduced probability of binging. Studies have revealed, using both self report measures and objective testing, that measures of stress and depression were predictive of binge eating in both an eating-disordered and a college student population.[45, 46]

It has been well-documented that bulimic individuals have mood disorders which may reflect a neurobiological component of the disorder.[47] Reduced serotonergic activity has also been implicated in the aetiology of depression.[48, 49] Evidence for reduced central serotonin activity in depressed patients has accumulated over the last decade.[50] Reduced T/LNAA ratios (see above) have been shown in depressed patients, a reflection of reduced tryptophan uptake into the brain[51, 52] and a correlation between the ratio and severity of depression has been demonstrated by De Meyer *et al.*[53] Furthermore, platelet 5HT2 receptor binding changes in correlation with changes in clinical state;[54] and, 5HT2 binding sites on the post-synaptic membrane increase in depressed individuals[55] but after corrective antidepressant treatment return to normal.

This 'up-regulation' of binding sites is suggested to occur due to reduced presynaptic output of serotonin and/or decreased innervation of the serotonin neurones.[56] Reduced CSF levels of HIAA have been shown in depressed patients[57, 58] but not all. More consistently an inverse relationship has been demonstrated between suicide attempt (i.e. impulsive behaviour) in unipolar depressed patients and HIAA levels.[58] It has been inferred from studies that serotonin deficiencies are a predisposing factor in depression and not a direct causal effect.[48] Depressed mood is therefore likely to reflect decreased serotonin function and could represent a common link between bulimia and depressive illness.

This has led to a considerable amount of research into a possible serotonergic link between depression and bulimia. Bulimics have a high lifetime rate of major affective disorders,[59] and a study by Vieselman and Rolg[60] showed that 79 per cent of their bulimic samples had concurrent depression. Walsh *et al.*[61] identified in their study that 75 per cent of their bulimic population developed mood disturbances at the onset (or shortly after) the first episode of bulimia. It has also been demonstrated that there is a higher than average likelihood of family depression.[62] There is good support, therefore, for a link between bulimia and depression. Further evidence comes from studies which have demonstrated that antidepressant drugs reduce the symptoms of bingeing and vomiting in bulimics. There has been a lively debate over the past decade concerning the link of depression and bulimia (reviewed by Swift *et al.*[63] and Jimmerson *et al.*[64]). Three views have been presented to date as follows.

1. That bulimia may be a variant expression of primary mood disturbance, i.e. bulimia is secondary to the depressive symptoms and that the binge/vomit behaviour is used to relieve depression (on the basis of 'self medication'). However, studies have shown that depression is not altered significantly after a binge although anxiety, guilt and tension were significantly reduced.[59]
2. That the mood disturbance is secondary to the eating disorder, and that mood will lift as the eating behaviour 'normalises'.[4] This approach is currently the most popular.
3. An alternative view has been proposed (e.g. by Garfinkel and Garner[65]). This eclectic model suggests that eating disorders such as bulimia are the result of an interplay of many forces (biological, psychological, familial and sociocultural) and not the result of a single determinant factor.

Although the evidence outlined above suggests a possible link between the affective disorders and bulimia, criticisms have been made which may not make the evidence conclusive.[66] For example, the raters who made the concurrent diagnoses in these studies were aware of the primary eating disorder and therefore may have biased the outcome. The positive response of antidepressant medication in bulimic symptoms[67] does not necessarily confirm a relationship since antidepressants have shown a positive response in a broad range of disorders. Finally, in addition, bulimics exhibit other psychopathological symptoms such as anxiety, alcohol and substance abuse that are not demonstrated in individuals with major affective disorders.

Bulimia has frequently been described as an impulsive-style behaviour. Descriptions of the binge eating episodes have been described by bulimics as unplanned and impulsive and 'out of control'. Studies have indicated that bulimic patients have increased frequencies of behaviours including suicidal attempts, self-injury, substance abuse and stealing.[13] These behaviours can all be distinguished by their core pathology of impulsivity, and it is only recently that impulsivity has been seen as a basic psychological trait. From a neurobiological view, impulsive style behaviours have been identified with lowered serotonin function.[68, 69] Apter *et al.*[70] suggest that low mood, aggression and impulsivity and anxiety may be linked by an common basic neurobiological component, i.e. reduced serotonergic function. However, correlation between impulsive ratings and degree of symptomology has not been corroborated.[71] Decreased central serotonin function could potentially contribute to impaired satiety and therefore to increased tendency to binging.[72]

The Effect of Dieting on Serotonergic Function

In recent years it has been suggested that dietary behaviour could be causal in the development of eating disorders *per se*.[73, 74] By definition dieting and eating disorders are correlated. There is some evidence which implicates a causal role for dieting. For example, occupations that entail low body weight such as dancers and models, do have a higher rate of eating disorders; bulimic tendencies frequently follow periods of dieting (although of course not all dieters binge, nor all bingers diet); bulimics often have been dieting shortly before or at the time of the development of their eating disorder. Prospective studies have also indicated that the actual activity of dieting led to the development of eating disorder.

The action of restricting food to lose weight brings about a wide range of physiological changes. Goodwin, Fairburn and Cowen[75] demonstrated that after a period of moderate dieting (for 3 weeks) an altered serotonin neuroendocrine response could be demonstrated in women but not men (a tryptophan load was given to both males and females and the prolactin response noted). All the subjects that participated in this study were healthy and had no known family history of affective disorder, and as such these results indicate that women may be more vulnerable to men to diet induced changes in brain serotonin function, an interesting finding considering the preponderance of women with eating disorders. This finding could be important since women frequently become bulimic after a period of successful dieting.

Bulimics could, therefore, self-perpetuate their reduced levels of tryptophan and hence serotonin levels through repetitive dieting behaviour. Studies have investigated the types of foods consumed during binging periods. There are problems inherent in investigating this; the majority of studies have been laboratory based and may therefore not be equivalent to a natural binge; and self-report measures may not be totally truthful. However, in spite of this the majority of studies are quite unanimous in revealing that binge foods are high in both fats and carbohydrates.[76–79] It has been suggested that binging on high carbohydrate type foods may represent a self-regulatory attempt to improve negative mood state, as has been suggested in other disorders, e.g. such as seasonal affective disorder.[80]

SUMMARY OF EVIDENCE FOR ALTERED SEROTONERGIC ACTIVITY IN BULIMIA

The role of serotonin has been extensively investigated and numerous studies indicate that decreased serotonin function exists in this disorder.[81, 82] It remains unclear whether the abnormal metabolism of serotonin predates the onset of the bulimic symptoms, whether it results from dietary abnormalities due to erratic eating patterns, or whether it could be due to other concurrent psychophysiological aspects of the disorder (anxiety, stress, etc).

A body of research has implicated altered serotonergic activity in bulimia. Decreased serotonin activity and function has been found to exist in active bulimic sufferers.[81, 82] The following findings are presented in support of this argument.

1. **Antidepressants** are an effective treatment in both depressed and non depressed bulimics,[83] by reducing binge frequency.[84] (However, the positive response of antidepressant medication does not in itself confirm a relationship since antidepressants have shown a positive response in a broad range of disorders.)

2. **CSF studies** – no studies have been performed on normal weight bulimics. However, administration of probenecid to bulimic anorectic and non-bulimic anorectic led to less accumulation of the serotonin metabolite, HIAA in bulimics; which is indicative of reduced serotonin activity.[85]

3. **Neuroendocrine studies** – in healthy individuals, the administration of a serotonin agonist will result in increased prolactin secretion which could be a reflection of increased serotonergic activity. However, the administration of the agonist mCPP to bulimic patients demonstrated a significant decrease in prolactin secretion compared to the controls.[86] There is considerable evidence suggesting that prolactin secretion by the anterior pituitary gland is regulated in part by the serotonergic system. Direct serotonin receptor agonists, as well as large doses of 5HTP or tryptophan, lead to increase in plasma prolactin in healthy humans. Delgado *et al.*[87] demonstrated that after normal subjects were depleted of tryptophan by dietary manipulation, later infusion of tryptophan led to enhanced prolactin response which may be an indication of increased post-synaptic serotonin receptor sensitivity. However, determining the role of serotonin in bulimia via the release of prolactin is complicated as the mechanisms

underlying serotonin stimulation in prolactin is not clearly defined.

4. **Platelet uptake of 5HT** – the rate of uptake of serotonin in blood platelets has been suggested to reflect synaptic serotonergic uptake and as such has been used as an indirect model for synaptic uptake.[42] Increased platelet serotonin uptake has been identified in bulimics.[55] In addition to this, Biegon *et al.*[54] demonstrated that changes in platelet 5HT2 receptor binding changed correlated with changes in clinical state.

5. **Precursor availability studies** – several studies have measured the ratio of tryptophan to other large neutral amino acids (T/LNAA) in bulimics as an index of tryptophan uptake across the blood–brain barrier both before and after a binge. This ratio was increased in those bulimics who felt satiated after one or more binges; no increase though was noted in those bulimics who did not feel satiated.[88]

CONCLUSION

A wide range of studies has clearly provided substantial evidence that serotoninergic function is altered in bulimia. What remains unclear is if this purported deficiency is a result of the behavior, a cause of the bulimic behaviour, or is it a predisposing factor? This and many other questions remain open to speculation. This review has highlighted the complex and numerous range of biological factors which appear to be involved in bulimia. Considering the very nature of bulimia, to increase our understanding of this distressing and complicated disorder the way forward in research is to adopt a multidisciplinary approach. The onset and continuation of bulimic behaviour cannot be solely a result of neurochemical changes. It is feasible that altered activity of neurochemical systems may be a trigger, but there needs to be a context in which the behaviour (i.e. eating) becomes so altered. Despite the mass of interactions of biological, social and psychological factors that all play a role in this disorder, continued analysis of the individual components and their integration into combined data sets will, hopefully, provide an insight into those aspects of bulimia which might be amenable for therapeutic exploitation.

FUTURE AREAS TO BE CONSIDERED FOR RESEARCH

Future research in the biological sciences could address some of the following aspects of serotonergic function in bulimia. The liver enzyme, tryptophan pyrrolase, could potentially be a regulatory factor in the synthesis of serotonin in bulimics, by (a) its ability to divert tryptophan from serotonin synthesis, and (b) by inhibiting the transport of tryptophan into the CNS, and could therefore be causal in the development of bulimia. However, to date, the role of the metabolites of this liver enzymic pathway in the pathogenesis of bulimia has received no attention.

A second area amenable for research is that of the effect of female gonadal hormones on the synthesis and production of serotonin. In spite of the fact that eating disorders occur most commonly in women, little attention has been paid to either its effect on reproductive status or, alternatively, the role female gonadal hormones could play in precipitating disordered eating. Anorexia, by definition, causes amenorrhoea, a fact known for over a century. However, the disturbance of reproductive function in bulimics has been only been investigated during the last decade and studies suggest that approximately 50 per cent of bulimic women have abnormal cycles. Recent studies have shown that unexplained infertility in women may sometimes be due to an undisclosed eating disorder or severe weight control.[89] In addition, exacerbation of binging during the premenstrual phase of bulimics with intact cycles has been demonstrated.[90, 91] Gonadal hormones could play a role in mediating serotonin synthesis and, therefore, by inference those specific behaviours in bulimia that are known to be disrupted, e.g. eating control and mood states.

NOTES

1. G. Russell, 'Bulimia Nervosa: An Ominant Variant of Anorexia Nervosa', *Psychological Medicine*, 9 (1979):429–48.
2. American Psychiatric Association (APA), *Diagnostic and Statistical Manual* (Washington, DC: APA, 1980).
3. American Psychiatric Association (APA), *Diagnostic and Statistical Manual* (Washington, DC: APA, 1987).
4. P. J. Cooper and C. G. Fairburn, 'The Depressive Symptoms of Bulimia Nervosa', *British Journal of Psychiatry*, 148 (1986):268–74.
5. C. G. Fairburn and P. J. Cooper, 'The Clinical Features of Bulimia Nervosa', *British Journal of Psychiatry*, 144 (1984):238–46.

6. H. G. Pope, J. I. Hudson and J. P. Mailet, 'Bulimia in the Late Nineteenth Century: The Observations of Pierre Janet', *Psychological Medicine*, 15 (1985):739–43.
7. J. H. Lacey, C. Chadbund, A. H. Crisp *et al.*, 'Variation in Energy Intake of Adolescent Schoolgirls', *Journal of Human Nutrition*, 32 (1978):419–26.
8. M. Vollrath, R. Koch and S. Angst, 'Binge Eating and Weight Concern Among Young Women', *British Journal of Psychiatry*, 160 (1992):498–503.
9. Eating Disorders Association, *Basic Factsheet* (1994), abstract.
10. J. E. Mitchell and G. Goff, 'Bulimia in Male Patients', *Psychosomatics*, 25 (1984):909–13.
11. T. Habermas, 'Possible Effects of the Popular and Medical Recognition of Bulimia Nervosa', *British Journal of Medical Psychology*, 65 (1992):59–66.
12. E. Hackmann, A. WirzJustice and M. Lichsteiner, 'The Uptake of Dopamine and Serotonin in the Rat Brain During Progesterone Decline', *Psychopharmacologia*, 32 (1973):183–91.
13. D. M. Garner, P. E. Garfinkel and M. O'Shaughnessy, 'The Validity of the Distinction between Bulimia with and without Anorexia Nervosa', *American Journal of Psychiatry*, 142 (1985):581–7.
14. J. H. Lacey, 'Self Damaging and Addictive Behaviour in Bulimia Nervosa: A Catchment Area Study', *British Journal of Psychiatry*, 163 (1993):190–4.
15. J. H. Lacey and C. D. Evans, 'The Impulsivist: A Multi-impulsive Personality Disorder', *British Journal of Addiction*, 81 (1986):715–23.
16. C. C. Holderness, J. Brooks-Gunn and M. P. Warren, 'Co-morbidity of Eating Disorders and Substance Abuse. Review of the Literature', *International Journal of Eating Disorders*, 16 (1994):1–34.
17. M. D. Beary, J. H. Lacey and J. Merry, 'Alcoholism and Eating Disorders in Women of Fertile Age', *British Journal of Addiction*, 81 (1986):685–9.
18. J. Brisman and M. Siegel, 'Bulimia and Alcoholism; Two Sides of the Same Coin?', *Journal of Substance Abuse*, 1 (1984):113–8.
19. W. J. Filstead, D. P. Parrella and J. Ebbitt, 'High Risk Situations for Engaging in Substance Abuse and Binge Eating Behaviours', *Journal of Studies on Alcohol*, 49 (1988):136–41.
20. J. I. Hudson, H. G. Pope, D. Yurgelun-Todd *et al.*, 'A Controlled Study of Lifetime Prevalence of Affective and other Psychiatric Disorders in Bulimic Outpatients', *American Journal of Psychiatry*, 144 (1987):1283–7.
21. J. E. Mitchell, R. Pyle, E. C. Eckert *et al.*, 'The Influence of Prior Alcohol and Drug Abuse Problems on Bulimia Nervosa Treatment Outcome', *Addictive Behaviours*, 15 (1990):169–73.
22. M. Strober, 'Family Genetic Studies of Eating Disorders', *Journal of Clinical Psychiatry*, 52 (1991):9–12.
23. A. S. Kaplan and D. B. Woodside, 'Biological Aspects of Anorexia Nervosa and Bulimia Nervosa', *Journal of Consulting and Clinical Psychology*, 55 (1987):645–53.
24. K. M. Pirke, M. B. Kellner, E. Frieb *et al.*, 'Satiety and Cholecystokinin', *International Journal of Eating Disorders*, 15 (1994):63–9.

25. T. L. Abel, 'Gastric Electromechanical and Neurohormonal Function in Anorexia Nervosa', *Gastroenterology*, 93 (1987):958–65.
26. S. F. Leibowitz and G. Shur Posner, 'Brain Serotonin and Eating Behaviour, *Appetite*, 7 (1986):1–14.
27. A. Heller, J. A. Harvey and R. Y. Moore, 'A Demonstration of a Fall in Brain Serotonin Following CNS Lesions in the Rat', *Biochemical Pharmacology*, 11 (1962):859–66.
28. N. E. Anden, K. Fuxe and K. Carsson, 'Effects of Large Mesencephalic–Diencephalic Lesions on Noradrenaline, Dopamine and Serotonin Neurones of the Central Nervous System', *Experientia*, 22 (1966):759–64.
29. G. Curzon and P. J. Knott, 'Effects on Plasma and Brain Tryptophan in the Rat, of Drugs and Hormones that Influence the Concentration on Unesterified Fatty acids in Plasma', *British Journal of Pharmacology*, 50 (1974):197–214.
30. J. D. Fernstrom and R. J. Wurtman, 'Brain Serotonin Content: Physiological Regulation by Plasma Neutral Amino Acids', *Science*, 178 (1972):414–6.
31. A. R. Green and G. Curzon, 'The Effect of Tryptophan Metabolites on Brain Serotonin Metabolism', *Biochemical Pharmacology*, 19 (1970):2061–8.
32. D. A. Bender, 'Oestrogens and Vitamin B6 – Actions and Interactions', *World Review of Nutrition and Dietetics*, 51 (1987):140–88.
33. R. Martin du Pon, C. Mauron, B. Glaeser *et al.*, 'Effects of Various Oral Glucose Doses on Plasma Neutral Amino Acid Levels', *Metabolism*, 31 (1982):937–43.
34. J. D. Fernstrom and R. J. Wurtman, 'Brain Serotonin Content: Increase Following Ingestion of Carbohydrate Diet', *Science*, 174 (1971):1023–5.
35. D. A. Bender, A. E. Laing, J. A. Vale *et al.*, 'Effects of Oestrogen Administration of Tryptophan Metabolism in Rats and in Menopausal Women Receiving Hormone Replacement Therapy', *Biochemical Pharmacology*, 32 (1983):843–8.
36. V. N. Luine and J. C. Rhodes, 'Gonadal Hormone Regulation of MAO and other Enzymes in Hypothalamic Area', *Neuroendocrinology*, 36 (1983):235–41.
37. V. N. Luine and B. S. McEwan, 'Effect of Oestradiol on the Turnover of Type A Monoamine Oxidase', *Journal of Neurochemistry*, 28 (1977):1221–7.
38. A. Biegon and B. S. McEwan, 'Modulation by Oestradiol of Serotonin-1 Receptors in Brain', *Journal of Neuroscience*, 2 (1982):199–205.
39. W. Ladisch, 'Effects of Progesterone on Regional Serotonin Metabolism in the Rat Brain', *Neuropharmacology*, 13 (1974):877–83.
40. W. Ladische, 'Influence of Progesterone on Serotonin Metabolism: A Possible Causal Factor for Mood Changes', *Psychoneuroendocrinology*, 2 (1977):257–66.
41. D. Hoyer and P. Scoeffter, 'Serotonin Receptors: Subtypes and Second Messengers', *Journal of Receptor Research*, 11 (1991):197–14.
42. M. Da Prada, A. M. Cesurs, J. M. Launay *et al.*, 'Platelets as a Model for Neurones', *Experientia*, 44 (1988):115–26.
43. R. Samaninin, O. Ghezzi, L. Valzelli *et al.*, 'The Effect of Selective

Lesioning of Brain Serotonin or Catecholamine Containing Neurones on the Anorectic Activity of Fenfluramine and Amphetamines', *European Journal of Pharmacology*, 19 (1972):318–22.
44. D. G. Schlundt, W. G. Johnson and M. P. Jarrell, 'A Naturalistic Functional Analysis of Eating Behaviour in Bulimia and Obesity', *Advances in Behaviour Research and Therapy*, 7 (1985):149–62.
45. E. C. Johnson Sabine, K. H. Wood and A. Wakeling, 'Mood Changes in Bulimia Nervosa', *British Journal of Psychiatry*, 145 (1984):521–6.
46. B. R. Greenberg, 'Predictors of Binge Eating in Bulimic and Non bulimic Women', *International Journal of Eating Disorders*, 5 (1986:269–84.
47. A. P. Levin and S. E. Hyler, 'DSM IIIR Personality Diagnosis in Bulimia', *Comparative Psychiatry*, 27 (1986):47–53.
48. H. M. van Praag and S. de Haan, 'Central Serotonin Metabolism and Frequency of Depression', *Psychiatric Research*, 1 (1979):219–24.
49. H. Meltzer, 'Serotonergic Dysfunction in Depression', *British Journal of Psychiatry*, 155 (1989):25–31.
50. H. Y. Meltzer, R. C. Arora, R. Babner et al., 'Serotonin Uptake in Blood Platelets of Psychiatric Patients', *Archives of General Psychiatry*, 38 (1981):1322–6.
51. M. S. Joseph, T. D. Brewerton, V. I. Rees et al., 'Plasma Tryptophan/ Large Neutral Amino Acid Ratio and the Dexamethasone Suppression Test in Depression', *Psychiatric Research*, 11 (1984):185–92.
52. M. J. Russ, S. H. Ackerman, M. Banay Schwartz et al., 'Plasma Tryptophan to Large Neutral Amino Acid Ratios in Depressed and Non Depressed Subjects', *Journal of Affective Disorders*, 19 (1990):19–24.
53. M. K. De Meyer, P. A. Shea, H. Hendrie et al., 'Plasma Tryptophan and Five other Amino Acids in Depressed and Normal Subjects', *Archives of General Psychiatry*, 38 (1981):642–6.
54. A. Biegon, N. Essar, M. Israeli et al., 'Serotonin 5HT2 Receptor Binding on Blood Platelets as a State Dependent Marker in Major Affective Disorder', *Psychopharmacology Berlin*, 102 (1990):73–5.
55. M. Stanley, J. Virgilio and S. Gershon, 'Tritiated Imipramine Binding Sites are Decreased in the Frontal Cortex of Suicides', *Science*, 216 (1982):1337–9.
56. O. S. Goldbloom, L. Hicks and P. E. Garfinkel, 'Platelet Serotonin Uptake in Bulimia Nervosa', *Biological Psychiatry*, 17 (1990):839–42.
57. M. Asberg, P. Thoren and L. Traskman, 'Serotonin Depression – A Biochemical Subgroup within the Affective Disorders', *Science*, 191 (1976):478–81.
58. M. Asberg, P. Thoren and L. Traskman, '5HIAA in CSF: A Biochemical Suicide Predictor', *Archives of General Psychiatry*, 33 (1976):1193–7.
59. J. I. Hudson, H. G. Pope and J. M. Jonas, 'Family History Study of Anorexia and Bulimia Nervosa', *British Journal of Psychiatry*, 142 (1983):133–8.
60. J. O. Viesselman and M. Roig, 'Depression and Suicidality in Eating Disorders', *Journal of Clinical Psychiatry*, 46 (1985):118–24.
61. B. T. Walsh, S. P. Roose and A. H. Glamman, 'Bulimia and Depression', *Psychosomatic Medicine*, 47 (1985):123–31.
62. H. G. Pyle, J. E. Mitchell and E. Eckert, 'Bulimia Nervosa: A Report of 34 Cases', *Clinical Psychiatry*, 42 (1981):60–4.

63. W. J. Swift, D. Andrews and N. E. Barklage, 'The Relationship Between Affective Disorders and Eating Disorders: A Review of the Literature', *American Journal of Psychiatry*, 143 (1986):290–9.
64. D. C. Jimerson, M. D. Lesem, W. H. Kaye *et al.*, 'Eating Disorders and Depression: Is there a Serotonin Connection', *Biological Psychiatry*, 28 (1990):443–54.
65. P. Garfinkel and D. Garner (eds), *Anorexia Nervosa: A Multidimensional Perspective* (New York: Bruner Mazel, 1982).
66. A. B. Levy, K. N. Dixon and S. L. Stern, 'How are Depression and Bulimia Related?', *American Journal of Psychiatry*, 146 (1989):162–9.
67. A. W. Brotman, D. B. Herzog and S. W. Woods, 'Antidepressant Treatment of Bulimia: The Relationship between Bingeing and Depressive Symptamology', *Journal of Clinical Symptomology*, 45 (1984):7–9.
68. E. F. Coccaro, L. J. Siever and H. M. Klar, 'Serotonergic Studies in Affective and Personality Disorder Patients: Correlates with Suicidal and Impulsive Aggressive Behaviour', *Archives of General Psychiatry*, 46 (1989):587–99.
69. T. D. Brewerton, E. A. Mueller, M. D. Lesem *et al.*, 'Neuroendocrine Responses to *m*-chlorophenylpiperazine and L-tryptophan in bulimia', *Archives of General Psychiatry*, 49 (1992):852–61.
70. A. Apter, H. M. van Praag, R. Plutchik *et al.*, 'Interrelationships among Anxiety, Aggression, Impulsivity and Mood: A Serotonergically Linked Cluster', *Psychiatry Research*, 32 (1990):191–9.
71. B. E. Wolfe, D. C. Jimerson and J. M. Levine, 'Impulsivity Ratings in Bulimia Nervosa: Relationship to Binge Eating Behaviours', *International Journal of Eating Disorders*, 15 (1994):289–92.
72. D. C. Jimerson, 'Low Serotonin and Dopamine Metabolite Concentrations in Cerebrospinal Fluid from Bulimic Patients with Frequent Binge Episodes', *Archives of General Psychiatry*, 49 (1992):132–8.
73. J. Polivy and C. P. Herman, 'Dieting and Binging: A Causal Analysis', *American Psychologist*, 40 (1985):193–201.
74. S. A. French and R. W. Jeffrey, 'Consequences of Dieting to Lose Weight: Effects on Physical and Mental Health', *Health Psychology*, 13 (1994):195–212.
75. G. M. Goodwin, C. G. Fairburn and P. J. Cowen, 'Dieting Changes Serotonergic Function in Women not Men; Implications for the Aetiology of Anorexia Nervosa', *Psychological Medicine*, 17 (1987):839–42.
76. S. F. Abraham and P. J. Beumont, 'How Patients Describe Bulimia or Binge Eating', *Psychological Medicine*, 12 (1982):632–5.
77. J. E. Mitchell, R. L. Pyle and E. D. Eckert, 'Frequency and Duration of Binge Eating Episodes in Patients with Bulimia', *American Journal of Psychiatry*, 138 (1981):835–6.
78. G. R. Leon, K. Carroll, B. Chernyk *et al.*, 'Binge Eating and Associated Habit Patterns within College Students and Identified Bulimic Populations', *International Journal of Eating Disorders*, 4 (1985):43–57.
79. J. C. Rosen, H. Leitenberg, C. Fisher *et al.*, 'Binge Eating Episodes in Bulimia Nervosa: The Amount and Type of Food Consumed', *International Journal of Eating Disorders*, 5 (1986):255–67.
80. N. E. Rosenthal, M. J. Genhart, B. Caballero *et al.*, 'Psychobiological

Effects of Carbohydrate and Protein Rich Meals in Patients with Seasonal Affective Disorder and Normal Controls', *Biological Psychiatry*, 25 (1989):1029–40.

81. D. Marazziti, E. Macchi, A. Rotondo *et al.*, 'The Involvement of the Serotonin System in Bulimia Nervosa', *Life Sciences*, 43 (1988):2123–6.

82. S. F. Liebowitz, 'The Role of Serotonin in Eating Disorders', *Drugs*, 39 (1990):33–48.

83. H. G. Pope, J. I. Hudson and I. M. Jonas, 'Bulimia Treated with Imipramine: A Placebo Controlled Double Blind Study', *American Journal of Psychiatry*, 140 (1983):554–8.

84. A. W. Brotman, D. B. Herzog and S. W. Woods, 'Antidepressant Treatment of Bulimia: The Relationship Between Bingeing and Depressive Symptomology', *Journal of Clinical Psychiatry*, 45 (1984):7–9.

85. W. H. Kaye, M. H. Ebert and H. E. Gwirtsman *et al.*, 'Differences in Brain Serotonergic Metabolism between Nonbulimic and Bulimic Patients with Anorexia Nervosa', *American Journal of Psychiatry*, 141 (1984):1598–601.

86. T. D. Brewerton, E. Mueller and T. E. George, 'Blunted Prolactin Response to the Serotonin Agonist mCPP in Bulimics', in *International Neuro-Psychopharmacological Congress*, San Juan, Puerto Rico, 1986, p. 186.

87. P. L. Delgado, D. S. Charney and L. H. Price *et al.*, 'Neuroendocrine and Behavioural Effects of Dietary Tryptophan Restriction in Healthy Subjects', *Life Sciences*, 45 (1989):2323–32.

88. W. H. Kaye, H. E. Gwirtsman, T. D. Brewerton *et al.*, 'Bingeing Behaviour and Plasma Amino Acids: A Possible Involvement of Brain Serotonin in Bulimia Nervosa', *Psychiatric Research*, 23 (1988):31–4.

89. G. B. Collins, M. Kotz and J. W. Janesz, 'Alcoholism in the Families of Bulimic Anorexics', *Cleveland Clinic Quarterly*, 52 (1985):65–7.

90. K. M. Pirke, M. Dogs and M. M. Fichter *et al.*, 'Gonadotrophins, Oestradiol and Progesterone during the Menstrual Cycle in Bulimia Nervosa', *Clinical Endocrinology*, 29 (1988):265–70.

91. D. Stewart, 'Reproductive Function in Eating Disorders', *Annals of Medicine*, 24 (1992):287–91.

13 Molecules, Brain and Addictive Behaviour

Adrian Bonner

INTRODUCTION

Studies on alcohol are providing an important view of the way in which disruption of cellular and regional organisation of brain activity result in specific behaviour changes. Many of these effects are mediated by the reward and punishment systems of the brain. This link between molecular events and overt behaviour suggests a common mechanism which might exist in a range of addictive behaviours.

Drinking alcohol is recognised as one of several consummatory behaviours which has a genetic infrastructure, is subject to learning and at any point in time is dependent on motivation. The consequences of excessive alcohol consumption are: the development of physiological and behaviour dependence, and pathological damage to body tissues.[1-3] Dependence results from increasing physiological tolerance and increased alcohol consumption thought to originate from self medication of alcohol, a compensatory mechanism directed at reducing the negative effects of the brain's punishment system. The central mechanisms underlying these effects will be discussed later in the chapter. Alcoholism is observed only in humans and so biological observations must be interpreted in the context of the society in which the individual exists and the individual's psychological uniqueness. There have been a considerable number of studies into the metabolism of ethanol, much of this work focusing on the enzyme systems responsible for the breakdown of ethanol[4] and on the importance of nutrition in alcoholic liver disease.[5] During recent years there has been an increasing interest in the cellular mechanisms of dependence and the neurobiological substrate of the behaviours involved in the development of alcohol dependence. These advances are complemented by increasing information on the biological aspects of dependence which are trait markers (inherited predisposition) and state markers (indicators of consumption). Assessments of the validity and reliability of such measures are essential for the improvement in the identification and treatments of individuals whose lives are wrecked by dependence on alcohol.

BIOLOGICAL MARKERS OF PREDISPOSITION TO ALCOHOLISM

The sons of alcoholics have a high risk of developing alcoholism. One explanation for this might be their increased sensitivity to alcohol during the ascending phase of the blood alcohol curve (BAC), when its positive effects are purportedly greatest, and lower than normal sensitivity during the descending phase, when alcohol's negative effects predominate. The greater subjective sensitivity of the sons of alcoholics during the ascending limb of the BAC reinforces their drinking and this is coupled with their relative resistance to alcohol's negative effects. Alternatively, the sons of alcoholics might be at more risk because they are less sensitive to alcohol effects after three to five drinks when compared to controls. If this is the case they fail to regulate their drinking owing to reduced internal feedback. Meta-analysis of eleven studies[6] clearly supports the later suggestion. The lower activity of monoamine oxidase B in families of alcoholics[7] would be expected to affect neurotransmission and neuronal tone in those susceptible individuals. An application of these finding is that biological sons of male alcoholics should be informed that they might not feel as affected or as 'high' (or intoxicated) as other individuals. This reduced awareness of the effects of alcohol might mitigate against the cessation of the bouts of drinking. This preventative approach is helpful but limited in that self-reported sensitivity to alcohol may be due to the effect of alcohol on cognitive abilities which affect proficiency in verbal communication or personality features. On the other hand, the lower subjective sensitivity might reflect hormonal or metabolic factors such as a reduced cortisol response to stressors[8] or P300 response. The validity of the P300 event related potentials (ERP) as a biological marker for alcoholism has been explored since the early 1980s. The importance of these measures relates to their association with cognitive aspects of information processing and the growing evidence that the ERP are under genetic control. The early studies, using auditory stimuli, were not easily replicated but the results for P300 using visual tasks are more consistent. The strongest evidence that P300 is a marker for alcoholism has been obtained in studies of prepubescent boys[9] in which children from high-risk backgrounds had been screened for absence of other psychopathology and control matched for socioeconomic background. The ERP test–retest has been shown to have a long-term reliability in both controls and alcoholic populations.[10] P300 studies are begining to uncover the neuropsychological processes attributable to tasks requiring attention to stimuli or controlled tasks that reflect neural processes that are preattentive or automatic.[11] The decreased amplitude of P300 in alcoholics and their sons suggests a deficit of perceptual, automatic and subsequent mis-match processes. Investigations of these robust electrophysiological markers are being paralleled by frontal brain pathology, neurochemical and imaging data. The question as to whether this psychophysiological deficit is inherited and predisposes individuals to particular behavioural and social activities, leading them into alcoholism or some other maladapted lifestyle, remains to be answered.

BIOLOGICAL MARKERS OF ALCOHOL CONSUMPTION

In view of the often reported lack of reliability of self-reporting by patients, there is a need for objective biological markers of alcohol consumption. Gamma-glutamyltranspeptidase (GGT), aspartate aminotranferase (AST), alanine aminotransferase (ALT), ß-hexosaminidase (ß-hex), high-density lipoprotein,[12] blood ethanol concentrations and mean red cell volume (MCV) have been used as markers of alcohol abuse. The usage of these tests relates to differences which, over many years, have been found between alcoholics and controls and largely reflect derangements of the liver and associated metabolism . However, these tests are non-specific and influenced by liver damage. Recently interest has focused on carbohydrate-deficient transferin (CDT), in serum, which provides a measure of accumulated alcohol consumption, appearing after an intake of >50–80 g of ethanol/day for at least one week and normalised during abstinence of two weeks.[13, 14] CDT is an isoform of transferrin and has been demonstrated to be at increased levels in the serum of a high percentage of alcoholics with a daily consumption greater than 60 g ethanol for some weeks.[15] CDT appears to be a more reliable indicator of abstention than GGT, AST and MCV in patients with alcoholic liver disease but has a deceased sensitivity for detecting recent heavy drinking. There appears to be no correlation between CDT and other markers such as GGT,AST,ALT and ALP, suggesting that these measures reflect different biological processes. On this basis the combination of CDT and GGT increased the detection of alcohol abuse from 61 to 98 per cent and combination of CDT and AST to 64 per cent. The confounding effect of liver disease probably accounts for the greater sensitivity of GGT and AST than CDT in abusing alcoholics.[13] A new biochemical approach employs the shift in breakdown of serotonin to 5-hydroxyindole-3-acetic acid (5-HIAA) to increased formation of 5-hydroxytrytophol (5-HTOL). The increased urinary excretion of 5-HTOL is observed for several hours after blood ethanol levels reach zero both in alcoholics and in healthy subjects. The 5-HTOL/5-HIAA ratio reflects blood ethanol concentration but the former is still detectable in urine several hours after ethanol concentration has reached zero. 5-HTOL measurements are therefore useful when recent alcohol intake monitoring is required. This approach could be employed to complement the markers of accumulated alcohol consumption during past weeks such as GGT and CDT.[14]

Whole blood associated acetaldehyde (WBAA) measurements appear to parallel peak blood levels of ethanol and might be expected to occur prior to the elevation of other markers that reflect tissue damage, as a result of ethanol exposure. Significant gender differences were found in WBAA, ß-hex, and GGT measurements.[16] Another suggested 'state marker' of alcoholism is blood aldehyde dehydrogenase (ALDH). The considrable overlap in ALDH values between alcoholics and social drinkers provides limited optimism for the use of this marker on its own. However, ALDH in erythrocytes and leukocytes might provide easily accessible *in-vitro* and *in-vivo* model systems to screen for drug treatments that cause ALDH inhibition.[17]

The limited specificity observed in many of the biochemical markers results from the confounding effect of liver disease. Currently, the only urinary tests by which hepatic disorders can be diagnosed are qualitative (e.g. bilirubin, urobilinogen). A new method suggests that the measurement of urinary L-fucose offers a precise diagnosis of alcoholic liver cirrhosis. L-fucose is important in the functioning of glycoconjugates. In patients with alcoholic liver disease, the terminal glycosylation of the glyocproteins in the Golgi apparatus is impaired, accompanied by the presence of a carbohydrate-deficient transferrin in serum. The altered glycoproteins may be the result of abnormal metabolism of L-fucose due to alteration in fucosyltransferase.[18] The proposal has therfore been made that L-fucose is a possible marker of alcoholic liver disease.[19] Using this approach it should be possible to classify patients into liver-damaged and non-liver-damaged alcoholics and provide more specificity for the available markers. It has been argued that the differential effects of ethanol in individuals of different ages[20] and between the sexes[21] suggest that the care should be taken in the use of 'state markers' in the absence of appropriate normalised values.

CELLULAR MECHANISMS

Explanations for the inhibitory acute action of ethanol, the development of tolerance to it, and the hyperexcitability commonly found in ethanol withdrawal have implicated the action of the neurotransmission of GABA. Ethanol has been reported to increase the movement of chloride ions through the $GABA_A$ receptor channel. Positron emission tomography (PET) scanning, using [18F]fluorodeoxyglucose (^{18}F-FDG) has been applied to investigate these receptors in humans. Measurement of brain metabolism by this means has demonstrated the sensitivity of various brain regions to pharmacological agents and thus permits investigations into specific brain receptors. The brain's metabolic response to a challenge with a benzodiazepine drug, lorazepam[22] was found to be decreased in alcoholics. This study provides good evidence that alcoholics have abnormal GABA–benzodiazepine receptor function in specific brain areas, primarily the occipital cortex, thalamus and cerebellum. Decreased receptor function would reduce the influx of Cl⁻ ions into neurons. Some of these areas form part of the neuronal circuit that regulates the initiation and termination of behaviours. When disrupted, this system can lead to the emergence of compulsive, repetitive behaviours. Decreased response to inhibitory neurotransmission has been implicated in the lack of control and compulsory alcohol intake seen in alcoholics.[23]

There have been many demonstrations that the $GABA_A$-receptor complex is involved in the action of ethanol, but the growing number of negative reports suggests that other cellular processes are also involved. Recent data has suggested that the primary locus of action of ethanol is more likely to be the N-methyl-D-aspartate (NMDA)-receptor-linked cation channel than the GABA-activated chloride channel (see Figure 13.1). Both humans and laboratory animals develop tolerance and physical dependence following chronic consumption of large amounts of ethanol, this is decribed as *ethanol withdrawal syndrome*. Evidence has recently been provided that demonstrates that a functional activation of glutamatergic synapses, rather than a decrease in $GABA_A$ receptor function, is a critical event during ethanol withdrawal.[24] Although ethanol appears to be associated with sensitisasation or subsensitivity of the GABA-coupled chloride channel, the effects could only be detected within 3 hours after last ethanol administration, that is, the animals were still intoxicated. Downregulation of the GABA-coupled chloride channel was not detected 9–24 hours after withdrawal. Conversely, binding studies, using the noncompetitive NMDA inhibitor ^{3}H-MK 801,

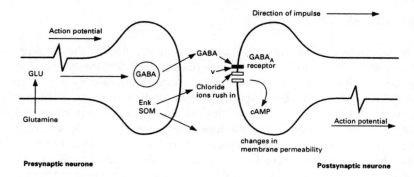

Figure 13.1 Schematic representation of the GABA receptor action

δ amino butyric acid (GABA) is synthesised from glutamine, co-released with a neuropeptide such enkephalin (Enk) or somatostatin (SOM) from presynaptic neurones. $GABA_A$ receptor is coupled to a chloride channel which, via the secondary messenger cAMP, causes a change in the membrane permeability of the postsynaptic membrane and the generation of an action potential. The $GABA_A$ receptor also has binding sites for benzodiazepines, such as valium (V).

indicate that withdrawl symptoms may be correlated with increased NMDA receptor-mediated transmission. The decrease of ^{3}H-MK 801 binding in rats 3–6 days after withdrawal suggests that a compensatory downregulation of the NMDA receptor complex occurs following overactivation during the withdrawal period (see Figure 13.2). The NMDA receptor is highly permeable to Ca^{2+} ions and over-stimulation results in neuronal death due to excitotoxicity. The effects are observed in stroke, trauma, hypoxic–ischaemia, and may be important in a number of neurodegenerative diseases. *In-vivo* and *in-vitro* studies have shown that non-competitive NMDA inhibitors, such as MK 801, protect against excitotoxic cell death. Using lactate dehydrogenase production as a measure of neurotoxicity in primary neuronal cultures Chandler[25] has demonstrated that ethanol also has a marked inhibitory effect on the NMDA receptor complex. Ethanol protects the neuronal cultures against externally provided NMDA and its agonists. This effect is explained by the reduction in neuropathological increases in intracellular calcium caused by ethanol. Apparently, glycine can reverse these effects of ethanol, *in vitro*, via influences on cGMP and Ca^{2+} flux. These *in-vitro* studies suggest that ethanol provides some degree of neuroprotection but, paradoxically, chronic ethanol is a risk factor for stroke. Although, it is not known whether acute ethanol exposure in the non-alcoholic is

The publishers regret the following error on page 219, for which the editors and the author concerned are not responsible: for the diagram printed, please substitute the one shown below.

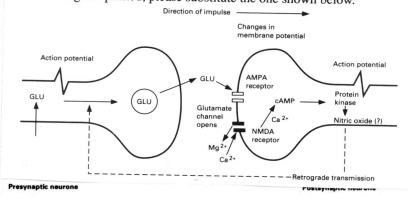

Figure 13.2 The glutamate receptor

Glutamate is synthesised from glutamine which is released from the presynaptic neurone. Several types of glutamate receptors exist, identified by specific antagonists, such as N-methyl-D-aspartate (NMDA). This receptor type is normally blocked by magnesium (Mg^{2+}) which becomes displaced when non-NMDA receptors (AMPA:alpha-amino-3-hydroxy-5-methyl-4-isoxazole-propionate) are stimulated. Release of magnesium from the NMDA receptor allows influx of calcium ions (Ca^{2+}) into the postsynaptic neuron and, following a cascade of reactions involving protein kinases, an action potential is generated. The importance of the generation of retrograde tranmitters (possibly nitric oxide?) by this process is thought to be important in 'cellular learning' in hippocampal cells. Here, coincidence of the presynaptic neurone facilitates the strengthening of the synapse via the generation of a Long-Term Potential (LTP).

also a risk factor, there is some data[25] to suggest that NMDA receptors are up-regulated in chronic ethanol consumption. This increased sensitivity of the receptors is interpreted as an adaptive response to the depressant actions of ethanol on the glutamatergic system. Up-regulation of NMDA receptors may contribute to seizure activity following withdrawal of ethanol from dependent animals.

The ongoing debate as to whether acute, rapid and chronic tolerance are related or separate processes continues. Neurochemical evidence suggests that chronic tolerance involves the actions of norepinephrine (NE) and serotonin (5-HT). 5-HT projections from the median raphe nucleus and projecting to the septum and hippocampus, play the same role in both acute and rapid tolerance.[26] The maintainance of chronic tolerance to ethanol if facilitated by the neuropeptide arginine vasopressin (AVP)[5-HT$_2$receptors are specifically involved in the interaction between AVP and 5-HT]. The excitatory amino acid glutamate is also implicated in the learned basis of tolerance. Acting via the NMDA subtype of the glutamate receptor, two receptor blockers (+MK-801, and ketamine) prevent the development of rapid tolerence to ethanol.[27, 28] The NMDA receptor appears to be specifically related to the learning component of tolerance. Bringing the data from these various systems together, Kalant[29] has produced a schema of the neural interconnections in the septum and hippocamus which provides an initial insight into the possible roles played by the various neurotransmitters and modulators in tolerance.

EFFECTS OF ETHANOL ON BRAIN FUNCTION

Structural alterations in the human brain were first reported in 1955 by Courville.[30] Since that time increasingly sophisticated studies have attempted to focus on the effects of ethanol on specific brain regions and to relate any structural changes to behaviours which are affected by acute and chronic ethanol consumption. Learning, memory, attention, higher reasoning and a range of neuropsychological deficits are affected by chronic consumption of alcoholic beverages. The hippocampus is considered to be important in the processes of learning and memory. Chronic ethanol treatment (CET) of laboratory rodents produces abnormalities in the hippocampus. Losses of 10–40 per cent of principle cells (hippocampal pyramidal and dentate gyrus granule cells) and internenurons occur, the extent of degeneration depending on the duration of the CET.[23] Studies of gross morphological changes, neurocytological and behaviour deficits in humans are problematic due to vitamin deficiencies and malnutrition, both of which commonly accompany alcohol consumption. Nutritionally controlled animal models, however, can obviate these confounding influences. The first study of this type in 1987[31] indicated that after 20 weeks of alcohol intake a significant loss of hippocampal tissue occurred. More recent studies have demonstrated that the hippocampus is capable of compensatory changes in response to neurotoxic damage produced by CET.[32] Furthermore, functional deficiencies appear to be related to influences on long-term potentiation (LTP). LTP is thought to be the mechanism whereby enduring memory is established. The synaptic efficacy produced by brief repetitive activation of afferents to and within the hippocampus is the contemporary view of the cellular mechanism underlying learning and memory. Electrophysiological studies have recently indicated that ethanol significantly decreases the LTP of spikes in populations of inhibitory synapses in the dentate gyrus.[33] This work suggests a major role for septal regulation and the first evidence that ethanol acts on specific hippocampal afferents, thus disrupting hippocampal physiology. This action is likely to underlie the mnemopathic actions of ethanol. A review of the influence of alcohol on memory is presented in Chapter 9.

Studies of the growth, development and degeneration of the brain structures involved in memory are beginning to provide an understanding of the molecular basis of the behavioural aspects of alcoholism. The relationship between hippocampal and basal forebrain atropy, septophippocampal cholinergic dysfunction, and impaired memory has been studied with regard to the role of neurotrophic factors.[32] Nerve growth factor (NGF) is a neurotrophic factor for the magnocellular cholinergic neurons of the basal forebrain. NGF plays a critical role in the development, survival and maintainence of these neurons. Target tissues synthesise NGF which acts on specific neuronal receptors, after which retrograde transport then causes the NGF/receptor complex to be moved towards the cell body where protein synthesis is stimulated. This process is necessary for the survival and expression of the neurotransmitter properties of the cells. Deficiencies in NGF production have been related to the morphological and functional changes which occur in the aging brain. Similar effects have been found in animals subject to chronic ethanol treatment in that significant reductions in hippocampal neurotrophic activity, induced by ethanol, occur.[32] Further work using mRNA probes is required to specifically implicate NGF in this processs and the relative importance of other neurotrophic factors such as bFGF, BDNF and neurotrophin-3 needs to be elucidated. The development of positron emission tomography (PET) using [^{18}F]fluorodeoxyglucose (^{18}F-FDG) has permitted assessments of brain atrophy, metabolic functioning and neuropsychological performance.[34, 35] Using this imaging technique performance on the Wisconsin Card Sorting Test (WCST) has been correlated with higher cerebral metabolic rates for glucose. Local rates of glucose metabolism were decreased in a sagittal strip of the medial frontal cortex in alcoholic patients compared to normals.These direct measures of metabolism are providing some insight into the effects of ethanol on specific brain mechanisms. The anterior cingulate and other parts of the medial frontal cortex are specifically affected and linked with deficits in inductive logic, abstraction, and problem solving found in patients suffering from chronic alcoholism. This approach opens up the possibility of monitoring 'cognitive remediation' during the use of neuropsychological strategies in alcoholic patients. This research will hopefully complement the cognitive approaches to treatment which are described in Chapter 10.

From the studies reviewed above the reader will be aware of the increasing evidence that cellular and brain mechanisms are involved in ethanol dependence. Some progress is being made in linking such neurobiological mechanisms to overt behaviour.

SEROTONIN AND ALCOHOL-SEEKING BEHAVIOUR

Reviews of the importance of serotonin metabolism in alcohol abuse and eating disorders have been provided in Chapters 4 and 12. Preclinical studies first indicated that central serotonin (5-HT) neurotransmission was linked with alcohol consumption. Current studies on 5-HT_3 receptors are beginning to provide a unifying theory of drug dependence.[36] This neurotransmitter system has also been implicated in other behaviours including mood, and eating disorders (see Chapter 12). The amino acid tryptophan (Trp) is the precurser of brain 5-HT. Some years ago Banki[37] reported that platelet 5-HT levels are decreased in alcoholics. This work had not been followed up until recently[38] when greater attention was paid to the behavioural descriptions of the alcoholics. In this study a more marked decrease in the level of platelet 5-HT was found in the *alcohol-dependent subgroup* (with ordinary personality) compared with the *alcoholic subgroup with antisocial behaviours* (acting out or suicidal tendancies, i.e. impulse control disorders). This data is important because the proportion of patients with lifetime diagnoses of impulse control disorders (25 per cent) was similar to that found by Cloninger who classified 24 per cent of his population as Type II (see Chapter 7). Type II alcoholics are thought to have a 5-HT deficiency. Evidence for a brain 5-HT deficiency in the control and possibly the predisposition to alcohol consumption and the development of alcoholism has been reviewed by Sellers and Higgins.[39]

Platelet serotonin and blood tryptophan levels are low in children diagnosed as having attention deficit hyperactivity disorder (ADHD) and also in their parents. The same families have also been found to be at increased risk of alcoholism. This insight into the spectrum of disorders with which 'alcoholism genes' may be associated provides a unique approach whereby the behavioural antecedents of alcoholism may be studied. Comings[40] has reviewed the numerous studies which suggest that ADHD has a strong genetic basis and that children with ADHD are at increased risk of developing problems with alcohol and drug abuse. A population survey of 1440 Tourette syndrome and ADHD individuals and their relatives showed significantly decreased levels of both serotonin and tryptophan in the affected groups compared with the controls. Genetic analysis of the populations predict that the frequency of the carriers of a single common gene (Gts) leading to these conditions would be 15–25 per cent. This is in line with predictions for the frequency of Type II alcoholism gene.[40] At a biochemical level, Comings suggests that the Gts gene might be a mutation of the tryptophan dioxygenase (TDO2) gene. Such a mutation would be expected to cause elevated levels of the enzyme and a resultant reduction in circulating tryptophan. The gene has been mapped on chromosome 4q3.1 and linkage with Type II alcoholism is likely. This suggestion is based on the possible linkage between Type II alcoholism and MNS blood group.[41] Sequencing over 6000 base pairs of the human TDO2 gene indicates a high degree of conservation (96 per cent) between rat and human TDO2 amino acid sequences. This observation complements the previously described work of Badawy (see Chapter 4) in which TDO2 has been demonstrated to be elevated in alcohol-preferring rats. This provides an indication that depletion of tryptophan in the circulation (due to the liver enzyme, TDO2) would result in lowered synthesis of serotonin in the brain, and the resultant effect on the modulation of behaviour as noted at the beginning of this section. The importance of this hepatic control over tryptophan concentrations, and resulting brain synthesis of serotonin, might possibly be a primary defect in the development and maintainance of alcoholism.

NEUROBIOLOGICAL SUBSTRATES FOR REWARD

Misuse of ethanol is probably sustained by its rewarding properties which are mediated by the mesolimbic dopamine pathway. In animal studies, ethanol administration activates neuronal firing in the ventral tegmental area (VTA) which, in turn, increases dopamine (DA) release in the terminal area (nucleus accumbens). In the place-preference paradigm experiments ethanol only becomes rewarding after a long period of conditioning, suggesting that it is necessary to develop tolerance to the aversive properties of ethanol before the rewarding influences of the drug becomes apparent. Using a combination of electrophysiological and microdialysis experiments Diana *et al.*[42] have demonstrated that tolerance to ethanol by the mesoaccumbens DA neurons and on DA output in the terminal field does not occur. This provides further evidence that the mesolimbic system may, at least in part, be a neuronal substrate for the reinforcing actions of ethanol. Further support for this is provided by studies using the techniques of microinjection and voltammetry.[43]

In alcohol-prefering rats (P line) there appears to be an abnormal 5-HT and/or DA abnormality in parts of the limbic structure (the nucleus accumbens, olfactory tubercles and medial prefrontal cortex) when compared to alcohol-non-preferring (NP) lines. The ventral tegmental area (VTA) is important in facilitating the rewarding actions of ethanol. From intracranial self-administration experiments, in which the P line, but not the NP line, will self-administer 50–150mg per cent ethanol directly into the VTA.[44] The dorsal raphe nucleus (DRN) 5-HT system appears to be involved in regulating the VTA DA projections to the nucleus accumbens such that suboptimmal 5-HT innervation in the central nervous system prevents the VTA and other limbic structures from operating normally. McBride[44] suggests that this situation causes the system to over-respond to the rewarding actions of ethanol, initiated by the VTA. Behavioural compensation attempting to normalise the hypo-functioning DA system thus results in P line rats consuming increased amounts of alcohol in order to maintain appropriate levels of neuronal activity in the brain-reward systems.

In view of the importance of the dopamine mesolimbic system as a central feature of the neurobiological basis of reward motivated behaviour, it is not surprising that attention has been paid to the genetic basis of DA receptor activity. A candidate gene approach, using the restriction fragment length polymorphism (RFLP), has been used to explore the DRD2 dopamine receptor gene association with alcoholism. Goldman[45] has reviewed the work in this area and found that three population studies, including two by one group, detected a higher Tacq1 A1 frequency of the gene in alcoholics compared to controls. However, six studies showed no association and one study was equivocal. The overall conclusion was that the finding in the original study[46] has not been replicated. This conclusion is challenged by Pato *et al.*[47] This meta-analysis of eight studies supported a statistically significant association between the A1 allele of DRD2 and alcoholism, with an apparent increased risk associated with increased severity of alcoholism. Both Pato *et al.* and Goldman suggest that the large intra-population variations, due to sampling error and varying distributions of the various ethnic subgroups, have given rise to the spurious population associations. Addressing the issue of heterogeneous populations, a population (*n* = 78) of Japanese has recently been studied.[48] This study revealed a highly significant difference in the frequence of the A1 allele of the D2/TaqIA RFLP in the Japanese unscreened controls compared with those in the unscreened white populations in the USA. Alcoholics aged 60 or over had significantly lower frequences of the A1 allele than the younger subjects suggesting a poorer outcome (i.e. longevity) for those with the A1 allele. This is consistent with the finding that the A1 allele was most frequently found in deceased alcoholics.[48] When the sample was partitioned into severe and less severe alcoholics, a highly significant difference was found between non-alcoholic controls and severe alcoholics. The total genetic variance associated with the D2/TaqI A RFLP contributed only 9.5 per cent to the total population variability. This detailed Japanese study suggests that the A1 allele does not have a major effect on susceptibility to alcoholism, and linkage between this allele and alcoholism was only found in late-onset individuals. The conclusion from this work is that the D2/TaqI A RFLP is related to or has a linkage disequilibrium with a genetic factor that has a modest and additive effect on the severity of alcoholism.

CONCLUSION

Advances in a range of biological sciences are providing a unique view into the mechanisms of alcohol dependence. Data collected from electrophysiology, neurochemistry, neuropsychology and imaging studies suggest that aspects of alcoholism might result from cognitive deficits and dysfunction of the reward and punishment systems. Research into the neurobiological substrate of these functions of the brain has begun to focus on the mesolimbic dopamine system. As with other approaches discussed within this volume, there are a large number of methodological pitfalls in investigations of the genetic basis of these mechanisms. Studies on brain dopamine receptors suggest a small but significant genetic influence on the development and maintenance of alcohol dependence. This is not surprising as alcohol dependence is multifactorial in its causation. Studies on alcohol dependence are contributing to our understanding of brain function. The commonality of these mechanisms with other the biological basis of other addictive behaviours remains to be explored in future years.

NOTES

1. E. M. Higgins, 'Alcohol and the Skin', *Alcohol and Alcoholism*, 27(6) (1992):595–602.
2. P. Peris, 'Reduced Spinal and Femoral Bone Mass and Deranged Bone Mineral Metabolites in Chronic Alcoholics', *Alcohol and Alcoholism*, 27(6) (1992):619–25.
3. V. R. Preedy, 'Mechanisms of Ethanol-induced Cardiac Damage', *British Heart Journal*, 69 (1993):197–200.
4. J. Panes and J. Caballeria, 'Determinants of Ethanol and Acetaldehyde Metabolism in Chronic Alcoholics', *Alcoholism: Clinical and Experimental Research*, 17 (1992):48–53.
5. S. W. French, 'Nutrition in the Pathogenesis of Alcoholic Liver Disease', *Alcohol and Alcoholism*, 28(1) (1993):97–109.
6. V. E. Pollock, 'Meta-analysis of Subjective Sensitivity to Alcohol in Sons of Alcoholics', *American Journal of Psychiatry*, 149(11) (1992):1534–8.
7. E. J. Devor, 'A Genetic Familial Study of Monoamine Oxidase B Activity and Concentrations in Alcoholics', *Alcoholism: Clinical and Experimental Research*, 17(2) (1993):263–7.
8. A. L. Errico, 'Attenuated Cortisol Response to Biobehavioural Stressors in Sober Alcoholics', *Journal of Studies on Alcohol*, 54 (1993):393–8.
9. S. Hill and S. Steinhauer, 'Assessment of Prepubertal and Postpubertal Boys and Girls at Risk of Developing Alcoholism with P300 from a Visual Discrimination Task', *Journal of Studies on Alcohol*, 54 (1993):350–8.
10. R. Sinha, N. Bernardy and O. A. Parsons, 'Long-term Test–Retest Reliability of Event-related Potentials in Normals and Alcoholics', *Biological Psychiatry*, 32 (1992):992–1003.
11. G. Realmuto, H. Begleiter, J. Odencrantz *et al.*, 'Event-related Potential Evidence of Dysfunction in Automatic Processing in Abstinent Alcoholics', *Biological Psychiatry*, 33 (1993):594–601.
12. H. Charng-Ming, R. Elin, M. Ruddel *et al.*, 'The Effect of Alcohol Withdrawal on Serum Concentrations of Lp(a), Apolipoproteins A-1 and B, and Lipids', *Alcoholism: Clinical and Experimental Research*, 16 (1992):895–8.
13. H. Bell, C. Tallakeim, T. Sjaheim *et al.*, 'Serum Carbohydrate-deficient Transferrin as a Marker of Alcohol Consumption in Patients with Chronic Liver Disease', *Alcoholism: Clinical and Experimental Research*, 17 (1993):246–52.
14. V. Voltaire Carlsson, A. J. Hiltunen, O. Beck *et al.*, 'Detection of Relapses in Alcohol-dependent Patients: Comparison of Carbohydrate-deficient

Transferrin in Serum, 5-Hydroxytryptphol in Urine, and Self-reports', *Alcoholism:Clinical and Experimental Research*, 17 (1993):703–8.
15. H. Stibler, 'Carbohydrate-deficient Transferrin in Serum: A New Marker of Potentially Harmful Alcohol Consumption Reviewed', *Clinical Chemistry*, 37 (1991):2029–37.
16. M. R. Halvorson, J. L. Campbell, G. Sprague *et al.*, 'Comparative Evaluation of the Clinical Utility of Three Markers of Ethanol Intake: The Effect of Gender', *Alcoholism: Clinical and Experimental Research*, 17 (1993):225–9.
17. A. Helander, 'Aldehyde Dehydrogenase in Blood: Distribution, Characteristics and Possible Use as a Marker of Alcohol Misuse', *Alcohol and Alcoholism*, 28 (1993):135–45.
18. W. L. Hutchinson, M. Q. Du, P. J. Johnson *et al.*, 'Fucosyltransferases: Differential Plasma and Tissue Alterations in Hepatocellular Carcinoma and cirrhosis', *Hepatology*, 13 (1991):683–8.
19. M. Yamauchi, K. Kimura, Y. Maezawa, *et al.*, 'Urinary Level of L-Fucose as a Marker of Alcoholic Liver Disease', *Alcoholism: Clinical and Experimental Research*, 17 (1993):268–71.
20. H. Mulford and J. L. Fitzgerald, 'Elderly versus Younger Problem Drinker Profiles: Do they Indicate a Need for a Special Programs for the Elderly?', *Journal of Studies of Alcohol* (November 1992):601–11.
21. K. Mann, A. Gunther and G. Schroth, 'Do Women Develop Alcoholic Brain Damage More Readily Than Men?', *Alcoholism: Clinical and Experimental Research*, 16 (1992):1052–56.
22. N. D. Volkow, M. D. Wang, R. Hitzemann *et al.*, 'Decreased Cerebral Response to Inhibitory Neurotransmission in Alcoholics', *American Journal of Psychiatry*, 150 (1993):417–22.
23. J. G. Modell, J. Mountz and T. P. Beresford, 'Basal Ganglia/Limbic Striatal and Thalamocortical Involvement in Craving and Loss of Control in Alcoholism', *Journal of Neuropsychiatry*, 2 (1990):123–44.
24. E. Sanna and D. Goldman, 'Chronic Ethanol Intoxication induces Differential Effects on GABAA and NMDA Receptor Function in the Rat Brain D2 Dopamine Receptor Genotype and Cerebrospinal Fluid Homovanillic Acid, 5-Hydroxyindoleacetic Acid and 3-Methoxy- 4-Hydroxyphenylglycol in Alcoholics in Finland and the United States', *Alcohol Clinical Research*, 86 (1992):351–57.
25. L. J. Chandler, C. Sumners and F. T. Crews, 'Ethanol Inhibits NMDA Receptor-mediated Excitotoxicity in Rat Primary Neuronal Cultures', *Alcoholism: Clinical and Experimental Research*, 17 (1993):54–60.
26. B. Tabakoff and P. L. Hoffman, 'Recent Advances in Alcohol Research – 1990', in H. Kalant, J. M. Khanna and Y. Isreal (eds), *Advances in Biomedical Alcohol Research: Proceedings of the Fifth ISBRA/RSA Congress* (1991), pp. 1–7.
27. J. M. Khanna, H. Kalant, G. Shah *et al.*, 'Effect of (+)MK801 and Ketamine on Rapid Tolerance to Ethanol', *Brain Research Bulletin*, 28 (1992):311–4.
28. P. H. Wu, J.-F. Liu, A. D. Mihic *et al.*, 'Blockade of the Development of Chronic Tolerance to Ethanol by (+)MK801', *Alcohol: Clinical and Experimental Research*, 16 (1992):638.

29. H. Kalant, 'Problems in the Search for Mechanisms of Tolerance', in P. V. Taberner and A. A. Badaway (eds), *Advances in Biomedical Alcohol Research* (Oxford: Pergamon Press, 1993), pp. 1–8.
30. C. B. Courvill, *Effects of Alcohol on the Nervous System* (Los Angeles: San Lucas Press, 1955).
31. J. N. Riley and D. Walker, 'Morphological Alterations in the Rat Hippocampus after Long-term Consumption of Ethanol in Mice', *Science*, 201 (1978):646–8.
32. D. Walker, N. Heaton, M. King *et al.*, 'Effect of Chronic Ethanol on the Septohippocampal System: A Role for Neurotrophic Factors?', *Alcoholism: Clinical and Experimental Research*, 17 (1993):12–18.
33. S. C. Steffensen, 'Ethanol-induced Suppression of Hippocampal Long-term Potentiation is Blocked by Lesions of the Septohippocampal Nucleus', *Alcohol Clinical Research*, 17(3) (1993):655–9.
34. K. Adams, S. Gilman, R. A. Koeppe *et al.*, 'Neuropsychological Deficits are Correlated with Frontal Hypometabolism in Positron Emission Tomography Studies of Older Alcoholic Patients', *Alcoholism: Clinical and Experimental Research* 17 (1993):205–10.
35. N. D. Volkow, 'Decreased Cerebral Response to Inhibitory Neurotransmission in Alcoholics' *American Journal of Psychiatry*, 150(3) (1993):417–22.
36. D. Nutt, 'The Neurochemistry of Alcohol', *Current Opinions in Psychiatry*, 6 (1993):395–402.
37. C. M. Banki, '5-Hydroxytryptamine Content of the Whole Blood in Psychiatric Illness and Alcoholism', *Acta Psychiatrica Scandinavica*, 57 (1978):232–8.
38. D. Bailly, 'Platelet Serotonin Levels in Alcoholic Patients: Changes Related to Physiological and Pathological Factors', *Psychiatry Research* 47 (1993):57–68.
39. E. Sellers, G. Higgins and M. Sobell, '5-HT and Alcohol Abuse', *Trends in Pharmaceutic Science*, 13 (1992):69–75.
40. D. E. Comings, 'Serotonin and the Biochemical Genetics of Alcoholism: Lessons from Studies of Attention Deficit Hyperactivity Disorder (ADHD) and Tourette Syndrome', in P. V. Taberner and A. A. Badawy (eds), *Advances in Biomedical Alcohol Research* (Oxford:Pergamon Press, 1993), pp. 237–45.
41. S. Y. Hill, C. Aston and B. Rabin, 'Suggestive Evidence of Genetic Linkage between Alcoholism and the MNS Blood Groups', *Alcoholism: Clinical and Experimental Research*, 12 (1988):811–4.
42. M. Diana, 'Lack of Tolerance to Ethanol-induced Stimulation of Mesolimbic Dopamine System', *Alcohol and Alcoholism*, 27 (1992):329–33.
43. H. H. Samson and C. W. Hodge, 'The Role of the Mesolimbic Dopamine System in the Ethanol Reinforcement: Studies Using the Techniques of Microinjection and Voltammetry', *Alcohol and Alcoholism*, (Suppl. 2 (1995):469–74.
44. W. J. McBride, J. M. Murphy, G. J. Gatto *et al.*, 'CNS Mechanisms of Alcohol Self-Administration', *Alcohol and Alcoholism*, 1993 (Suppl. 2 (1993):463–7.
45. D. Goldman, 'The DRD2 Dopamine Receptor and the Candidate Gene

Approach in Alcoholism', in P. V. Taberner and A. A. Badawy (eds), *Advances in Biomedical Alcohol Research* (Oxford: Pergamon Press, 1993), pp. 27–30.

46. K. Blum, E. P. Noble and P. J. Sheridan, 'Allelic Association of Human Dopamine D2 Receptor Gene in Alcoholism', *Journal of the American Medical Association*, 263 (1960):2055–60.

47. C. N. Pato, 'Review of the Putative Association of Dopamine D2 Receptor and Alcoholism: A Meta-analysis', *American Journal of Medical Genetics (Neuropsychiatric Genetics)*, 48 (1993):78–82.

48. T. Arinami, 'Association Between Severity of Alcoholism and the A1 Allele of the Dopamine D2 Receptor Gene Taq1 A RFLP', *Society of Biological Psychiatry*, 33 (1993):108–14.

Part V
Alcohol Abuse in Society

14 Estimating the Prevalence of Alcohol-related Conditions: The Use of Routine Health Data

Gerry Waldron

DEFINING THE PROBLEM

Alcohol-related problems represent such a varied and complex interaction between a multiplicity of medical and social factors that this initial step is in itself a daunting task. A good definition, however, improves communication between workers and allows comparisons over time and between areas. Those with a medical background will consider physical conditions such as liver disease. Others will concentrate on the psychiatric aspects. More will look at the broader social consequences to the drinker, his family and perhaps to society at large. The last group may often decry the use of the 'medical model' as irrelevant, nevertheless it is important that workers in different areas learn to speak each others' languages when they meet to discuss a common interest. It will then quickly become apparent that the medical model is appropriate in some situations and the social model in others. What is most important is that when we communicate with each other we are talking about the same problem.

For the purposes of this chapter, 'medical' diagnoses are used. This allows clarification of the information on routine hospital statistics that follows.

Table 14.1 shows a selection of alcohol related diagnoses taken from the ninth revision of the International Classification of Diseases (ICD9).[1] The corresponding numbers from the most recent revision (ICD 10)[2] are also given.

These diagnoses may be divided into psychological and physical conditions. The most commonly diagnosed single condition is alcohol dependence, which ICD9 more fully defines as:

TABLE 14.1   *International Classification of Diseases, ICD9 and ICD10*

Diagnosis	ICD 9 No.	ICD 10 code
Alcohol dependence	303	F10.2
Alcoholic psychosis	291	F10.5
Nondependent alcohol abuse	305	F10.0
Alcoholic liver disease	571.0–571.3	K70.9
Alcoholic gastritis	535.3	K29.2
Alcoholic cardiomyopathy	425.5	I42.6

A state, psychic and usually also physical resulting from taking alcohol, characterised by behavioral and other responses that always include a compulsion to take alcohol on a continuous or periodic basis in order to experience its psychic effects and sometimes to avoid the discomfort of its absence.

A similar definition was used by the Royal College of Physicians in its report on alcohol-related problems – *A Great and Growing Evil.*[3] The 'dependent drinker' was defined as:

Someone who has a compulsion to drink; takes roughly the same amount each day; has increased tolerance to alcohol in the early stages and reduced tolerance later; suffers withdrawal symptoms if alcohol is stopped which are relieved by consuming more; in whom drinking takes precedence over other activities and who tends to resume drinking after a period of abstinence

These definitions reflect the complexity of the condition. The Royal College of Psychiatrists' guidelines for sensible drinking[4] are well known – less than 21 units per week for men and less than 14 units per week for women. (A unit of alcohol is half a pint of normal strength beer or lager, a standard measure of spirits or a glass of wine.) By their very nature, these divisions are arbitrary and could conceivably be set at higher or lower levels. However, those who drink more than the recommended limits are more likely to suffer from physical and psychological alcohol-related conditions than those whose alcohol consumption remains within the limits. This is not to say that everyone who drinks above the limits will definitely suffer from an alcohol related conditions. It is a question of risks.

A Great and Growing Evil suggests two further categories for drinkers who exceed these limits but have not yet progressed to the stage of dependent drinking: heavy drinking and problem drinking.

TABLE 14.2   *Categories of alcohol consumption*

Level of consumption	Male (UNITS)	Female (UNITS)
Fairly high	22–35	15–25
High	36–50	26–35
Very high	Over 50	Over 35

Heavy drinking may be defined as consumption of alcohol resulting in a measurable biochemical abnormality (e.g. raised liver enzymes), without apparent harm to the drinker.

Problem drinking is drinking resulting in harm to the drinker or to others.

This establishes a hierarchy of severity of conditions related to excessive use of alcohol. However, although appropriate to individual drinkers, the definitions are not suited to the task of estimating the extent of the problem in the general population. The identification of 'dependent drinkers' depends on the availability of a comprehensive drinking history, that of 'heavy drinkers' on a clinical test and 'problem drinkers' on a social judgement of the meaning of harm.

At a population level, it is possible to approximate the number of drinkers in each of the three categories by the somewhat simplistic, though appropriate, consideration of the amount of alcohol consumed.

An approach used in the General Household Survey[5] may overcome the problem. Three levels of drinking are defined according to the weekly consumption level. These are shown in Table 14.2.

It is not making too unreasonable an assumption to equate these three levels to those of heavy drinking, problem drinking and alcohol dependence. Drinkers regularly consuming amounts in the 'fairly high' range must have a greater likelihood of becoming 'problem drinkers' than those keeping within the recommended limits. Those in the 'high' range are at greater risk of physical harm and are thus more likely to be classified as 'heavy drinkers'. Finally, those in the 'very high' range are very likely to be physically dependent on alcohol.

If this assumption is valid, information on the drinking habits of the population may be used to give a tentative estimate of the likely numbers of drinkers in an area whose consumption of alcohol is likely to cause problems for themselves or their families.

It should be noted that the above suggestion of linkage of the amount consumed with the types of drinking problems is the author's own suggestion.[6] However, a similar pragmatic classification has subsequently been independently developed by Edwards and Unnithan.[7]

GETTING THE INFORMATION

Information on alcohol-related problems in the community may be obtained from two sources: routine data collection and special surveys.

The following are the most relevant sources of information with regard to health services:

Routine data collection
    Mortality statistics
    Hospital admission statistics
    Regional Substance Use databases

Special surveys
    Lifestyle surveys
    Ad hoc surveys
    Literature reviews

In the long-term, routine statistics are likely to be the more useful as they allow comparisons to be made over time and within a larger geographical area than is usually possible with special surveys. The main advantages of special surveys are that the subject may be examined in greater depth and errors of data entry are less likely.

The advantages and disadvantages of the various sources will now be considered.

Routine Data Collection

Mortality statistics
In theory, these are the most relevant routinely available statistics. Studies have shown the inverse relationship between the price of alcohol and the mortality rates from alcoholic liver disease.[8,] However, in practice, the number of deaths as a result of alcohol-related diseases is likely to be grossly underestimated if identified on death notification data alone. It is likely that many certifying doctors do not register excessive alcohol as a chief or contributory factor to a death either owing to lack of recognition or a wish to spare the family of the deceased from the stigma of such a diagnosis.

Hospital admission statistics
These may be expected to vary widely owing to differences in medical care between areas. This is particularly true for psychological diag-

noses such as alcohol dependence. Areas which have a policy of admitting all people with severe alcohol-related problems will evidently have higher admission rates than those where most problem drinkers are managed in a community setting and will therefore be absent from the inpatient statistics. However, it is likely that admission policies for 'physical' conditions will be more uniform. For instance, most patients with alcoholic liver disease will require a hospital admission. Therefore, the admission rates for these conditions may be a closer reflection of the extent of these conditions diagnosed in the population.

A more general problem with the use of hospital inpatient statistics is that the figures are based upon episodes of care rather than actual patients – a large number of episodes in a year could reflect individual patients or several repeat admissions of a smaller group of patients. Given the chronic recurring nature of most alcohol-related conditions the latter is the more likely.

Patient identification numbers are usually unique within a district but not between districts. Thus, patients admitted to hospitals in two or more districts will have different patient identification numbers.

Examination of the regional admissions dataset will not take account of admissions outside the region. At the time of this study the national admissions database was not fully developed. Neither system could take account of admissions to non-NHS units.

Substance use databases

Most regions in England have set up a structure to record contacts of drug users with voluntary and statutory agencies. In many instances an attempt has been made to include people whose problems are solely alcohol related. The system obviously depends on accurate reporting. Given the large scale of alcohol-related problems, relative to those of the use of illicit substances, an accurate recording of all contacts made by problem drinkers would probably overwhelm the database. However, what is much more likely is that the bulk of such contacts will remain unrecorded and the best that may be expected is that the database will give a picture of multiple substance users who also have drinking problems.

In conclusion, of the routinely available statistics analysis of mortality data and any existing substance use database is unlikely to be of value in their present state. Hospital inpatient statistics are also of little use in determining the absolute amount of alcohol-related problems in an area. However, they may be of value in estimating the workload that alcohol-related problems place on the health services and when examined at a regional level may highlight variations between different districts.

Special Surveys

Special surveys may be most useful when they have actually taken place within the district or region itself. The generalisation of rates found in studies conducted elsewhere may be of little value. For example, the General Household Survey provides estimates of the amount of alcohol consumed per week for a sample throughout Britain. It is well-known that there are marked regional variations in the weekly consumption of alcohol with people in Northern England and Scotland reporting higher consumption levels than those in Southern England. Simple extrapolation of national rates to the local population may therefore seriously under- or overestimate the extent of the problem. Even where regional rates are known their application at district level may be misleading. The presence within that district of ethnic minority populations in whom the use of alcohol is frowned upon or forbidden may greatly reduce the prevalence of problem drinking.

Lifestyle surveys

Many districts and regions have conducted lifestyle surveys to determine the extent of 'healthy behaviours' among their populations. Lifestyle surveys invariably contain some questions on alcohol use. As the alcohol-related questions are only a small part of the survey, there may be a greater degree of honesty than with a dedicated alcohol questionnaire. It also has the advantage of approaching people who have not necessarily sought help for alcohol-related problems, and thus an estimate of the unmet need in the population may be made. There are obvious problems with the inferences that may be drawn from this method but where the results of a lifestyle survey exist this is a cheap 'quick and dirty' approach to estimate the amount of excessive drinking in an area. The use of similar questions in different surveys may allow some comparisons between areas to be drawn.

A major disadvantage is that most lifestyle surveys do not achieve a high response rate. A rate of 60 per cent is regarded as an excellent result. The sheer bulk of the questionnaire may well be a deterrent to many. It is also likely that those with the most unhealthy lifestyle behaviours are least likely to complete the questionnaire. Thus, in the case of alcohol-related questions, those drinking heavily would be least likely to reply. Any figure for the prevalence of alcohol-related prob-

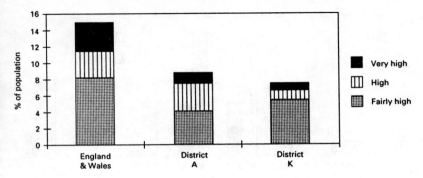

Figure 14.1 Alcohol consumption patterns

lems based on the result of a lifestyle survey alone would be a gross underestimation.

The main advantage of such surveys may be comparative. A similar survey in another district may be assumed to be subject to the same constraints. Therefore, differences between the districts in the proportion of the population admitting to drinking to excess may be an indication that real differences exist. This would assume that the questions asked in the different surveys were very similar, if not identical.

EXAMPLES OF THE USE OF AVAILABLE DATA

Lifestyle Surveys

Figure 14.1 shows data on alcohol consumption from two separate lifestyle surveys conducted in neighbouring Health Authority areas. Identical questions on alcohol consumption were used in both surveys.

This may have implications on the type of service required in a district. For example, where the 'fairly high' levels are predominant (District K) there may be a greater need for population-based health-promotion activities to encourage sensible drinking, whereas in areas with a relatively large amount of 'high' and 'very high' drinking (District A) a more intensive, individually centred approach may be more appropriate. Note that, as expected from their location in Southern England, the total proportion of the population drinking more than the recommended limits in the two South-West Thames districts is less than that for England and Wales.

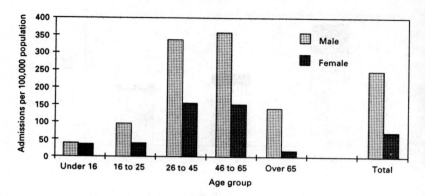

Figure 14.2   Alcohol-related admissions by age group and sex.

Routine Hospital Admission Statistics

The following is an example of the use of routine hospital admission statistics. This is presented to give a 'taste' of what may be achieved by looking at the data.

Data on admissions in South-West Thames region for all alcohol-related conditions listed in Table 14.1 have been examined for 1991 and 1992. In interpreting these data the caveats mentioned above should be borne in mind. In 1991/2 there were 2975 admissions classified as alcohol dependence – 2072 male and 903 female, representing a male: female ratio of over two to one. A similar ratio was observed in almost 5000 all-cause alcohol-related admissions during the same period.

The more than two to one male : female ratio is maintained in each age group, with the exception of the under-16-year-olds – most of whom were admitted for the non-dependent abuse of alcohol (deliberate or accidental ingestion of large amounts of alcohol in a single drinking session). The majority of admissions take place among those aged 26–65 – the economically active section of the population.

The data may also be examined by looking at the numbers admitted in each of the 13 districts. Figure 14.3 shows the admission rates of residents of each district admitted to any hospital in the region for any alcohol related diagnosis.There is a wide variation in admission rates with District A having rates of almost double the lowest district.

Figure 14.4 shows the number of admissions for each of the individual diagnoses – both psychological and physical. Alcohol dependence is by far the most common single diagnosis, the overall admission

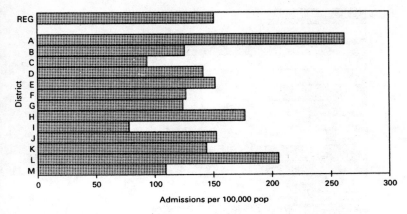

Figure 14.3   Alcohol-related admission by district of residence

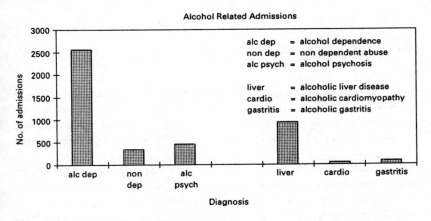

Figure 14.4   Alcohol-related admissions for each of the individual diagnoses

rates may be seen as largely dependent on the rates for this condition.

There are three possible explanations for the wide variation in admission rates between districts.

1. There is a real difference in the incidence of alcohol-related conditions in the districts with the highest admission rates (**epidemiology**).

2. There is better recognition of the conditions in some districts resulting in more accurate coding, or, conversely, overdiagnosis of alcohol-related conditions occurs (**artefact**).

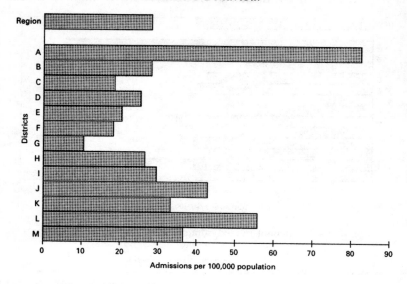

Figure 14.5 Alcohol-related admissions by physical diagnoses

3. There are different admission policies in the districts resulting in more people with a diagnosis of alcohol-related conditions being admitted in some districts with more being treated as out-patients in others and therefore not appearing on the admission data (**treatment**).

Using routinely collected data alone, it is not possible to determine which explanation is most likely. However, all these conditions should be relatively easy to diagnose making the artefact explanation unlikely. A difference in admission policies would be most apparent in the psychological diagnoses such as alcohol dependence but, in theory, if the treatment explanation is the cause of the variation we should not expect a major difference in admission rates for physical diagnoses such as alcoholic liver disease.

Figure 14.5 shows the admission rates by district for physical diagnoses alone.

It is evident that there is still a large variation in admission rates, which is even greater than the combined figures. Moreover, those districts with a high admission rate for psychological diagnoses tend to also have a high rate of admission for physical diagnosis. As Figure 14.6 shows, this relationship is positively correlated. It is also statistically significant ($r = 0.56$, 95 per cent confidence intervals 0.01–0.85).

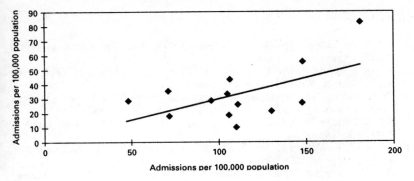

Figure 14.6 Physical and psychological admissions

Does this mean that there is a real difference in the incidence of alcohol-related conditions between the districts? We cannot say for certain but it must be considered a strong possibility.

This positive correlation between physical and psychological admission rates is interesting. We know that the districts with lower psychological admission rates have community alcohol teams rather than a residential facility. The average age of admission for the most common psychological diagnosis – alcohol dependence is 45; that for the most common physical diagnosis is 65. It is therefore tempting to conclude that the districts with a residential treatment policy are failing to prevent the development of physical problems at a later stage. However, this cannot be proven by this relatively crude analysis of routinely available data.

CONCLUSION

Routine health service data can not give the full picture of alcohol-related conditions in a region or district and it would be unfair to expect them to do so. However, they may provide reasonably accurate estimates of the extent of the problem. In a climate where resources are restricted it may often be better to use these estimates than to develop more accurate and more expensive systems.

NOTES

1. *International Classification of Diseases*, 1975 Revision (Geneva: World Health Organisation, 1975).
2. *International Statistical Classification of Disease and Related Health Problems* (Geneva: World Health Organisation, 1992).
3. Royal College of Physicians, *A Great and Growing Evil – The Medical Consequences of Alcohol Abuse* (London: Tavistock, 1987).
4. Royal College of Psychiatrists, *Alcohol – Our Favourite Drug* (London: Tavistock, 1986).
5. Office of Population Censuses and Surveys, *The General Household Survey* (London: HMSO, 1992).
6. G. Edwards and S. Unnithan, 'Alcohol Misuse', in A. Stevens and J. Raftery (eds), *Health Care Needs Assessment* (Oxford: Radcliffe Medical Press, 1994).
7. R. E. Kendall, M. de Roumanie, and E. B. Ritson, 'Effect of Economic Changes on Scottish Drinking Habits 1978–82', *British Journal of Addiction*, 78 (1983):365–79.
8. E. Goddard, *Drinking in England and Wales in the late 1980s* (London: HMSO, 1991).

15 Alcohol and Traumatic Brain Injury

Chris Eberhardie and Adrian Bonner

INTRODUCTION TO THE SCALE OF THE PROBLEM

It is estimated that alcohol is a contributory factor in 50 per cent of murders, 40 per cent of road traffic accidents, 30 per cent of fatal accidents and 65 per cent of all serious traumatic brain injuries in the United Kingdom.[1] Among the 65 per cent of serious head injuries there will be those who have been the victims of violent crime, falls and road traffic accidents. The costs to the individual, the family, the health service and society are considerable. In these alcohol-related injuries, the underlying pathophysiology is likely to have an important impact on the subsequent recovery and rehabilitation of the brain injured patient. The distinction between the role of ethanol as a contributory cause of the injury, and its effects during treatment, care and outcome, is rarely noted in the literature. The figures quoted above are now over 10 years old. Estimates of the true impact of alcohol on traumatic brain injury are difficult to obtain as the statistics are fragmentary. Recording of alcohol-related incidents is carried out by agencies such as the Home Office, the police, the NHS and the alcohol-related voluntary bodies. However, it is usual to assess alcohol consumption in head-injured patients, a factor which undoubtedly will have an influence on outcome. The exception is where a brain-injured patient also has liver damage, here alcohol intake will have been recorded in relation to the latter only.

Clinically , the number of tests carried out on patients should be minimised, both in the interests of the patient and of the hospital budget. However, it could be argued that there is a need for more research into the alcohol and drug history of the patient and alcohol and drug status at the time of the trauma. The following hypothetical case histories illustrate the difficulties facing the clinician and the researcher.

Case 1

A two-car accident involving two drivers and six passengers occurs. The two drivers were sober and the six passengers had consumed more than 4 units of alcohol each. Four passengers had severe traumatic brain injury requiring admission to an accident and emergency department where one died and two needed to be transferred to a regional neurosurgical unit.

Case 2
The host at a family lunch-time barbecue tripped over a flagstone, fell on to a barbecue fork and suffered a penetrating traumatic brain injury as a result. He had consumed 2 units of alcohol as wine immediately before the accident and 5 units at a party the previous evening.

Case 3
A middle-aged vagrant was alcohol-dependent and had liver and neurological damage. He staggered into the path of a car and suffered a moderately severe traumatic brain injury

Case 4
A young man, whose father and grandfather were alcohol-dependent, drank heavily, was involved in a fight and suffered mild traumatic brain injury. He showed no obvious clinical signs of liver damage.

INADEQUACY OF RECORDS OF ALCOHOL INTAKE

The researcher trying to gain a picture of the relationship between alcohol and traumatic brain injury is confronted with a lack of data. In the case of the two-car accident, police statistics will record only the fact that there had been an accident. But the head-injured passengers will not have been breathalysed and, unless they had clinical complications, it is unlikely that blood alcohol levels or liver function tests will have been undertaken.

In the case of the barbecue fork incident, it is unlikely that records on alcohol intake will have been made. There was no police involvement and it will have been entered in the hospital records as a frontal craniocerebral injury using the International Classification of Diseases or Read coding systems. The individual concerned had consumed moderate quantities of alcohol during the previous twenty-four hours. Even if blood alcohol levels had been measured, these would be unreliable as actual ethanol concentration in the blood is only detectable for a limited number of hours after consumption, see below. The current means of acquiring this information is by careful history taking and this is known to be unreliable. The conclusion from this is that there is a need for objective biological markers of alcohol consumption. In Case 3, where alcohol dependence is known to be an aspect of case management, there may be existing information about the alcoholism but there may be no link recorded between this and the brain injury statistics. As far as the police are concerned the accident to the pedestrian will be recorded but not necessarily as being alcohol related. Another factor in the management of this patient is the presence of liver disease and related neurological problems. Wernicke–Korsakoff syndrome and/ or polyneuropathies are nutritional disorders which result from the combination of alcoholism, liver disease and malnutrition.[2] This is an important factor but if this had been recorded at all, it will not necessarily have been related to head injury but to the general state of the patient. The psychopathological aspects of Wernicke–Korsakoff syndrome are discussed in Chapter 9.

In Case 4 there are no clinical signs of alcohol abuse but there was a family history of alcoholism, the problem may only manifest itself after the acute stage of injury. There appears to be little research into the effects of traumatic brain injury on young men with a genetic predisposition to alcoholism as described by Scukitt.[3] The possibility of developing biochemical markers has been discussed by Thompson and McMillan[4] with regard to ratios of tryptophan metabolites. The hypermetabolic state following trauma will presumably disturb these metabolic pathways. The changes in such ratios during recovery and rehabilitation might provide a useful index of physiological homeostasis and more specific differences between alcohol-abusers and non-alcoholic patients.

MEASURING ALCOHOL CONSUMPTION

A range of biological tests is available which can be used to detect alcohol useage. Many of these are purely research tools which would be of limited use to the clinician.

Gamma-glutamyltranspeptidase (GGT), aspartate aminotransferase (AST) alanine aminotransferase (ALT) and mean red cell volume (MCV) are all commonly used in clinical tests of liver function. GGT is found to be above 40 IU/l in 80 per cent of problem drinkers;[5] even before there is demonstrable liver damage MCV is raised in alcoholism.

In a Finnish study, university students, aged between 20 and 28 years, were investigated with regard to their drinking activity and subsequent measurements of serum carbohydrate-deficient transferrin (CDT) indicated that this was a useful marker for detecting heavy drinking.[2] Recent alcohol consumption appears to be reliably monitored using CDT and is more specific than GGT, MCV, high density lipoprotein and β-hexosaminidase. As many traumatic brain injuries occur in young males aged 17–30 years, CDT may be a marker which deserves further study in this group of patients. Other markers of alcohol-related liver damaged such as urinary L-fucose have been proposed.[6]

Although more research is required to develop more objective markers of alcohol consumption, the importance of tolerance, chronic abuse and the potential effects of alcohol and its metabolites on blood vessels, the liver and the central nervous system itself must be recognised. Alcohol use and abuse is an important secondary insult to the already damaged brain and clinical profiling should reflect this.

SUBCLINICAL EFFECTS OF ALCOHOL

From animal studies there is increasing evidence that alcohol influences brain activity via neurotransmitters and their receptors. Inhibitory Gamma-aminobutyric acid (GABA) transmission appears to be enhanced by alcohol, inducing anti-convulsant activity. With repeated alcohol use, tolerance develops and there is a reduction in GABAergic neurotransmission and, if alcohol is then withdrawn, seizures ensue.[7] During the traumatic phases of head injury, seizure occurrence may be due the brain injury and also to alcohol withdrawal. This area of research should be explored further in the hope that such seizures could be minimised by treating the alcoholism as well as the traumatic brain injury. N-methyl-D-aspartate (NMDA) receptors have been studied during the past ten to twenty years. Alcohol inhibits the NMDA receptor at low concentrations but the chronic effects on these receptors is not fully understood.[8] Research on the effects of alcohol on NMDA receptors and ischaemia has resulted in the development of NMDA-protective compounds such as MK801.[9] This an area of interest in neurosurgery where secondary brain damage is being addressed. Work on the interaction of alcohol, NMDA-protective agents and secondary brain damage is in its infancy, but studies on neurodegeneration suggest that this an important area for future research.[10]

DOES ALCOHOL AFFECT THE OUTCOME OF TREATMENT?

Researchers in the United States[11] have examined the relationship between alcohol abuse and the outcome of traumatic brain injury using 407 subjects from the Traumatic Coma Data Bank assessed by the Glasgow Outcome Score (GOS).[12] Levels of blood alcohol were evaluated to determine whether there was a relationship between the level of alcohol in the blood and the severity of the head injury.The pathophysiology of the brain injury was evaluated in relation to the preinjury alcohol history and the initial severity of the head injury. The patient's age and blood alcohol levels were controlled. The subjects were divided into two groups: those with a reported history of alcohol abuse and those with a reported history of abstinence or moderate occasional drinking. To assess intoxication for the two groups, blood alcohol levels (BAL) were recorded. The subject was deemed to be sober if the BAL was less than 100 mg per cent and to be intoxicated if it was over 100 mg per cent.

The results from this work indicated that (for similar initial severities of head injury) there is a strong correlation between alcohol history and poor outcome. Alcohol abusers tended to have a greater risk of mass lesions because they are more likely to have friable vessels due to alcohol-related cerebral atrophy. Overall they have a poorer outcome as measured by GOS than non-abusers. Nearly half the alcohol abusers died, which, the researchers concluded, was due in part to a generalised reduction in ability to survive the stress of traumatic brain injury. Various factors are implicated here such as a reduction in circulating platelets and clotting factors caused by alcohol. This will increase the risk of intracranial haemorrhage. More work is required to provide explanations of these observations.

Intoxication of the patient at the time of a severe traumatic brain injury appears to be irrelevant to the outcome, duration and level of the alcohol abuse that existed prior to the accident are the predominate factors which affect outcome. The chronic use of alcohol will affect several organs and physiological processes as discussed in Chapter 6. Following head injury a report of moderate to high levels of alcohol in the blood is only an initial indication that there has been a history of alcohol abuse prior to trauma. Further investigations should be undertaken to ascertain the extent of tissue damage caused by chronic use of alcohol.

CLINICAL MANAGEMENT AND REHABILITATION

There are three groups of patients who have different treatment needs:

A. individuals who have had a drink but are not intoxicated and have no liver damage;

B. heavy drinkers who may have early liver damage without the clinical signs and symptoms;

C. alcohol abusers who may have neurological, cardiac and liver damage.

The first group present no serious management problem but, as discussed Chapter 4, there is evidence that even small amounts of alcohol can cause major changes in brain function. It is conceiveable that even small amounts of alcohol should be taken into consideration for treatment purposes. Presently, special attention is only paid to the other two groups. The assessment of these patients on admission is very important. Whilst neurological and cardio-respiratory assessment will remain at the top of the list of priorities, the nutritional, functional and social assessments should follow as soon as possible afterwards. A careful history of the patient's eating and drinking habits should be recorded. If the patient is unconscious, this information should be gained from family and/or friends. This information can be unreliable for many reasons. The family may not know the patient's current habits or the patient may have eating and drinking habits of the family disapproves of and therefore prefers not to disclose. In many cases, families fear that any record of an alcohol history may attract the attention of the police or affect insurance claims. It is important for the family to realise the importance of this information to clinical outcome and treatment. The current trend for nurses to give a brief dietary history using terms such as 'normal diet' or 'poor diet' does not meet the requirements of a short but effective nutritional assessment. There is a need for such a tool to be developed which not only assesses the patient's nutritional status on admission but continues to monitor it regularly thereafter. Such a nutrition assessment tool needs to be more cohesive so that it can be used by various members of the team including the medical staff, dieticians , speech and language therapists, pharmacists and nurses. There is evidence to suggest that early appropriate feeding of head-injured patients reduces the effects of hypermetabolism and hypercatabolism.[13]

The progress of treatment has frequently relied on the Glasgow Coma

Scale (GCS)[14] which is a valid and reliable tool for assessing arousal and awareness but it does not present the whole picture of neurological deficits. A Glasgow Coma score of 15 (the maximum possible score) may seem to be very good but the patient may be restless, aggressive, dysarthric and have an array of cranial nerve deficits. Psychologists have made attempts to assess patients in the early acute phase of injury.[15] They are trying to assist those working in the intensive care unit to assess patient progress using measures other than the GCS. Neuropsychological deficits found in alcoholics (see Chapters 9 and 12) suggest specific approaches should be developed for head-injured patients who have chronically abused alcohol. It is unlikely that these assessments will be used routinely in clinical management but there is a need for research tools which can measure changes in behaviour which are too 'fine grain' for the Glasgow Coma Scale. Used in conjunction with biological markers and other objective monitoring these assessments should give clinicians more help in formulating treatment and anticipating its outcome in future.

CONCLUSIONS

Although an increasing amount of research has been carried out on the effects of alcohol on the brain, very little attention has been paid to the relationship between alcohol consumption, prior to the injury, and the effects of pre-existing, alcohol-related pathology in the recovery phase. There are indications from incomplete and unsystematic research that pre-injury alcohol levels and abuse can measurably impair outcome and are susceptible to nutritional and other treatment.[13] Cost-effective ways of gathering the data need to be developed in order to estimate the true size of the problem before proceeding with further work on clinical management and predicting outcomes. In an age of medical and nursing audit, when the quality and cost-effectiveness of clinical treatment and care is under constant review, it is time to have a closer look at the role played by alcohol in the treatment and outcome of traumatic brain injury.

NOTES

1. A. Paton, *ABC of Alcohol* (London: British Medical Association, 1988).
2. K. Lindsay and M. Nystrom, 'Neurology and Neurosurgery Illustrated Carbohydrate-deficient Transferrin (CDT) in Serum as a Possible Indicator of Heavy Drinking in Young University Students', *Alcohol: Clinical Experimental Research*, 16 (1992):93–7.
3. M. A. Schukit, 'Responses of Sons of Alcoholics', *Alcohol*, 12 (1995):1.
4. S. M. Thomson and B. A. Mcmillen, 'Test for Decreased Serotonin/ Tryptophan Metabolite Ratios in Abstinent Alcoholics', *Alcohol*, 4 (1987):1–5.
5. K. O. Lewis, 'Tools of Detection', *British Medical Journal*, 283 (1981):1531–2.
6. M. Yamauchi, K. Kimura, M. Ohata, *et al.*, 'Urinary Level of L-Fucose as a Marker of Alcoholic Disease', *Alcohol: Clinical and Experimental Research*, 17 (1993):268–71.
7. J. Peris, *Differential Sensitivity of Nigrotectal GABA Neurons to Alcohol and Alcohol Withdrawal Seizures* (Boca Raton: CRC Press, 1992).
8. L. J. Chandler, C. Summers and F. T. Crews, 'Ethanol Inhibits NMDA Receptor-mediated Excitotoxicity in Rat Primary Neuronal Cultures', *Alcohol: Clinical and Experimental Research*, 17 (1993):54–60.
9. J. M. Khanna, H. Kalant, G. Shah *et al.*, '(+)MK801 and Ketamine on Rapid Tolerance to Ethanol', *Brain Research Bulletin*, 28 (1992):311–4.
10. A. Freese, K. L. Schwartz, M. During *et al.*, 'Kynurenine metabolites of Tryptophan: Implications for Neurologic Disease', *Neurology*, 9 (1990):691–5.
11. R. M. Ruff, 'Alcohol Abuse and Neurological Outcome of the Severely Head Injured', *Journal of Head Trauma Rehabilitation*, 5 (1990):21–31.
12. B. Jennett, 'Assessment of Outcome after Severe Brain Damage: A Practical Scale', *Lancet*, i (1975):480–4.
13. J. W. D. Dickerson, 'Nutritional Factors: Recovery of Function', in F. D. Rose and D. A. Johnson (eds), *Recovery from Brain Damage* (New York: Plenum Press, 1992).
14. G. Teasdale and B. Jennett, 'Assessment of Coma and Impaired Consciousness', *Lancet*, ii (1974):81.
15. S. Horn, 'A Review of Behavioural Assessment Scales for Monitoring Recovery in and after Coma with Pilot Data on a New Scale of Visual Awareness', *Neuropsychological Rehabilitation*, 3 (1993):121–37.

16 The Role of Clinical Forensic Medicine in the Assessment of Alcohol Misuse in the Community

J. J. Payne-James

INTRODUCTION

In the United Kingdom, general practitioners (GPs or primary care physicians) are often the first point of contact for individuals seeking help for problems of alcohol misuse. Many individuals, however, do not seek help, either because they are unaware that they have a problem, or because of denial of the problem. Many individuals with, or at risk of, alcoholism may fail to get help until the alcohol misuse is much more severe.

Clearly if it were possible to identify such individuals and direct them to appropriate treatment or counselling agencies, a certain proportion may benefit from earlier intervention.

CLINICAL FORENSIC MEDICINE

Clinicians who specialise in clinical forensic medicine (variously known as police surgeons, forensic physicians or forensic medical examiners) are responsible for the medical care of detainees in police stations.[1] Detainees may be held in custody in a number of circumstances. For example, some may be under arrest, some may be detained while investigations into offences are being undertaken, some may be 'wanted on warrant', whilst others may be on remand. Under s66 of the Police and Criminal Evidene Act (1984),[2] 'Codes of Practice'[3] were issued. Code C deals with the detention, treatment and questioning of suspects by police officers and also addresses medical issues. The Codes instruct the custody officer (the police officer responsible for the care of the detainee) to call a police surgeon if the detainee appears to be:

1. suffering from physical or mental illness;
2. injured;
3. showing no signs of sensibility and awareness or fails to respond normally to questions or conversation, other than through drunkenness;
4. in need of medical attention.

A detainee may also specifically request medical attention, in which case a police surgeon must also be summoned. There is thus a considerable number of circumstances in which a police surgeon may attend a detainee. The purpose(s) of the examination may include:

1. determining a detainee's 'fitness to be detained' which may require one or more of the following:
   (a) assessment of illness/injuries/drug-related problems/alcohol misuse,
   (b) advice to the custody officer on general care,
   (c) prescribing medication,
   (d) referral to hospital,
   (e) admission to hospital under the Mental Health Act 1983;
2. determining a detainee's 'fitness to be interviewed' which may require one or more of the following:
   (a) assessment of competence to understand and answer questions.
   (b) assessment of the need for an 'appropriate adult' in the vulnerable or mentally ill,
   (c) assessment of a substance misuser;
3. taking of samples:
   (a) blood for alcohol estimation under the Road Traffic Act 1988,
   (b) intimate samples (e.g. for murder or sexual assault cases),
4. assessment in relation to injuries and allegations of police assault.

In the Metropolitan Police area almost 100 000 doctor/detainee contacts are made every year.

Consultation Types

A study of the work patterns of a forensic medical examiner (see Figure 16.1) showed that assessment of drunk or alcoholic detainees was the primary reason for examination in 16 per cent, whilst drink-

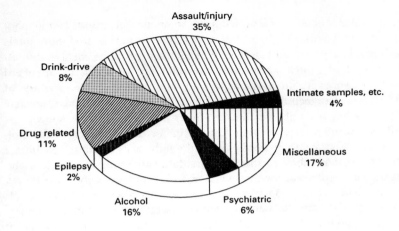

Figure 16.1 Primary reason for examination

drive offences under the Road Traffic Act 1988 constituted a further 8 per cent. Thus almost one-quarter of examinations were primarily alcohol initiated.

The majority of the alcohol-related consultations were assessments for fitness to be detained in chronic alcoholics (41 per cent) whilst 36 per cent were for non-alcoholics who were drunk. The remainder of this group had mixed pathology (e.g. ulcer, epilepsy, asthma) of which alcohol misuse was the main contributing factor for the reason for being in custody. It is a concern of many forensic practitioners that custody in a police cell is not the most appropriate place to care for such individuals and that special centres should be made available for their immediate[1, 4] care.

Unrecognised Alcohol Misuse

The identification of individuals with previously unrecognised or treated alcoholism or alcohol dependence has been the subject of a number of studies in different settings. In a study of patients attending an accident and emergency department[5] 13.5 per cent of males and 2.6 per cent of females exceeded the 'safe limits' advised by the Health Education Council (the forerunner of the Health Education Authority, and these figures were similar to those in other such units.[6] These figures were consistent with nationwide drinking habits.[7] These figures may, however, be an underestimate of true alcohol misuse and in more recent studies where the relationship between assault, injury and alcohol have been examined it has been shown that 33 per cent of individuals seen in an accident and emergency department for assessment and treatment of head injury were under the influence of alcohol.[8] Shepherd *et al.*'s data were in agreement with this finding.[9,10] In a study of individuals examined for assault and injury in the clinical forensic medical setting it has been shown that in 36 per cent of cases the alleged assailant appeared (to the victim) to be under the influence of alcohol, with only 8 per cent apparently under the influence of drugs.[10] Redmond and colleagues[11] showed that of individuals attending an accident and emergency department with alcohol misuse problems only a small proportion had sought help from professional agencies. A recent study[12] reported an attempt to identify individuals presenting with an alcohol-related problem to an accident department, to assess the severity of the problem and to attempt to refer those with serious problems to the appropriate agencies. In order to establish the presence of an alcohol problem, CAGE and modified Michigan Alcoholism Screening Tests (MAST) were completed. These indicators of alcohol abuse[13,14] established that there was a high number of individuals with untreated alcohol problems. Of those so identified, 46 per cent attended subsequently to discuss these problems further.

ALCOHOL MISUSE IN CLINICAL FORENSIC MEDICINE

No attempt has previously been made to quantify the relevance of alcohol misuse in clinical forensic medicine, although the links between alcohol and crime are recognised. Indeed the Government has recently set up an enquiry – the 'All Party Group on Alcohol Misuse – Alcohol and Crime', the aims of which are:

1. to consider the link between alcohol and crime from the practical perspective of professionals involved in dealing with alcohol-related offences and offenders, and of those involved in the drink trade;
2. to consider current difficulties and to identify recommendations for action in order to reduce the incidence and costs of crime.

A recent study attempted to determine the prevalence of alcohol misuse in clinical forensic medical practice.[15]

In this prospective study a questionnaire survey of all individuals seen in the clinical forensic setting of police stations in East and Central London was undertaken. Individuals were asked to complete an anonymised structured questionnaire, after history-taking and examination by a Forensic Medical Examiner. Basic demographic details, and details of drinking habits (frequency and amount) were recorded. CAGE & Brief MAST were also completed. Of 180 consecutive individuals asked to complete the survey, 20.4 per cent ($n = 47$) did not, because of refusal or inability to give consent to participate in the study, the purposes of which were explained prior to examination. Of those who did not participate, 15/47 were in custody having been arrested either for alcohol-related offences (e.g. being drunk and disorderly, drunk and incapable, or who had been arrested under the provisions of the Road Traffic Act 1988) or were too incapacitated by alcohol to give consent. Of the 133 individuals who gave consent, 2 per cent ($n = 37$) admitted to having had current or previous alcohol dependence or alcoholism or had been treated for such problems in the past. Those individuals were not asked to continue the questionnaire. Of the remaining 96 respondents, 81 per cent drank alcohol regularly. The mean number of days per week on which alcohol was drunk was 2.3, with a mean of 6.4 units of alcohol on each occasion. The estimated mean weekly consumption of alcohol for these individuals ranged from 0 to 140 units. Twenty-five per cent of those respondents ($n = 24$) exceeded the 'safe' levels of intake of alcohol recommended by the Health Education Authority[16] (per week, 21 U – male, 14 U – female). 22 per cent ($n = 21$) had positive CAGE scores ($1 - n = 4$, $2 - n = 7$, $3 - n = 4$, $4 - n = 1$); 7.3 per cent ($n = 7$) had Brief MAST scores >10.

If all those individuals arrested for alcohol offences or being incapable through alcohol, those with self-admitted prior or current alcohol problems, and those who exceed 'safe' weekly alcohol intakes, are considered together, then 42 per cent (76/180) of those examined had potential or actual alcoholism or alcohol dependence.

IMPLICATIONS

The fact that almost half of individuals seen in police custody by forensic physicians may be or have been at risk for alcohol misuse is alarming. These figures are considerably higher than those identified in accident and emergency departments, and considerably higher than would be expected from considering purely alcohol-related offences. It is apparent that the forensic physician is in a good position to elicit an appropriate alcohol history from a detainee in police custody, and at least to inform the examinee of the risks to their health and to advise them to take further advice from their own general practitioner or an appropriate counselling agency. As with drug misusers[17] many individuals have not recognised that they have a problem or have not sought help through ignorance or lack of information. Clearly, even if only a small percentage of examinees so identified subsequently seek help there are potential benefits not only to the individual themself, but also to their families, the police and judicial system. It must be hoped that in the UK the All Party Group on Alcohol Misuse recognises the potential for identification and treatment of alcohol misusers seen in police custody and identifies clear routes by which treatment or counselling of such individuals may be expedited.

ACKNOWLEDGEMENTS

I am grateful to my colleagues Derek Keys, Peter Dean, Peter Jerreat and Ian Wall for their input into our research studies and to the Metropolitan Police Service and its personnel for their cooperation in enabling us to undertake this research.

Opinions expressed in this manuscript are the author's and do not in any way represent the opinion of the Metropolitan Police Service.

NOTES

1. BMA Medical Ethics Committee/Association of Police Surgeons, *Health Care of Detainees in Police Stations* (London: BMA Publishing, 1994).
2. Police and Criminal Evidence Act 1984 (London: HMSO).
3. Police and Criminal Evidence Act 1984 (s66) Codes of Practice, revised edn (London: HMSO, 1991).
4. J. J. Payne-James, 'Work Patterns of a Forensic Medical Examiner', *The Police Surgeon*, 42 (1992):21–4.
5. T. G. Barrett and C. M. Vaughan Williams, 'Use of a Questionnaire to Obtain an Alcohol History from those Attending an Inner City Accident and Emergency Department', *Archives of Emergency Medicine*, 6 (1989):3–40.
6. D. W. Yates, J. M. Hadfield and K. Peters, 'The Detection of Problem Drinkers in the Accident and Emergency Department', *British Journal of Addiction*, 82 (1987):163–7.

7. P. Wilson, 'Drinking Habits in the United Kingdom', *Population Trends*, 22 (1980):14–18.
8. M. J. Boyle, L. Vella and E. Moloney, 'Role of Drugs and Alcohol in Patients with Head Injury', *Journal of the Royal Society of Medicine*, 81 (1991):223–4.
9. J. J. Payne-James and P. J. Dean, 'Assault and Injury in Clinical Forensic Medical Practice', *Medicine, Science & the Law*, 34 (1994):202–6.
10. J. Shepherd, C. Scully, M. Shapland, M. Irish and I. J. Leslie, 'Assault: Characteristics of Victims Attending an Inner-city Hospital', *Injury*, 19 (1988):185–90.
11. A. D. Redmond, S. Richards and P. K. Plunkett, 'The Significance of Random Breath Alcohol Sampling in the Accident and Emergency Department', *Alcohol and Alcoholism*, 22 (1987):341–3.
12. M. Green, J. Setchell and P. Hames *et al.*, 'Management of Alcohol Abusing Patients in Accident and Emergency Departments', *Journal of the Royal Society of Medicine*, 86 (1993):393–5.
13. D. Mayfield, G. McLeod and P. Hall, 'The CAGE Questionnaire: Validation of a New Alcohol Screening Instrument', *American Journal of Psychiatry*, 131 (1974):1121–3.
14. A. D. Pokorny, B. A. Miller and H. B. Kaplan, 'The Brief MAST: A Shortened Version of the Michigan Alcoholism Screening Test', *American Journal of Psychiatry*, 129 (1972):118–21.
15. J. J. Payne-James, D. W. Keys, I. Wall, P. G. Jerreat and P. J. Dean, 'Prevalence of Alcohol Misuse in Clinical Forensic Medicine', *Journal of Clinical Forensic Medicine* (1995, in press).
16. Health Education Authority, *That's the Limit: A Guide to Sensible Drinking* (London: HMSO, 1992).
17. J. J. Payne-James, D. Keys and P. Dean, 'Drug Custody: A Prospective Survey', *Journal of the Royal Society of Medicine*, 87 (1994):13–14.

17 Alcohol Abuse in Society: Case Studies

The last three chapters have demonstrated how routine data may be collected from the health service and forensic medicine. These data present a view of the occurrence of alcohol and drug abuse in society which is generated from a 'medical model'. As useful as this approach is, it does not take into account the nature and needs of specific groups. To do this a more 'socially appropriate perspective' can be used. The following case studies illustrate some of the problems resulting from methodological issues in this area of investigation and, in particular, from studies undertaken in short-term projects undertaken by graduate students. Important discussions relating to: 'what level of consumption constitutes *abuse*', 'alcohol usage by the elderly', and 'the effectiveness of health education' will be introduced.

Case Study I
Identifying Women at Risk of Alcohol Dependency
Margaret Millar

As part of its strategy for health one of the targets in the Government's White Paper *The Health of the Nation* (Department of Health, 1992) is 'to reduce . . . the proportion of women drinking more than 14 units of alcohol per week from 11% in 1990 to 7% by 2005'. This target is based on guidelines of sensible drinking levels for women derived from reports of the Royal College of Physicians,[1] Royal College of Psychiatrists,[2] and the Royal College of General Practitioners.[3] These guidelines for sensible drinking of less than 14 units of alcohol per week have been acknowledged as being arbitrary,[4] but are used to present the conceptual relationship between alcohol consumption and alcohol-related harm including dependency as linear. Thus increasing consumption of alcohol above the sensible limits is linked to increasing risk of alcohol-related harm. However, is this a valid model upon which to identify women at risk of alcohol dependency? It is possible that women are being put at risk of alcohol dependency by the message given out by health professionals who use these arbitrary sensible drinking limits in health education leaflets on alcohol (e.g. Health Education Authority, 1992).

Gorman *et al.*[5] investigated the relationship between measures of alcohol consumption and alcohol dependence. The Severity of Alcohol Dependence Questionnaire (SADQ *r* = 0.72) and the Short Alcohol Dependence Data Questionnaire (SADD *r* = 0.69) were most highly correlated with alcohol consumption (range 42–420 units/week) in women. The SADQ does include a measure of alcohol consumption. Both these questionnaires were also compared with the Alcohol Related Problems Questionnaire with a correlation of *r* = 0.30. Gorman *et al.* argue that this weak association supports the view that alcohol dependence is conceptually distinct from other alcohol-related problems. Thus a straight quantity–frequency measure, that is, amount of alcohol consumed in the measured week, may be insufficient to identify women who are at risk of alcohol dependency particularly at sensible drinking levels.

From the OPCS study Drinking in England and Wales in the late 1980s,[6] the adult male average consumption is 14.1 units/week and for adult women 4.2 units/week. When only drinkers of alcohol in the measured week are looked at, the adult male average consumption per drinker is 18.5 units/week and for adult women is 7.2 units/week. Between 1978 and 1987, alcohol consumption by women in England and Wales showed a statistically significant rise from 4.2 to 4.8 units per week. However, this rise is accounted for by an increase in the actual proportion of women drinking along with a small rise in the amount drunk by the majority of women drinkers who fall into the sensible or 14 units or less of alcohol per week category.[7] This apparent picture of alcohol consumption at sensible levels by women is also reflected in a survey carried out by Breeze.[8] The study found that 70 per cent of women drank 5 units or less in the week that was measured. Of the remaining 30 per cent, 22 per cent drank 5–15 units, 3 per cent had 15–20 units, 4 per cent drank 20–30 units and less than 1 per cent drank more than 35 units. Recent mortality figures[9] on deaths from alcohol related causes show that women make up a substantial percentage (38 per cent) of these deaths. When specifically looking at deaths from alcohol dependence syndrome the ratio of one woman to two men is obtained. However, the limitations of mortality figures in providing an accurate overall picture are acknowledged. Alcohol Concern[10] collated several relevant reports from 1976 to the mid-1980s to provide a summary of trends in alcohol-related problems including hospital treatment for alcohol dependence. Although in gross terms men far out number women, apart from liver damage, the trend is for a greater percentage rise in women than in men. However, Shaw reviewing similar statistical trends on women from the mid-1960s to the mid-1970s suggests a degree of caution in their interpretation since the prevalence of alcohol-related problems may not have changed.[11]

Rather, he argues that changes within society and education with respect to alcohol and related problems have enabled women to request help more easily. Also the police and the medical profession have become more aware of alcohol misuse in women and are therefore more ready to label it as such. Nevertheless Shaw does consider that the trends taken together rather than separately are making a valid point.[11] Perhaps a decade later, the expectation would have been for these social effects to have stabilised and thus the increasing rate of change with respect to women to have levelled with men. Nevertheless, societal influences remain in the increasing earning power of women through employment, facilitating the purchase of alcohol, and also through targeting by advertisement from the brewing industry.

Current trends can also be supported by the more recent evidence that more women, despite a lack of facilities, are using counselling services as well as in hospital treatment.[12] Allan carried out a study in Scotland comparing clients using counselling services and alcohol treatment units.[13] Both groups had men and women who were heavily dependent on alcohol as measured by the SADQ. Thus women attending non-statutory community based facilities have an alcohol dependency problem of similar magnitude to those attending in-hospital treatment.

How is it that alcohol dependency appears to be on the increase in women when reports of alcohol consumption indicate that a vast majority of women drink (if at all) within the sensible drinking limits? Possible explanations for this may be inaccurate self-reporting of alcohol consumption on the part of women, or that it is alcohol consumption and drinking patterns together which is important with respect to alcohol dependency in women, or that understanding of alcohol dependency in relation to consumption is based primarily on research into men rather than women. It is not possible to explore these arguments in detail here; however, what is common to these explanations are the two essential features of any self-reporting instrument – reliability and validity.

The reliability of an instrument is the degree of consistency with which it measures the attribute it is supposed to be measuring.[14] Reliability can be addressed in a variety of ways. Different alcoholic beverages contain different amounts of alcohol. The unit system has attempted to increase the objectivity of measurement of alcohol consumption. One unit of alcohol is equivalent to 10 ml or approximately 8 g of alcohol. In terms of beverages this is equivalent to a half pint of beer or cider, 1 glass of wine or 1 measure of spirit (England). However, drinks taken at home may not exactly conform to these volumes and measurement error be introduced in equating a glass of an alcoholic beverage with a pub measure.

Measurement error may occur from social desirability leading to underreporting by women of alcohol consumption. However, if social desirability is a source of measurement error than it is likely to be constant rather than random, since over the years alcohol surveys consistently report average adult female consumption of around 4.5 units per week.

Using the test–retest method, the stability of self reports of quantity frequency measures of alcohol consumption has been investigated in both pregnant and non-pregnant female social drinkers.[15–16] Time periods from test to retest were 6 months and 5 years. Both studies indicated a high degree of consistency between pretest and post test. Waterson & Murray Lyon also found a quantity frequency measure of alcohol consumption to be more reliable than either the CAGE questions or the Brief Michigan Alcoholism Screening Test (BMAST) in women attending the antenatal clinic.[17] This is probably due to the low alcohol consumptions, 93 per cent of the women ($n = 893$) falling within the sensible drinking limits, the CAGE questions and BMAST being insensitive at this level of alcohol consumption.

It appears that overall not much confidence can be placed in the reliability of self-reports of quantity frequency measures of alcohol consumption by women who drink within sensible drinking limits. Thus inaccurate reporting seems an unlikely explanation for the increasing alcohol dependency in women.

Validity refers to the degree to which an instrument measures what it is supposed to be measuring.[14] It is more difficult to demonstrate this in self reports than reliability. One method is criterion-related validity where a comparison is made of the measure under scrutiny with a known objective measure. Thus drawing on the linear model the comparison is made between alcohol consumption and accepted measures of alcohol related harm.

Kranzler *et al.* carried out a cross-sectional study of both male and female hospital patients.[18] A quantity frequency measure was used to calculate total alcohol consumption. Women were also classified according to the number of occasions on which they had 6 or more units to drink labelled frequency of intoxication.

Both measures, alcohol consumption and frequency of intoxication, were associated with alcohol-related harm, but frequency of intoxication was a greater risk factor than alcohol consumption in relation to alcohol-related harm including dependency.

Thus, a reliable and valid measure of alcohol consumption, to identify women at risk from alcohol dependency, needs to include the number of occasions on which 6 units or more are consumed as well as total weekly alcohol consumption. That is, the drinking pattern may be of greater significance than total alcohol consumption in identifying women at risk of alcohol dependency. I would like to illustrate this point through looking at a set of results from my own research into women and drinking.[19]

The sample comprised of 39 female social drinkers who completed a quantity–frequency measure of alcohol consumption using a grid based on the days of the week. The week prior to the completion of the grid was assumed to be representative of the drinking pattern of the women. The total units of alcohol consumed per week and the pattern of drinking during the measured week was obtained. Women who drank more than 6 units on any one day were identifiable although the total units per week was 14 or less, that is it fell within the sensible drinking limits.

Of the 39 women, 35 drank 14 units or less in the measured week. However 3 (8.6 per cent) of these women drank 6 units or more on at least one day of the week. Waterson and Murray Lyon found 10 per cent of women usually drinking with 14 units a week admitted to occasions of being more than 14 units at a sitting varying from less than once a month to at least once a month but not weekly.[12] In her women and drinking survey Breeze looked at drinking patterns by daily consumption level.[8] An intensive day was defined as having more than 6 units in a day. Of those women drinking 5–10 units per week 8 per cent had one intensive drinking day and of those drinking 10.5–15 units per week 24 per cent had one intensive drinking day. Using Kranzler *et al.*'s results these women would seem to be at greater risk of alcohol dependency than would at first seem from their total weekly alcohol consumption.[18]

The model of the association between increasing total alcohol consumption per week and increasing risk of alcohol dependency might require revision with respect to women, the vast majority of whom drink within the sensible drinking limit of 14 units/week. Self-reports of alcohol consumption used in screening for alcohol-related harm and identification of women at risk of alcohol-dependency require to include questions which will permit the number of occasions on which 6 units or more are consumed as well as total weekly alcohol consumption. It will be of interest in 2005 to see that if reducing the percentage of women drinking more than 14 units per week has a significant effect on alcohol-related harm. As to whether harm is more related to total drinking or total bouts of drinking remains to be seen.

NOTES

1. Royal College of Physicians, *A Great and Growing Evil: The Medical Consequences of Alcohol Abuse* (London: Tavistock, 1987).
2. Royal College of Psychiatrists, *Alcohol Our Favourite Drug* (London: Tavistock, 1986).
3. Royal College of General Practitioners, *Alcohol – A Balanced View: Reports from General Practice* (London: RCGP, 1986).
4. Royal College of Physicians, *Alcohol and the Public Health* (London: Macmillan, 1991) p. 226.
5. D. M. Gorman *et al.*, 'Level of Agreement between Questionnaire Measures of Alcohol Dependence, Alcoholism and Problem-Drinking in a Sample Presenting at a Specialist Alcohol Treatment Service', *Drug and Alcohol Dependence*, 24 (1989):227–32.
6. E. Goddard, *Drinking in England and Wales in the late 1980s* (London: OPCS, HMSO, 1991).
7. E. Goddard and C. Ikin, *Drinking in England and Wales in 1987* (London: HMSO, 1988).
8. E. Breeze, *Women and Drinking* (London: HMSO, 1985).
9. *OPCS: Mortality Statistics – Cause (England & Wales) 1990*, no. 17 (London: Department of Health, 1991).
10. *Women and Drinking* (London: Alcohol Concern Report, 1988).
11. S. Shaw, 'The Cause of Increasing Drinking Problems Amongst Women', in *Camberwell Council on Alcoholism: Women and Alcohol* (London: Tavistock, 1980).
12. E. J. Waterson, 'Screening for Alcohol-Related Problems in the Antenatal Clinic: an Assessment of Different Methods', *Alcohol & Alcoholism*, 24 (1989):21–30.
13. C. A. Allan, 'Characteristics and Help-seeking Patterns of Attenders at a Community-based Voluntary Agency and an Alcohol- and Drug-Treatment Unit', *British Journal of Addiction*, 84 (1989):73–80.
14. P. F. Polit, *Essentials of Nursing Research Methods and Applications* (Philadelphia, PA: Lippincott, 1985).
15. N. L. Fox, 'The Reliability of Self Reports of Smoking and Alcohol Consumption by Pregnant Women', *Addictive Behaviour*, 14 (1989):187–95.

16. D. M. Czarnecki, 'Five-Year Reliability of Self-Reported Alcohol Consumption', *Journal of Studies on Alcohol*, 51 (1990):68–76.
17. J. Waterson, 'Providing Services for Women with Difficulties with Alcohol or Other Drugs: The Current UK Situation as Seen by Women Practitioners, Researchers and Policy-Makers in the Field', *Drug and Alcohol Dependence*, 24 (1989):119–25.
18. H. R. Kranzler, 'Problems Associated with Average Alcohol Consumption and Frequency of Intoxication in Medical Population', *Alcoholism: Clinical and Experimental Research*, 14 (1990):119–26.
19. M. Millar, 'An Exploratory Study of the Coping Styles of Women Drinkers and Non-Drinkers of Alcohol', thesis, University of Surrey (Roehampton Institute London, 1990).

REFERENCES

Alcohol Concern (1988) *Women and Drinking* (Alcohol Concern Report).
Allan, C. A. (1989) 'Characteristics and Help-seeking Patterns of Attenders at a Community-based Voluntary Agency and an Alcohol and Drug Treatment Unit', *British Journal of Addiction*, 84(1):pp. 73–80.
Breeze, E. (1985) *Women and Drinking* (London: HMSO).
Czarnecki, D. M., Russell, M., Cooper, M. L. and Salter, D. (1990) 'Five Year Reliability of Self Reported Alcohol Consumption', *Journal of Studies on Alcohol*, 51(1):pp. 68–76.
Department of Health (1992) *The Health of the Nation: A Strategy for Health in England* (London: HMSO).
Fox, N. L., Sexton, M., Hebel, J. R. and Thompson, B. (1989) 'The Reliability of Self Reports of Smoking and Alcohol Consumption by Pregnant Women', *Addictive Behaviour*, 14(2):pp. 187–95.
Goddard, E. (1991) *Drinking in England and Wales in the late 1980s* (OPCS London: HMSO).
Goddard, E. and Ikin, C. (1988) *Drinking in England and Wales in 1987* (London: HMSO).
Gorman, D. M., Duffy, S. W., Raine, S. and Taylor, C. L. (1989) 'Level of Agreement between Questionnaire Measures of Alcohol Dependence, Alcoholism and Problem Drinking in a Sample Presenting at a Specialist Alcohol Treatment Service', *Drug and Alcohol Dependence*, 24: pp. 227–232.
Health Education Authority (HEA) (1992) *That's the Limit: A Guide to Sensible Drinking* (London: HEA).
Kranzler, H. R., Babor, T. F. and Laverman, R. J. (1990) 'Problems Associated with Average Alcohol Consumption and Frequency of Intoxication in Medical Population', *Alcoholism: Clinical and Experimental Research*, 14(1):pp. 119–26.
Millar, M. (1990) 'An Exploratory Study of the Coping Styles of Women Drinkers and Non-Drinkers of Alcohol', unpublished Masters dissertation, University of Surrey.
OPCS (1991) *Mortality Statistics – Cause (England & Wales) 1990*, Series DH2 No. 17 (London: OPCS).

Polit, P. F. and Hungler, B. P. (1985) *Essentials of Nursing Research Methods and Applications* (Philadelphia: Lippincott).

Royal College of General Practitioners (1986) *Alcohol – A Balanced View*, Reports from General Practice 24 (London: RCGP).

Royal College of Physicians (1987) *A Great and Growing Evil. The Medical Consequences of Alcohol Abuse* (London: Tavistock).

Royal College of Physicians (1991) *Alcohol and the Public Health* (London: Macmillan).

Royal College of Psychiatrists (1986) *Alcohol Our Favourite Drug* (London: Tavistock).

Shaw, S. (1980) 'The Cause of Increasing Drinking Problems Amongst Women', in Camberwell Council on Alcoholism, *Women and Alcohol* (London: Tavistock Publications).

Waterson, J. and Ettore, B. (1989) 'Providing Services for Women with Difficulties with Alcohol or Other Drugs: The Current U.K. Situation as seen by Women Practitioners, Researchers and Policy Makers in the Field', *Drug and Alcohol Dependence*, 24(2):pp. 119–25.

Waterson, E. J. and Murray Lyon, I. M. (1989) 'Screening for Alcohol Related Problems in the Antenatal Clinic: An Assessment of Different Methods', *Alcohol and Alcoholism*, 24(1):pp. 21–30.

Case Study II
Alcohol Abuse in the Elderly
Mary Chad

INTRODUCTION

By the year 2001 it is estimated that 18 per cent of the UK population will be over 65 (OPCS, 1991). As the nation's fastest growing age group there is growing concern about the effect of the use of alcohol on their physical, social and psychological well-being.

In recent years a number of investigations by health and social researchers has indicated an increase in alcohol abuse among elders (Bridgewater *et al.*, 1987; Illiffe *et al.*, 1991). Although an age-related decline in the number of elderly abusers has been identified (Adams *et al.*, 1990), and elderly male alcohol abusers are consistently recognised as the predominant group (OPCS, 1988; Lichtenberg, 1993), some studies indicate that the number of female drinkers has been steadily rising (OPCS, 1988; Goddard, 1991). It is also suggested that there are two types of elderly drinkers, those who are described as late-onset (LO) and those who are termed early-onset (EO) alcohol abusers. EO abusers have frequently experienced problems with alcohol abuse over their life-time and continue to do so in old age. In comparison, LO abusers have no history of drinking problems, but develop an abusive pattern in response to physical and psychosocial factors associated with aging such as depression, loneliness, marital stress, physical illnesses, the stresses of aging and the loss of social support networks (Gurnack and Hoffman, 1992; Jennison, 1992).

Prevalence of Alcohol Abuse

The extent of alcohol abuse among the elderly remains controversial as estimates of prevalence vary between 10 and 15 per cent and definitions of alcohol abuse and what constitutes aging or aged are inconsistent (Barnes, 1982; Brody, 1982; Wood, 1982). Graham (1986) suggests that owing to the elderly persons' increased sensitivity to alcohol and other influential variables such as age, sex, weight and absorption levels, different recommended maximum levels are required. Some reports based on the subjects' physical and psychosocial problems (Zimberg, 1984; Bienenfeld, 1987) frequently fail to take into account the older person's decreased tolerance to alcohol and the more extreme behavioural and psychological effects of intoxication they may present with (Hahn and Burch, 1983; Jaques *et al.*, 1989).

Alcohol-related Problems in the Elderly

Variations in estimates of the prevalence of alcohol-related problems may reflect the difficulties in separating the alcohol-related health problems in the elderly from chronic illness and medication effects. For example, falls and other accidents, musculoskeletal pain, insomnia, depression and anxiety are particularly common in the elderly alcoholic (Colsher and Wallace, 1990; Illife *et al.*, 1991).

In the ageing body the central nervous system (Hurt *et al.*, 1988), cardiovascular system (Atkinson, 1984; Jackson *et al.*, 1991) and the gastrointestinal tract (Payne, 1990) are particularly vulnerable to excessive drinking. Other effects on the sleep–wake cycle and interactions with drugs have been noted (Atkinson, 1984).

Assessing Alcohol Consumption in the Elderly

Medical practitioners, clinically and community based, are in a prime position to identify those 'at risk' of alcohol abuse and actual abusers (Gulino and Kadin, 1986; Illife *et al.*, 1991). Yet studies have shown many fail to do so, or if they diagnose the problem, are often at a loss as to how to manage the elderly alcohol issue (Anderson, 1985; Curtis *et al.*, 1989). Likewise, there are few studies which have investigated the function of community nurses, social workers and health visitors in the management of elderly alcohol abusers. Parette *et al.* (1990) found that negative attitudes of the nursing staff towards aging alcohol abusers interfered with assessment and diagnostic procedures. It was suggested that by having such an attitude nurses overlooked symptoms of alcoholism and failed to refer patients whom they did identify as an abuser. These findings appear somewhat similar to results found in doctors.

The White Paper *Caring for People* (Department of Health, 1989) and the *NHS and Community Care Act* (1990) have placed considerable accountability for the health needs of the aging community in the hands of the Primary Health Care Team. Health assessment programmes and annual check-up among the elderly are imminent. Alcohol screening questionnaires offer a method of assessment which can be used by all relevant professional as part of a generalised health screening format. The adequacy of self-reporting is well researched (Babor *et al.*, 1987), but this is particularly evident when applied to elders who may have a poor recall memory, and where difficulty in distinguishing between alcohol and age-related problems can arise (Graham, 1986).

CAGE , an acroynym formed from its four questions, is an alcohol screening test developed by Ewing and Rouse (1970). A score of two affirmative answers suggests a degree of alcohol abuse. SMAST is a 12-item questionnaire which enquires about drinking-related behaviour and its effect on social relationships (Pokorny *et al.*, 1972). It is scored by applying a unit of one to each positive answer. Studies by Ewing (1984) and Willenbring *et al.* (1988) showed that CAGE and SMAST have sensitivities of 97 per cent and 89 per cent respectively. Tucker *et al.* (1989) and Buchsbaum *et al.* (1992) found that the CAGE can effectively discriminate elderly alcohol abusers, when compare with moderate drinkers. Whilst Beresford (1990) found that CAGE correlated well with biochemical measures such as blood alcohol levels.

The Aims of the Study

The purpose of this investigation was to:

1. identify the extent of alcohol abuse among the elderly within an inner-city setting;
2. compare the methods of assessment used by the community health care team;
3. Look for relationships between alcohol abuse and biopsychosocial variables within an aging cohort.

METHODOLOGY

Subjects

The sample ($n = 79$) was selected from the target population residing within the three health and social service catchments of an inner city area. The cohort was recruited in a variety of ways, for example via warden-controlled apartments, house-to-house calls in elderly neighbourhoods and street interviews.

In order to gain consent the investigator, wearing a prominent identification badge, verbally explained the nature of the interview and outlined the purpose of the questionnaire. Assurances of anonymity and confidentiality were also given.

Criteria of inclusion into the survey were:

1. the subject must be over the age of 65;
2. the subject must have resided within the city for at least 5 years;
3. the subject must not be a member of a nursing or rest home or any other form of institutionalised care setting;
4. the subject must be able to make their responses known.

A total of 85 elderly men and women were invited to participate in the study from which four refused, one failed to complete the questionnaire, and 1 person was excluded as they had not yet reached the age of 65. Thirty of the subjects were from the central area of the city, 25 from the south and 24 from the north of the city. This was an attempt to avoid age bias as the 1989 population figures for the region showed a preponderance of elderly within the south of the city.

Data Collection

For this descriptive study two quantitative methods of data collection were used:

1. The *Health and Social Service Questionnaire,* devised and named by the investigator, was a six-item closed-question device which was posted to a randomised sample of general practitioners, social workers and community nurses working with the aged 65 and over groups within the three areas of the city of Portsmouth.

   The purpose of the form was to gather information about the age range, sex and number of alcohol abusers within the aging cohort so that the incidence of abuse could be compared with prevalence of abuse. Questions were also asked about the methods of alcohol assessment and referral systems used by the health and social service agents.

2. An *Interview Questionnaire,* formulated and entitled 'Life-Styles and the Elderly' by the investigator, was designed to ascertain the prevalence of abuse and any associated biopsychosocial variables. It was divided into four sections:

   Section 1 enquired about biographical details, e.g. age, area lived in and ethnicity. These were inserted into the study because the literature suggests they may influence alcohol consumption.

   Section 2 was concerned with the type and amount of social support received, the regularity of visiting and attendance at social engagements. Such questions were considered pertinent to the study because limited social support and social isolation have been identified as factors associated with increased alcohol consumption among the elderly.

   Section 3 listed questions about the subject's mental and physical health. These were asked as there is a plethora of objective data which relates alcohol abuse to a number of biopsychological disorders in the elderly.

   Section 4 considered the extent to which tobacco, smoking, certain prescribed medications and alcohol consumption were used or abused.

   Validated alcohol screening instruments were also contained within the questionnaire design and included the CAGE (Ewing and Rouse, 1970) and Short Michigan Alcoholic Screening Questionnaire

(SMAST) questions (Pokorny *et al.*, 1972). Estimations of alcohol consumption, measured by frequency and quantity per week were also identified and provided the basis for determining alcohol abuse as defined by the Royal Colleges of Psychiatrists (1979), General Practitioners (1986) and Physcians (1987).

All statistical computations were carried out using the Social Science Statistical Package Mark 10 (SPSSX) on a Vax 7 computer (Dec Digital). The non-parametric Mann–Whitney U test was used to assess the significance between alcohol consumption and other variables. Relationships between estimated units of alcohol per week and other variables were examined by means of the Spearman's rank correlation. The probability used was the two-tailed probability of obtaining a particular value and the level taken as statistically significant was <0.05. The significance test used to decide on the degree of association between nominal variables such as CAGE and SMAST was chi-squared. Fisher's exact test was also used.

RESULTS

Health and Social Service Questionnaire

A total of 47 Health and Social Service Agents took part in the study. These included General Practitioners (GP), Community Nurses (CN) and were Social Workers (SW).

GPs used more patient/family reported measures of assessment compared to blood alcohol levels or alcohol screening questionnaires. SW and CN used the same means of assessment as those most frequently used by GP, i.e. non-invasive tools of assessment.

The general trend is that the SW and CN referred clients to the GP, and to a lesser extent to a psychiatric unit or a voluntary agency, e.g. Alcoholic Anonymous. Clients are most likely to be referred by GPs to the psychiatric unit (72.0 per cent) than any other agency. However, some GPs did use other members of the primary care team as referring agents, i.e. CN (36.3 per cent) and SW (13.6 per cent).

Incidence of Alcohol Abuse

A total of 105 alcohol abusers over the age of 65 were reported by the 47 agents. Of these, 69.5 per cent were reported by GPs, (males outnumbering females by 2 : 1). SW and CN reported 16.2 per cent and 14.2 per cent, respectively. In these groups the data showed an age-related decline in alcohol abuse. This was similar for both males and females. The overall incidence was 2.3 per cent for males and 0.9 per cent for females. In total this gave a recorded incidence of 1.4 per cent.

Prevalence of Alcohol Abuse

Using Fisher's exact test there was no statistical significance between the either the number of abusers in each area, or the gender. Thus the estimated prevalence of alcohol abuse was 10.1 per cent.

Analysis of data from the CAGE questionnaire revealed that 13 per cent of the sample were classified as alcohol abusers. This compared with an estimate of 20.4 per cent obtained using the SMAST questionnaire.

Male alcohol consumption correlated (Spearmans' rank) well with values from CAGE ($r = 0.570$; $P = 0.001$) and SMAST ($r = 0.462$; $P = 0.003$). However, this high level of significance was not reflected in female data obtained from SMAST ($r = 0.380$; $P = 0.050$). The CAGE scores for females showed the dame degree of association ($r = 0.519$; $P = 0.009$) with alcohol consumption as seen in the males.

Relationship Studies

A comparison between alcohol consumption and a number of social and psychological factors, tested by the Mann–Whitney U test, indicated that boredom ($P = 0.060$), lack of sleep ($P = 0.070$), self-directed anger ($P = 0.046$) and loneliness ($P = 0.080$) were linked with increased drinking. Whereas social drinking was significantly associated with decreased consumption of alcohol ($P = 0.003$). This was also indicated in those taking of prescribed drugs ($P = 0.060$). Although approximately 60 per cent of the clients are visited by friends or relatives the other 40 per cent might be socially isolated unless they visit churches, pubs, or clubs for the elderly. There was a tendency ($P = 0.070$) for those who did not visit their GP or hospital to consume more alcohol.

DISCUSSION

Identifying alcohol abuse in the elderly is fraught with difficulties, mainly related to issues concerning definition, inappropriate assessments and problems of sampling (Wood, 1982; Zimberg, 1984; Graham, 1986). In view of the White Paper *Caring for People* (1990) and the *NHS and Community Care Act* (1989) there is a growing need for health screening. The *NHS and Community Care Act* (1990) requires Social Service assessments to be made whilst elderly people are in a clinical setting in order for their needs to be met on discharge. To date, many health and social service assessments do not address the issue of alcohol use or abuse.

This report shows a mismatch between the incidence of 1.4 per cent reported by the Health and Social Service Agencies and the prevalence of 10.1 per cent estimated from a personal survey. This estimate is comparable to the national average of 11 per cent reported by Goddard (1991), but higher than local figures provided by the Alcohol Unit (5.2 per cent) and the Alcohol Advisory Centre (0.8 per cent).

The study revealed that only a limited degree of objective testing was used by the agencies. Of the various agencies involved with potential alcohol abusers, blood alcohol and questionnaires were employed by only a small number of GPs (13.7 per cent). There is a small number of haematological and biochemical objective tests available for assessing alcohol abuse. These include carbohydrate transferase and gamma-glutamyltranspeptidase (GGT). The latter has been used for sometime but has recently been shown to have limited reliability as a community screening tool (Vanclay *et al.*, 1991). A promising method for detecting recent drinking is the urinary 5-HIAA/5-hydroxytryptophol ratio which reflects blood-ethanol concentrations (Carlsson *et al.*, 1993). However, these tests are not readily available in the community and generally are not validated for elderly populations. In this survey, only a small number of GPs considered using a biochemical approach and this was restricted to measurements of blood alcohol concentration (BAC) measurements, which are of limited potential .

Additionally the use of objective testing by SWs and CNs was also restricted, reliance being place on 'intuitive methods'. Although there are some concerns about memory recall in the elderly, there is some support from this study to suggest that a questionnaire would be helpful in the primary screening for alcohol abuse in the community. The CAGE is an inexpensive and easily applied assessment tool and correlated well with alcohol consumption in both males and females. Consideration of more widespread use of this questionnaire should be give by the community team.

Some important causal factors in alcohol consumption and abuse in the elderly were highlighted. The data indicated that the changing pattern of alcohol abuse in the elderly is related to loneliness. The loss of peers appears to be compensated to some extent by relatives and friends, but in many old people a variety of physical and medical problems limits the number of outings. This increasing social isolation is compounded for some by negative psychological feelings including sadness and self-directed anger. Suicide is not uncommon in the elderly and such variables have been associated with it (De Leo and Ormskerk, 1991). Although there is an age-related decline in the number of alcohol abusers reported by the agencies, 8.9 per cent of those who survived into the late years began to drink after the age of 84. Increasing alcohol consumption in the elderly appears to be linked with greater social isolation.

The early identification of this self-medication by the Primary Health Care Team, perhaps using the CAGE might help to identify the specific needs of the individual and offset the need for increased consumption. Although specific maximum recommended levels are not available at present it is important to contain trends in consumption in order to minimise the harmful effects of alcohol on the aging physiological systems.

CONCLUSION

As a result of demographical changes it is expected that the health and social care needs of those over the age of 65 will increase dramatically during the next decade. An important aspect of the healthcare provision relates to alcohol-related illnesses; however, data on alcohol abuse in the elderly is limited and even less information on alcohol-related diseases is available. This is largely due to the lack of objective testing and insufficient research on the acceptable levels of alcohol consumption buy elderly people. Additionally, in view of recent legislation more attention to this area of need is required. A positive alcohol screening tool, such as the CAGE questionnaire, used by the Primary Health Care Team will help identify those who may be at risk. This should then be followed by non-invasive, non-threatening, more detailed psychosocial and physical tools. Further follow-up assessment would then consist of more objective measures which might include biochemical assays.

REFERENCES

Anderson, P. (1985) 'Managing Alcohol Problems in General Practice', *British Medical Journal*, 290:pp. 1873–5.

Atkinson, R. M. (1984) *Alcohol and Drug Abuse in Old Age* (Washington, DC: American Psychiatric Press), pp. 1–21.

Atkinson, R. M. and Kofoed, L. L. (1982) 'Alcohol and Drug Abuse in Old Age: A Clinical Perspective', *Substance and Alcohol Actions/Misuse*, 3:pp. 353–68.

Barnes, G. (1979) 'Alcohol Use among Older Persons – Findings from a Western New York State General Population Survey', *Journal of the American Geriatric Society*, 27:p. 244.

Barnes, G. M. (1982) in W. G. Woods and M. F. Elias (eds), *Alcoholism and Aging: Advances in Research* (Florida: CRC Press).

Bienenfeld, D. (1987) 'Alcoholism in the Elderly', *American Family Physician*, 36:pp. 163–9.

Brody, J. A. (1982) 'Aging and Alcohol Abuse', *Journal of the American Geriatric Society*, 38:pp. 123–6.

Butler, R. and Lewis, M. (1982) *Aging and Mental Health* (St Louis, MO: CV Mosby).

Cartwright, A. and Anderson, R. (1979) 'Patients and their Doctors', *Occasional Paper No. 8* (London: RCGP).

Drew, L. R. H. (1968) 'Alcoholism as a Self-limiting Disease', *Quarterly Journal of Studies on Alcoholism*, 29:pp. 956–67.

De Leo, D. and Ormskerk, S. C. (1991) 'Suicide in the Elderly: General Characteristics', *Crisis*, 12(2):pp. 3–17.

Ewing, J. A. and Rouse, B. A. (1970) 'Identifying the Hidden Alcoholic', presented at the 29th International Congress on Alcohol and Drug Dependence, Sydney, Australia, 3 February 1970.

Graham, K. (1986) 'Identifying and Measuring Alcohol Abuse among the Elderly: Serious Problems with Existing Instrumentation', *Journal of Studies on Alcohol*, 47(4):pp. 322–6.

Goddard, E. (1991) *OPCS: Drinking in England and Wales in the late 1980s* (London: HMSO).

Hahn, H. K. and Burch, R. E. (1983) 'Impaired Ethanol Metabolism with Advancing Age', *Alcoholism: Clinical and Experimental Research*, 7:pp. 299–304.

Hampshire County Council (1989) *Population and Dwelling Forecasts for 1987–1994: Parishes and Urban Wards* (Portsmouth: Hampshire County Planning Department).

Hartford, J. T. and Samorajski, T. (1982) 'Alcoholism in the Geriatric Population', *Journal of the American Geriatric Society*, 30:pp. 18–24.

Hurt, R. D., Finlayson, R. E., Morse, R. M. and Davis, L. J., Jr (1988)

'Alcoholism in Elderly Persons: Medical Aspects and Prognosis of 216 Patients', *Mayo Clinical Procedures*, 63:pp. 753–60.

Jackson, R., Scragg, R. and Beaglehole, R. (1991) 'Alcohol Consumption and Risk of Coronary Heart Disease', *British Medical Journal*, 303:pp. 211–16.

Jaques, P. F., Sulsky, S., Hartz, S. C. and Russell, R. M. (1989) 'Moderate Alcohol Intake and Nutritional Status in Non-alcoholic Elderly Subjects', *American Journal of Clinical Nutrition*, 50:pp. 875–83.

Kinney, J., Bergen, B. J. and Price, T. R. P. (1982) 'A Perspective on Medical Students Perceptions of Alcoholics and Alcoholism', *Journal of Studies on Alcoholism*, 43:pp. 488–96.

Mishara, B. L. and Kastenbaum, R. (1980) *Alcohol and Old Age* (New York: Grune & Stratton).

OPCS (1988) *General Household Survey* (London: HMSO).

OPCS (1991) *Social Trends 23* (London: HMSO).

Parette, H. W., Hourcade, J. J. and Parette, P. C. (1990) 'Nursing Attitudes Towards Geriatric Alcoholism', *Journal of Gerontological Nursing*, 16(1): pp. 26–31.

Payne, J. E. (1990) 'Colorectal Carcinogenesis', *Australian Journal of Surgery*, 60: pp. 11–16.

Pokorny, A.D., Miller, B. A. and Kaplan, H. B. (1972) 'The Brief Mast: A Shortened Version of the Michigan Alcoholism Screening Test', *American Journal of Psychiatry*, 129: pp. 342–7.

Royal College of General Practitioners (1986) *Alcohol – A Balanced View* (London: Royal College of General Practitioners).

Royal College of Psychiatrists (1979) *Alcohol and Alcoholism: A Report by the Special Committee of the RCP* (London: Tavistock).

Royal College of Physicians (1987) *A Great and Growing Evil: The Medical Consequences of Alcohol Abuse* (London: Tavistock).

Schuckit, M. A. (1979) 'Alcoholism and Affective Disorders: Diagnostic Confusion', in D. W. Goodwin and C. K. Erikson (eds), *Alcoholism and Affective Disorders* (New York: Spectrum), pp. 9–91.

Schuckit, M. A. and Pastor, P. A. (1978) 'The Elderly as a Unique Population: Alcoholism', *Alcohol: Clinical Experimental Research*, 2:pp. 31–8.

Simon, A. (1980) 'The Neuroses, Personality Disorders, Alcoholism, Drug Use and Misuse, and Crime in the Aged', in J. E. Birren and R. B. Sloane (eds), *Handbook of Mental Health and Aging* (Englewood Cliffs, NJ: Prentice Hall).

Skinner, H. A. and Holt, S. (1983) 'Early Interventions for Alcohol Problems', *Journal of the Royal College of General Practioners*, 33: pp. 787–91.

Wilson, P. (1980) *Survey on Drinking in England and Wales, OPCS* (London: HMSO).

Wood, W. G. (1982) 'Theoretical and Methodological Issues Associated with Aging Research', in W. G. Wood and M. F. Elias (eds), *Alcoholism and Aging: Advances in Research* (New York: CRC Press).

Yen, P. K. (1983) 'Alcohol – The Drug that's also a Nutrient', *Geriatric Nursing* (November/December):pp. 390–7.

Zimberg, S. (1974) 'The Elderly Alcoholic', *Gerontologist*, 14:pp. 221–4.

Zimberg, S. (1984) 'Diagnosis and Management of the Elderly Alcoholic', in R. Atkinson (ed.), *Alcohol and Drug Abuse in Old Age* (Washington, DC: American Psychiatric Press).

Case Study III
Therapeutic Use of Alcohol in the Elderly

Penny Simpson

Identifying the incidence and quantity of alcohol consumption by elderly people is not an exact science. Bridgewater *et al.* (1987) in their study of elderly people and alcohol consumption in a UK urban community identified that subjects under the age of 75 drank more than those over the age of 75.

General population surveys from 1970 to 1980, cited in Wood and Elias (1982) show that people over the age of 65 have higher rates of abstention and lower rates of heavy drinking than younger adults in the same populations. Adams *et al.* (1990) identified a true age-related decline in alcohol intake with consumption falling with increasing age. Longitudinal analysis showed a statistically significant decline in the percentage of subjects consuming alcohol over time. (The slope was -2 per cent per year). This was confirmed by McKim and Quinlan (1991) who showed that the age-related decline in total alcohol consumption was the result of changes in the amount of alcohol consumed per drinking session rather than a decrease in the number of drinking occasions. 'Health and happiness were not related to alcohol consumption' (McKim and Quinlan, 1991). The studies indicate that there is a decline in drinking across time in the elderly. The reasons may be related to cost, changed social values or decreased tolerance.

There are as many potential advantages to moderate alcohol consumption as there are disadvantages. These include:

1. increased bone mineral density,
2. enhanced nutritional benefit, including
    (a) calorie intake,
    (b) increased iron storage, and
    (c) appetite stimulation and increased digestive secretions;
3. increased longevity, due to effects on the cardiovascular system;
4. improved sleep induction;
5. enhanced personal and social benefits.

See below for references.

It is, therefore, worth exploring the benefits of including alcohol in the diet of elderly people. Hill (1983) underlined the theoretical possibility that some level of alcohol consumption by the elderly person may not be harmful to the brain; that the beneficial effects of light-to-moderate drinking social drinking (up to 21 units per week for men, 14 for women) was possible, although this had not yet been fully explored. The process of ageing decreases the relative contribution of body water to total body weight, but increases the relative contribution of body fat to total body weight. This higher fat to fluid ratio means that they therefore have less fluid in which to distribute drugs such as alcohol. Ethanol is distributed, preferentially, into body water compartments, including the blood and cerebrospinal fluid, but very little into fat, mineral or cell solids. It then follows that there will be higher peak blood concentrations of ethanol in the elderly person, than will be apparent in younger subjects of a similar weight and body type (Wood and Elias, 1982).

BONE MINERAL DENSITY

Holbrook and Barrett-Connor's (1993) study suggests that moderate social drinking is associated with higher bone mineral density in both men and women. They state that 'Although alcohol consumption cannot be recommended as a preventative for osteoporosis, it is reassuring that social drinking appears to have no negative effect on bone density.'

NUTRITIONAL STATUS

There is often an inverse relationship between calories derived from ethanol and those derived from carbohydrates, although surveys have found that alcohol calories are added to the diet rather than replacing calories from other foodstuffs. Thus Gruch'w's (1985) study found that drinkers had significantly higher calorie intakes than non-drinkers. Their intake of non-alcoholic calories decreased, as alcohol intake increased, and it was estimated that between 15 and 41 per cent of energy from alcohol replaced non-alcoholic calories. The most salient difference in nutritional intake between drinkers and non-drinkers was the substantially lower carbohydrate intake of drinkers.

By contrast, De Castro and Orozco (1990) suggest, in their study of moderate alcohol intake and spontaneous eating patterns in humans, that alcohol supplements rather than displaces macronutrient-supplied energy.

The calorific value of ethanol as fuel may be dose-related. Most evidence suggests that at moderate intake levels of alcohol, less than 45 g per day (three drinks) ethanol is efficiently utilized as fuel by the liver.

Davies and Holdsworth (1985) studied nutrition and health at retirement age in the UK, and stated that the 3 per cent contribution by alcohol, to the energy of the diet of the elderly person is within National Advisory Committee on Nutrition and Education (NACNE) guidelines. Yen (1983) indicates that a nutritional benefit of wine is its iron content. Shaper *et al.* (1985) found that alcohol has highly significant positive associations with haemoglobin. Passmore and Eastwood (1986) also suggest that iron absorption may be promoted by alcohol. Further studies would be needed to clarify the effects of alcohol on iron absorption.

Alcohol is a potent stimulant of gastric juices and appetite and can make meals more enjoyable (Mishihara and Kastelbaum, 1980; Yen, 1983). De Castro and Orozco (1990) found that alcohol consumption was associated with prolonged meal durations.

MODERATE ALCOHOL INTAKE AND THE CARDIOVASCULAR SYSTEM

The well-documented relationship between light drinking and increases in high density lipoprotein (HDL-C), a protective factor in heart disease, illustrates this point. Enhanced HDL-C levels are related to reductions in heart disease. Shaper *et al.* (1985) demonstrated that high density lipoprotein cholesterol (HDL-C) showed substantial direct association with alcohol intake. The effect of alcohol consumption on HDL-C is now established and has aroused considerable interest because of the possible protective effects in coronary heart disease. This fact was also identified by Ernst *et al.* (1980). It was noted that those who never drank had lower mean HDL-C levels than those who did drink but had not done so in the past week. The association of ethanol and HDL-C was strongest at age 60 and older. This makes it of particular interest to those studying alcohol and the elderly person.

Moderate drinking, i.e. that below current advised safe limits of 14/21 units, thus not only appears to be a positive potential factor against coronary heart disease but also against stroke. In support of this view a Newcastle study funded by Research into Ageing showed that being a teetotaller was a positive risk factor for stroke (James, 1992). Also mild alcohol consumption may be considered as a therapeutic regimen for selected persons at high risk of coronary heart disease (Krepostman and Borzak, 1993).

ALCOHOL AND SLEEP

A popular use of alcohol is as a hypnotic drug, to relax the subject and induce sleep. Alcohol appears to decrease sleep latency, even if consumed some hours beforehand, so that there is rapid onset of sleep (Mendelson, 1987). These findings are supported by Erman (1986), who also stated that large amounts of alcohol are not recommended as they interfere with deep sleep, and act as a diuretic.

In individuals in whom sleep pathophysiology has been investigated and ruled out, it becomes reasonable to consider the use of wine as an aid to inducing sleep. Mishihara and Kastelbaum (1980) studied long-term elderly care patients in a psychogeriatric ward, and found that, when wine was made available, chloral hydrate use decreased significantly.

Professor James in Newcastle has banned the use of sleeping tablets from his elderly care wards, except for those who have become addicted to them. The evening medicine trolley now contains beers, sherry and whisky, which is popularly known as Glen Pharmacy. In Professor James' own words 'A little tot at bedtime works wonders!' (James, 1992).

A conclusion may therefore be drawn from these findings that alcohol has a place in the promotion of sleep, but should be confined to those elderly people with sleep onset difficulties, i.e. most of them.

PERSONAL AND SOCIAL BENEFITS

Another popular effect ascribed to alcohol by the lay person is that of alterations in mood, in order to induce relaxation, increase sociability and reduce anxiety. Kalin, McLelland and Kahn (1965) found that alcohol ingestion produced a significant reduction in fear-anxiety; alcohol generally produces a decrease in 'inhibitory thoughts' after four or five drinks. Williams (1966) produced a similar study which tested the hypothesis that alcohol decreased anxiety and depression. This was found to be so after 4 ounces of a commercial alcoholic beverage. In Sayette, Wilson and Carpenter's (1989) study, the interpretation of the results could also indicate an anxiolytic effect of alcohol on heart rate. Cloninger's abstinent Type 1 alcoholics (mature onset) at rest are hypervigilant and apprehensive (see Chapter 7). In response to alcohol these individuals show a marked increase in alpha activity, and subjectively report a sense of calm alertness that they regard as a pleasant relief of tension (Cloninger, 1987).

However, much of the evidence for the tension-relieving effects of alcohol has been identified as being negative, equivocal and often contradictory (Capell and Herman, 1972). Individuals apparently will develop their own perceptions of what alcohol 'does' for them, and an elderly person may be inflexible in this belief, despite evidence to the contrary. It is reasonable to ask, therefore, and to suggest research to investigate whether the relief is real or illusionary – or even potentially dangerous?

Drinking among elderly people in the population is a deeply rooted behaviour, developed over the course of a lifetime, in response to social norms, as well as from numerous other psychosocial and biological factors. Alcohol is most likely to be consumed by socially active older people who consider themselves to be in good health (Lamy, 1984). It is less likely that the elderly person will suddenly begin problematic drinking in response to the stress of ageing if they have not previously used this coping mechanism in their younger years to deal with life crises (Wood and Elias, 1982). Elderly people with lower incomes consume less alcohol than those with higher incomes (Liberto *et al.*, 1992).

Nevertheless, the image of alcohol as a harmless social lubricant may be offset by concerns about its effects upon mental functioning. Goodwin (1989) reviewed the conflicting evidence for and against the amount of alcohol that produces significant and permanent impairments in cognitive function. His study of alcohol use by 70 healthy elderly people found no association between alcohol intake and psychological status or cognition (Goodwin *et al.*, 1987; see also Chapter 9).

The last words could be those of James (1992) who believes that alcohol in moderation is everybody's friend, particularly the old person's friend. Moderation is the right advice for alcohol and ageing.

REFERENCES

Adams, W. L., Garry, P. J., Rhyne, R., Hunt, W.C. and Goodwin, J. S. (1990) 'Alcohol Intake in the Healthy Elderly: Changes with Age in a Cross Sectional and Longitudinal Study', *Journal of the American Gerontological Society*, 38:pp. 211-6.

Bridgewater, R., Leigh, S., James, O. F. W. and Potter, J. F. (1987) 'Alcohol Consumption and Dependence in Elderly Patients in an Urban Community', *British Medical Journal*, 295:pp. 884–5.

Cappell, H. and Herman, C. P. (1972) 'Alcohol and Tension Reduction: A Review', *Quarterly Journal of Studies on Alcohol*, 33:pp. 33–64.

Cloninger, C. R. (1987) 'Neurogenetic Adaptive Mechanisms in Alcoholism', *Science*, 236:pp. 410–15.

Davies, L. and Holdsworth, M. D. (1979) 'Nutritional Investigation on Residents in Old People's Homes', *Journal of Human Nutrition*, 33:pp. 165–9.

de Castro, J. M. and Orozco, S. (1990) 'Moderate Alcohol Intake and Spontaneous Eating Patterns of Humans: Evidence of Unregulated Supplementation', *American Journal of Clinical Nutrition*, 52:pp. 246–53.

Erman, M. K. (1986) 'Sound Sleep: Alcohol not an Ingredient', *American Association of Occupational Health Nurses Journal*, 34(6):pp. 294–5.

Ernst, N., Fisher, M., Smith, W., Gordon, T., Rifkind, B. M., Little, J. A., Mishkel, M. A. and Williams, O. D. (1980) 'The Association of Plasma High-density Lipoprotein Cholesterol with Dietary Intake and Alcohol Consumption. The Lipid Research Clinics Program Prevalence Study', *Circulation*, 62(IV):pp. 41–52.

Goodwin, J. S. (1989) 'Social, Psychological and Physical Factors Affecting the Nutritional Status of Elderly Subjects: Separating Cause and Effect', *American Journal of Clinical Nutrition*, 50(5):pp. 1201–9.

Goodwin, J. S., Sanchez, C. J., Thomas, P. and Goodwin, J. M. (1987) 'Alcohol Intake in a Healthy Elderly Population', *American Journal of Public Health*, 77:pp. 173–7.

Gruchow, H. W., Sobociski, K. A., Barboriak, J. J. and Scheller, J. G. (1985) 'Alcohol Consumption, Nutrient Intake and Relative Body Weight among U.S. Adults', *American Journal of Clinical Nutrition*, 42:pp. 289–95.

Hill, S. Y. (1983) 'Alcohol and Brain Damage: Cause or Association?', *American Journal of Public Health*, 73:pp. 487–9.

Holbrook, T. L. and Barrett-Connor, E. (1993) 'A Prospective Study of Alcohol Consumption and Bone Mineral Density', *British Medical Journal*, 306:pp. 1506–9.

James, O. (1992) *Research into Ageing: Briefing Paper* (London: CIBA Foundation).

Kalin, R., Mclelland, D. C. and Kahn, M. (1966) 'The Effects of Male Social Drinking on Fantasy', *Journal of Personality and Social Psychology*, 1:pp. 441–52.

Krepostman, A. and Borzak, S. (1993) 'Coronary Heart Disease . . . Seven Steps to Primary Prevention', *Consultant*, 33 (6):pp. 33–5, 39–40, 49.

Lamy, P. P. (1984) 'Alcohol Misuse and Abuse Among the Elderly', *Drug Intelligence and Clinical Pharmacy*, 18:pp. 649–51.

Liberto, J. G., Oslin, D. W. and Ruskin, P. E. (1992) 'Alcoholism in Older

Persons: A Review of the Literature', *Hospital and Community Psychiatry*, 43(10):pp. 975–84.

Mendelson, W. B. (1987) *Human Sleep: Research and Clinical Care* (New York: Plenum Press).

McKim, W. A. and Quinlan, L. T. (1991) 'Changes in Alcohol Consumption with Age', *Canadian Journal of Public Health*, 82(4):pp. 231–4.

Mishihara, B. L. and Kastelbaum, R. (1980) *Alcohol and Old Age* (New York and London: Grune and Stratton).

Passmore, R. and Eastwood, M. A. (1986) *Human Nutrition and Dietetics* (Edinburgh: Churchill Livingstone).

Sayette, M. A., Wilson, G. T. and Carpenter, J. A. (1989) 'Cognitive Moderators of Alcohol's Effect on Anxiety', *Behaviour, Research and Therapy*, 27(6):pp. 685–90.

Shaper, A. G., Pocock, S. J., Ashby, D., Walker, M. and Whitehead, T. P. (1985) 'Biochemical and Haematological Response to Alcohol Intake', *Annals of Clinical Biochemistry*, 22:pp. 50–61.

Williams, A. F. (1966) 'Social Drinking, Anxiety and Depression', *Journal of Personality and Social Psychology*, 3:pp. 689–93.

Wood, W. G. and Elias, M. F. (1982) *Alcoholism and Ageing: Advances in Research* (Los Angeles: CRC Press).

Yen, P. K. (1983) 'Alcohol – The Drug that's also a Nutrient', *Geriatric Nursing* (November/December): 390–7.

Case Study IV
An Investigation into the Drinking Behaviour of Students

Margaret Cooksey

This study was designed specifically to look at the patterns of drinking of alcohol by student nurses and whether health education had any effect on their behaviour.

The author's interest in the use of alcohol by young people grew from experiences as a nurse teacher. Student nurses openly discuss drinking large amounts of alcohol on regular occasions and admit to feeling 'hung over' both in the classroom and in the clinical areas.

Many previous studies have been undertaken on drinking behaviour by young people in general: a report by the Royal College of Practitioners (1986) stated that the heaviest drinkers were to be found in the 18–24-year-old group. In a study of general practice patients, Wallace,

Brennan and Haines (1987) found that the greatest number of men drinking in excess were the 20–29-year-old age group, whilst among women it was the 17–20-year-olds who were drinking most. In a study at London University, West *et al.* (1990) found that 26.6 per cent of male students and 14.5 per cent of female students were drinking more than the recommended safe limits of alcohol per week. This study produced similar findings to those of Weschler and McFadden (1979), Anderson (1984) and Saltz and Elandt (1986).

Very few reports on nurses and alcohol have been published and most of those studies were from America and Australia. Hutchison (1986) indicated that one in ten Americans is chemically dependent (on drugs and/or alcohol) and that nurses have a rate of dependency 50 per cent higher than non-nurses. Haack and Harford (1984) indicated that 13 per cent of student nurses in America reported alcohol-related problems either at school or at work, whilst Haack (1988) demonstrated that a majority of student nurses experienced burn-out symptoms with an increasing frequency of alcohol use during their training.

In a Scottish study, Plant *et al.* (1991) indicated that general levels of alcohol use amongst qualified nurses were not exceptional although female psychiatric nurses were significantly more likely to drink heavily and experience adverse alcohol-related consequences than female nurses working on general wards. Plant (1991) also indicated the high number of cases of misconduct referred to in the United Kingdom Central Council which involved alcohol- or drug-related offences. This links with evidence which suggests that binge drinking tends to result in short-term consequences such as accidents, injuries, public disorder and family and social conflict, whilst long-term consequences for heavy drinkers, besides physical damage, have been shown to indicate a strong correlation with illicit drug use.

A literature search of the outcomes of health education in relation to alcohol showed that it was relatively easy to increase young people's knowledge (Grant, 1981; Cyster and McEwan, 1987) but that it is much more difficult to show any change in drinking behaviour as a result of this knowledge (Mauss *et al.*, 1988; Hopkins *et al.*, 1988; Roberts, 1988). Evidence is also available to show that even given the amount of health education available there remain serious omissions of knowledge in relation to alcohol (Black and Weare, 1989).

METHOD

Student nurses were recruited from two Colleges of Nurse Education in South-West London. The Colleges of Nursing were in the process of amalgamating, but when the study was planned they had not implemented a joint pre-registration programme and students on their courses were still being employed by two Health Authorities, being taught on separate sites by different teachers using a different curriculum.

A higher-education institution was chosen for comparision because of its long standing links with one of the colleges of nursing. It is a multi-site college based in South-West London. The students from the nursing and non-nursing organisations were matched for age, ratio of males to females, numbers of mature students and accommodation arrangements. Traditionally, nursing and teaching have both been considered to be vocational, and as this college of higher education is responsible for training large numbers of teachers, the students here were seen to be a valid control group.

The researcher planned to use a questionnaire which was designed to obtain information about the student's factual knowledge, previous health education and attitudes towards alcohol. This was to be followed up by a number of group interviews.

Questionnaires were administered to 148 students in the college of higher education; 140 were completed; 104 questionnaires were administered to student nurses with 102 completed – a return rate of 96 per cent. Two general students and six student nurses were interviewed following random sampling.

RESULTS

A summary of the general results can be found in Table 17.1. There was no significant difference between nurses and non-nurses in respect of the weekly amount of alcohol consumed, frequency of drinking and amounts drunk at one session. One area of difference proved to be where drinking took place with 34.8 per cent of student nurses admitting to drinking most alcohol at their residential address compared with 14 per cent of non-nurses. This difference was highly significant (P <0 .001).

Overall, the findings indicated that the incidence of 'binge' drinking was high. The general level of students drinking more than the weekly safe limits agree with the findings of West (1990). The 8.4 per cent of females drinking more than 7 units at a session and the 25.9 per cent of males drinking more than 10 units at a session can be considered to be 'heavy drinkers' in respect of guidelines by Plant (1991).

The results in relation to health education were of concern: 191 students admitted to having received health education about alcohol. The difference in response between nurses and non-nurses was significant; 93 nurses (92.1 per cent) had received health education in relation to alcohol compared with 98 non-nurses (70 per cent; $P > 0.001$, using chi-squared test). When asked if the education received about alcohol had changed their drinking habits, 57 (23.6 per cent) said 'yes', with 156 (64.5 per cent) saying 'no' and 29 (12 per cent) indicating that it was not applicable. There was no significant difference between nurses and non-nurses ($P = 0.130$): 30 of the 'yes' responses (25.9 per cent) were from non-nurses and 27 (27.8 per cent) from nurses ($P = 0.476$).

When asked for the safe limits per week 56 (23.1 per cent) had no idea of the figure in relation to women and 67 (27.7 per cent) had no idea in relation to men. Only 94 students gave the correct figure for women and 68 responded correctly in relation to men. Table 17.2 gives student responses in relation to the number of units of alcohol that the body can metabolise in one hour. There was no significant difference between nurses and non-nurses ($P = 0.130$).

The majority of students reported finding the health education they had received informative, helpful, interesting and enlightening. However, one student provided a telling comment:

I think too much health education about alcohol, etc., can have the adverse effect on young people, i.e. they get fed up with it and no longer take it seriously.

The general level of knowledge in relation to alcohol was poor across both groups. The student nurses acknowledged having received more health education than non-nurses but the pattern of drinking and the amounts drunk did not vary between the groups.

The hypothesis 'that students' drinking behaviour is not altered by their knowledge of the dangers associated with alcohol or by its adverse effects on them personally' was held to be true.

Additional Data from Interviews

Students who were interviewed had diverse views about the health education they had received:

> Well, it was, you know, (boring) ... they didn't actually give us any reasons why or what it does to you or anything like that.

> It was a long time ago, but I remember at the time that it kept me interested and it was relevant to everyday life.

However, the effects of the information received on themselves and their friends was discussed in negative terms by them all:

> whether you're told that drinking is good for you or not, you just want to be one of the crowd or one of the group and you're going to do it anyway. ... it won't make any difference.

> you're more inclined to be influenced by being with your friends than by what teachers tell you.

These students suggested a variety of methods by which they thought that an effective message in relation to alcohol could be put across. These included class discussions, use of controlled experiments within the classroom, use of video and the media. They all agreed that the most potent message would be through actually showing the effects that excessive amounts of alcohol could have on the individual:

> programmes I think, just sort of warning us, things that can happen ... the effects that alcohol has on everybody ... just so that you know what it does to you if you drink too much.

The respondents were also in agreement about the methods which would not be successful:

> I think a sort of lecture-type programme, just one person saying this happens and this happens, would be so boring.

Overall, the students were quite cynical about health education and one quote sums up the underlying feelings expressed during the interviews:

I don't really think when people go out they think of the effect of alcohol. They just think, you know, I'm having a good night, and, you know, it's all hyped up [health education] and it doesn't really matter anyhow . . . it's not going to happen to me and it won't happen for a few years yet if anything, you know, if drink does harm me. So I might as well, you know, have a good time whilst I can.

DISCUSSION

Davies (1991) suggests that people do not learn to drink in the sense that they strive to perfect it, like learning to ride a bike, but rather they learn it socially. People don't drink as a reaction to outside forces, they do it on purpose because they like doing it. As a result of this view that learning to drink is conditioned through the social context in which it is learned, Davies (1991) maintains that the problems will not go away through the use of education. Gillies (1991) is of the view that rather than being aimed at changing behaviour, health education in relation to alcohol should concentrate on improving the knowledge base and on attitude formation. If these two can be achieved the change in behaviour may follow.

In the case of student nurses, the education should also include attitudes towards their responsibility to patients and the establishments in which they are being educated. Student levels of knowledge need to be assessed, as accurate knowledge is required in order to educate others.

The result from this study would suggest that for this sample, there has been a failure in all three areas, which, particularly in the case of student nurses is not only disappointing in respect of their own health and well-being, but perhaps more disappointing in respect of their own role as future health educators. This is, of course, also a role for future teachers, as they may be involved in teaching health education within the National Curriculum. One student made a potent comment in relation to attitudes towards drinking alcohol. The student said that:

I think you have got to somehow make it socially unacceptable to get drunk.

This brings us back to Davies' (1991) view that learning to drink is conditioned by the social context in which it is learned. If it is socially acceptable to become drunk then young people will 'binge' drink irre-

TABLE 17.1 *Summary of findings*

Response	Number	Percentage
Never drunk alcohol	10	4.35
Drink 2–3 times per week	90	39.24
Drink more than 4 times per week	22	9.1
Females drinking a maximum of 14 units per week	30	13.9
Females drinking in excess of 21 units per week	9	4.2
5–6 units drunk at a session	38	15.8
7–9 units drunk at a session	14	5.8
10 or more units drunk at a session	11	4.5
Taken time off work due to alcohol	35	14.4
Work or studies suffered as a result of alcohol	22	9.1

None of these results show any significant difference between nurses and non-nurses.

TABLE 17.2 *Subject responding to the question of how many units of alcohol are metabolised per hour*

Response	Number	Percentage
No response	46	19.0
1 unit	119	49.2
2 units	51	21.1
3 units	17	7.0
4 units	4	1.7
5 units	4	1.7
Over 5 units	1	0.4

spective of the information they have been given, unless that information can be given in some way which will change their attitudes towards the drunken state.

REFERENCES

Anderson, P. (1984) 'Alcohol Consumption of Undergraduates at Oxford University', *Alcohol and Alcoholism*, 19:pp. 77–84.

Black, D. and Weare, K. (1989) 'Knowledge and Attitudes about Alcohol in 17- and 18-Year-Olds', *Health Education Journal*, 48(2):pp. 69–73.

Cyster, R. and McEwen, J. (1987) 'Alcohol Education in the Workplace', *Health Education Journal*, 46(4):pp. 156–61.

Davies, J. (1991) 'Learning to Drink', paper presented at a national conference on 'Alcohol and Young People', 8 October 1991, Queen Mother Conference Centre, Royal College of Physicians, Edinburgh.

Gillies, P. (1991) 'What Can Education Achieve?', paper presented at a national conference on 'Alcohol and Young People', 8 October 1991, Queen Mother Conference Centre, Royal College of Physicians, Edinburgh.

Grant, M. (1981) 'Aims, Form and Content: First Steps in Developing a Taxonomy of Preventative Education in Drug and Alcohol Abuse', in L. R. H. Drew *et al.* (eds), *Man, Drugs, and Society: Current Perspectives* (Canberra: Australian Foundation on Alcoholism and Drug Dependence).

Haack, M. (1988) 'Stress and Impairment among Nursing Students', *Research in Nursing and Health*, 11:pp. 125–34.

Haack, M. and Harford, T. (1984) 'Drinking Patterns among Student Nurses', *The International Journal of the Addictions*, 19(5):pp. 577–83.

Hopkins, R., Maussa, A., Kearney, K. and Weisheit, R. (1988) 'Comprehensive Evaluation of a Model Alcohol Education Curriculum', *Journal of Studies on Alcohol*, 49(1):pp. 38–50.

Hutchison, S. (1986) 'Chemically Dependent Nurses: The Trajectory towards Self Annihilation', *Nursing Research*, 35 (July/August):pp. 196–201.

Maussa, A., Hopkins, R., Weisheit, R., and Kearney, K. (1988) 'The Problematic Prospects for Prevention in the Classroom: Should Alcohol Education Programmes be Expected to Reduce Drinking by Youth?', *Journal of Studies in Alcohol*, 49(1):pp. 51–61.

Plant, M. (1991) 'Heavy Drinkers: Are They Distinctive?', paper presented at a national conference on 'Alcohol and Young People', 8 October 1991, Queen Mother Conference Centre, Royal College of Physicians, Edinburgh.

Plant, M. L., Plant, M. A. and Foster, J. (1991) 'Alcohol, Tobacco and Illicit Drug Use Amongst Nurses: A Scottish Study', *Drug and Alcohol Dependence*, 28:pp. 195–202.

Roberts, R. (1988) 'Hiccups in Alcohol Education', *Health Education Journal*, 47(213):pp. 73–5.

Royal College of General Practitioners (1986) *Alcohol: A Balanced View* (London: Tavistock).

Saltz, R., and Elandt, D. (1986) 'College Students Drinking Studies 1976–1985', *Contemporary Drug Problems* (Spring):pp. 117–59.

Wallace, P., Brennan, P., and Haines, A. (1987) 'Drinking Patterns in General Practice Patients', *Journal of the Royal College of General Practitioners*, 37:pp. 354–7.

Weichsler, H. and McFadden, M. (1979) 'Drinking among College Students in New England; Extent, Social Correlates and Consequences of Alcohol', *Journal of Studies on Alcohol*, 40:pp. 969–99.

West, R., Drummond, C., and Eames, K. (1990) 'Alcohol Consumption, Problem Drinking and Anti-Social Behaviour in a Sample of College Students', *British Journal of Addiction*, 85:pp. 479–86.

18 Methodology and Interpretive Problems: Do Studies on Shiftwork show a Parallel with Studies on Addiction?

James Waterhouse and Adrian Bonner

The preceding chapters indicate the breadth of studies in addiction: from biochemical and physiological to psychological and sociological approaches; from acute effects to chronic effects; and from factors predicting a predisposition to becoming addicted to those changes that result from the addiction. Accepting that advances can come when there is a cross-fertilisation between different areas, we can consider the possibility that there are certain parallels between addiction and shift work with regard to the methods used and the interpretive problems that arise. In the following account these parallels will be considered. It is left to the reader to decide the extent to which the parallel exists and then the degree to which the problems have been solved in studies of addiction.

USING QUESTIONNAIRES

Since these play a large part in studies of addiction it is appropriate to consider, first, some of the difficulties that are associated with the preparation, administration and assessment of them.

Devising and Validating Questionnaires

The factor being investigated will indicate the kind of question to be asked, but will the form of words that is produced be the best one? One method is to incorporate into the questionnaire several questions that approach the same factor from different angles. A consistent response to this set would be expected; failure to achieve this would cast doubt on the reliability of the set *or* the individual responding. Some external standard is required also. If a widely used questionnaire is this standard then the reliability of the individual can be assessed and, from this, the internal consistency of the set of questions can be inferred. But showing that the questions give rise to consistent replies is not sufficient to indicate that they measure what is required: an accepted standard is required for this, preferably (if not necessarily) an objective one. For example, the results from a questionnaire asking about subjective estimates of sleep quality can be compared with the sleep EEG.

Cultural differences might exist also according to the perceived norms of the group being studied. Such groups might show national differences or more local ones according to their position in society. National differences can be important in studies designed to test if the habits of those who tolerate night work differ from those who do not. One questionnaire investigated if the sleeping and activity habits of those who tolerated night work were phased later (evening types or 'owls') than of those who found it particular difficult (morning types or 'larks'). In assessing this, preferred hours of rising and retiring were asked. Whereas, in the UK it is uncommon to wish to rise before 7 a.m., this is not the case in some countries in Southern Europe. (This might be connected with the fact that the latter inhabitants often take an afternoon siesta). The proportion of 'larks' in Southern Europe was higher, and of 'owls' was lower than in a comparable UK workforce. The disparity was resolved by changing the questionnaire to take into account the norms for the population as a whole.

Choosing the Subjects

In comparing night and day workers, both groups are equally clearly defined and it presents no great problem to get a random sample from each sub-group. Moreover, if interindividual variation is to be removed, then rotating shift workers can be chosen, their responses to the different shifts being compared. With addiction, these issues are more complex. The whole population, rather than just a workforce, is the group from whom the sample has to be taken. The size of the problem can be greatly reduced and made more manageable if only restricted parts of the population are monitored, particularly in areas where the incidence of addiction will be, or can be expected to be, higher than for the population as a whole. Examples would be GPs' records, addiction centres and the appropriate units in hospital. Whilst such methods will find more subjects of interest, two problems are raised. First, it will be less certain that information about the population as a whole can be deduced from such records and, second, it is not even certain that the subjects will be representative of the addicts themselves. For example, some addicts will not come for treatment, and so escape the 'net', and (see later) there will be a dependency upon the policy of the medical and social personnel who are involved.

There is also the difficulty that, unlike the case with workers on rotating shift systems in whom intraindividual comparisons can be made (see above), the nature of addiction is such that a regular alternation between addicted and non-addicted states is not possible.

In shiftwork, interest is centred on those who respond particularly badly to the demands of night work and have to 'drop out'. These are unrepresentative of the workforce as a whole but, presumably, they show extreme examples of what happens to all night workers to some extent. Following up the 'drop-outs' after transfer to day work enables the reversibility of the effects to be assessed. It is argued, further, that the attributes of the drop-out enable those factors to be determined that predispose an individual to difficulties with night work. This need not be so; workers need to develop coping mechanisms to deal with the altered lifestyle and physiology demanded by night work. The size of these will depend upon the predisposition of the individual (thus 'larks' will have to alter their sleeping habits more than 'owls'). The 'drop-out' is an individual whose *combination* of predisposition and coping mechanisms has proved inadequate.

With studies on addiction, different sub-groups are being measured according to whether one chooses individuals who: are in the process of becoming addicted; have become addicted; are being treated for addiction; or have finished successful treatment. The differences arise not only because of the degree of dependency currently being shown but also because of any changes that might be irreversible in spite of successful treatment.

In both areas of research, there is not a single 'correct' source of subjects but rather a number of sources suitable for particular investigations. Related to this, since night work and addiction affect an individual's interactions with family and friends, these also are potentially useful subjects. The problem when addicts are being considered, and here there is not a parallel with night workers, is that family and friends might be scarce or unreliable, might show considerable reticence to answer questions due to the stigma of addiction.

Asking the Questions

Assuming the subject to be *compos mentis*, a double-blind study is not possible. A single-blind study, with the questioner unaware of whether the respondent is a day worker or night worker (or is or is not addicted to a drug), requires the questioner not to be able to ascertain the status of the subject. This is not always possible in practice and, anyway, restricts considerably the kind of question that can be asked.

Answering a written questionnaire has much to commend it, therefore, anonymity supposedly giving rise to more accurate answers. However, this prevents individuals being followed up, either to gain clarification of some of their answers or to extend the survey if a particularly 'interesting' or 'anomalous' subject is found.

Validating the Answers

Can the researcher be sure the answers are truthful? The issues of reliability and checking against an external standard (if such exists) have been considered already. Even these safeguards cannot obviate another difficulty which arises because of the subjects' perceived role of the questioner or questionnaire. If it is perceived to be a sympathetic one (for example, more support for the night worker or drug addict) then an exaggeration of the problems, even unintentionally so, is always a possibility. By contrast, if it is perceived that there might be negative consequences (loss of a job, for instance) then an under-emphasis is much more likely. The stigma associated with addiction (but absent from night work) might also affect responses, of the addict as well as of family and friends who might be questioned. Some assessment of the stigma as perceived by the respondent might also be made as part of the questionnaire, and this might then be used in some way to establish its effect upon answers to other questions. However, this is not simple since many statistical methods (such as partial correlation and multiple regression analysis) assume the factors to be independent, a condition that is unlikely to hold.

INTERPRETING RESULTS

All the rigour associated with standard scientific investigation is called for, of course, but some problems are particularly likely because of the nature of many investigations carried out in research into addiction.

The Conduct of the Survey

Multicentre trials and trials making use of more than one doctor or assessor have the advantage of allowing the experimenter access to more subjects in a shorter space of time. They have the disadvantage that the different centres and assessors must be shown to be comparable. With accident statistics during night and day shifts, for example, a comparison will be valid only if the work, the conditions of work and the mechanisms for reporting accidents are all equal. If this concept is applied to a proposed study on addiction, then the use of a common set of criteria for deciding upon a patient's eligibility for the study is recommended.

With retrospective data or accident statistics, and with data on the prevalence of addiction in different areas of the country, for example, such requirements are unlikely to have been met. The prevalence will be affected by the awareness of the problem of those in primary health care, by referral procedures, by treatment policy, etc. Differences in these factors and in the effects they might produce are very difficult to deal with satisfactorily.

Time-course Effects

The current position with regard to studies on individuals' response to night work can be summarized as follows.

Acutely, there are advantages (more money, more time off) and disadvantages (fatigue, loss of social life), and individuals differ in the severity of any problems and their response to them. The differences are based upon pre-existing factors ('larks' versus 'owls' and ability to nap) and upon current circumstances (the family, the mortgage and friends).

Chronically, problems can arise; these include health problems and difficulties with interpersonal relationships. Again, individuals differ both in the size of their problems and the facility with which they deal with them. For some, those who are susceptible, the problems force them to leave nightwork; for others the problems are overcome by the development of 'coping mechanisms'. As with acute exposure to night work, interindividual differences are believed to reflect pre-existing, even genetic factors and social (environmental) factors.

Importantly, an individual's ability to deal with the demands of night work will depend, at any moment, on all these factors. An individual who is tolerating night work at the time of study might have developed the coping strategies after great effort or with no difficulty; the individual who is experiencing difficulty might have a 'predisposition' which did not suit him to night work, a 'susceptibility' to its adverse effects, or poorly developed 'coping mechanisms' (this lack of development reflecting personal ability or willingness, or the force of external factors). Moreover, any factor might have a genetic or environmental component, or both.

The parallelism between night work and drug addiction can be made quite close if the development of coping mechanism and of drug tolerance are both seen as responses to chronic exposure. Both situations have a mixture of advantageous and disadvantageous effects, the balance between them being perceived differently by different individuals. The differences are believed to have genetic and environmental components and alter with time and amount of exposure.

There are similarities also when interpretive difficulties and experimental results are considered. If a factor X exists only in an individual shown to have developed tolerance to a drug after chronic exposure to it (and X might be a social, psychological, physiological, biochemical or genetic factor) then, amongst other possibilities, X might be:

a marker of addiction;
a marker of chronic exposure, but not addiction;
a marker of exposure to the drug, regardless of the length of exposure;
a marker of a predisposition to seek out the drug (or the effect it produces).

It will be noted that some of these possibilities are often considered but in a slightly different way. Thus we can have:

a 'state' or 'trait' marker;
the distinction between the pre-existing condition and those due to the acute and chronic effects of a drug;
differences between the desire for, handling of, and effects of a drug.

A distinction between these possibilities, however described, generally requires several measurements made at different stages of the disease process; unfortunately such longitudinal studies are time-consuming and measurements *before* drug abuse are rare. In effect, very little is known about predisposing and trait factors, therefore. In this respect, studies of night work are easier because it is generally known in advance of the event that workers will start night work; and so measurements can be made before the first exposure. Nevertheless, as indicated in this book, the study of individuals whose family history indicates that they are 'at risk' as potential drug users is one way of tackling this problem.

Establishing Causal Links

It is accepted that if A and B are linked in some way then there must be a correlation between them, either in an individual at different times or in different individuals taking part in a transverse study. The reverse argument – that a correlation measure between two variables implies a causal link – is logically suspect. Establishing causal links will require experimental manipulation of one of the variables, as by giving, for example, controlled exposure to the drug. This is ethically unacceptable with human subjects but is the basis of much work on rats and ethanol. However, all the problems associated with species differences are raised by this approach. For example, while it might be accepted that the biochemistry and pharmacology of drug exposure are very similar, the psychological and sociological effects are most certainly not. This is not as trivial as it might at first appear, since some interaction between all these effects is often proposed; if this is correct, then even the pharmacological and biochemical changes observed in the rat might not represent those occurring in humans. It must always be remembered that an individual's desire for night work or a drug, and the responses to acute and chronic exposure, can all have psychological and sociological components as well as pharmacological and biochemical ones.

Going Round in Circles or Refining Hypotheses?

One aim of many studies is to establish the presence of 'predisposing' factors or traits that enable it to be predicted if an individual is likely to experience undue difficulty with night work or if he/she is more likely to resort to drug abuse. In some cases, the results are based upon some degree of circularity of reasoning. Consider, for example, the frequently reported finding that 'larks' find night work more difficult to deal with than do 'owls'. In practice this is hardly surprising due to the nature of the questionnaires used to establish if an individual is a 'lark' or 'owl'. Thus, 'larks' are individuals who dislike going to bed late, have difficulty sleeping late into the day, and prefer to organise their activates to fall early in their waking span – all characteristics that are *the opposite* of what is required by night work and daytime sleep. Similarly, 'owls' prefer to organise their lifestyle in a way that is far more akin to the demands of night work. The findings – that 'owls' have less difficulty with night work – is not only predictable, therefore, but amount to little more than restating the criteria used to establish the existence of the 'owls' in the first place. Similarly, the demonstration that individuals who are assessed as 'unsociable' and 'excitement seeking' will be a circularity in reasoning unless the means of assessing 'unsociable' and 'excitement seeking' make no direct or indirect reference to drug taking. In practice, this might be very difficult to achieve since the individual who responds affirmatively to 'Do you like to surprise people?' or 'Do you like new experiences?' might be tacitly assuming that the questions refer to unsociable behaviour or drug-taking respectively.

The aim of experiments is to test hypotheses that are derived from theoretical constructs. Results that come out 'wrong' require the hypothesis to be rejected or modified; results that support the original hypothesis require it to be refined in such a way that tests to distinguish between various refinements can be made. The problem is that after several such refinements, the hypothesis can have several factors built into it that make it virtually worthless as a basis for scientific testing. Consider the propositions that:

Night work will, in 'susceptible' individuals, or in those who develop inadequate 'coping mechanisms' lead to severe problems

or that:

In individuals with the appropriate genetic and/or cultural backgrounds, the exigencies of normal life will lead them to become involved in drug abuse.

The difficulty is that the propositions have become unfocused – to accommodate all the interindividual variation that is normally found –

and as a result, have become all-embracing. Any individual case can be accommodated by such propositions, and, as such, they have lost any power of discrimination. Such a position is 'unscientific', since it cannot be refuted. It is not useless, however, provided that it is then focused more clearly.

Possible areas for focusing, and hence scientific testing would be:

for the first proposition, to define what are 'susceptible' individuals and 'coping mechanisms';

for the second proposition, to define what are 'inappropriate' genetic and/or cultural backgrounds and what exactly are the 'exigencies' of normal life.

Developed this way, both propositions become the subject of further experimentation which could provide further insight into the detailed mechanisms involved.

There are some useful parallels between the studies of addictive behaviours and shiftwork, but perhaps the most important is the issue of motivation. The reasons why people undertake shiftwork are complex and multifactorial but, it might be argued, in some ways motivations to addictive behaviours are not only complex from a scientific viewpoint but also are perceived in a different theoretical domain which has no parallel in the study of shiftwork. What is referred to here is that whilst physiological, psychological and sociological explanations might be used in studies of both addiction and shiftwork, deeper issues of morality and spirituality have been suggested as being significant in the onset and maintenance of addictive behaviour. Support for this view comes from the neo-religious approach employed by Alcohol-Anonymous-based therapeutic strategies and other *non-scientific* approaches to treatment which are used quite widely by many sufferers around the world, and probably as effective as medico-social approaches to treatment. The confounding variables of morality and spirituality cannot easily be incorporated into a reductionist explanation of the issues.

Cognitive behaviour approaches to therapy (see Chapter 10) take account of *belief systems* and childhood events in the application of behaviour modification. In this approach *labelling* is avoided as the social stigmata linked with addictions has strongly negative influences on self-esteem. Shiftworking does not have such profound effects on self-image. Breaking the cycle of relapse and recovery in the immediate to long term is difficulty to achieve for many clients; the therapy approaches described in Chapter 10 are 'effective for some people for some of the time'. Greater sucess would be derived by 'matching treatments more closely to a client's needs'. Problems relating to life-history taking and other methods relying on recall are fraught with difficulties relating to psychological factors (Chapter 7), memory (Chapter 9) and neurochemical events (Chapter 13) either present prior to, or as a result of the chronic consumption of addictive substances. On the other hand, there is strong evidence that genetic factors are important in the addictions. A large body of literature on alcohol biochemistry indicates that part of the variance between individuals is accounted for by genetic control over ethanol metabolism. There is a growing understanding of inherited differences in the neurobiological substrates of behaviour, although the evidence for genetic factors concerned with the receptors in the nervous system is more problematic. Pathological changes (such as gastrointestinal tract disturbances) might result from long periods of shiftwork, but it is unlikely that the clinical severity of these will be of the same magnitude of severity and have the same impact on behaviour as found in chronic substance misusers. Nevertheless, basic research into the psychophysiology of both shiftwork and dependence is essential if a good understanding of the dysregulation of motivated behaviours is to be understood.

FURTHER READING

MRC Field Review, *The Basis of Drug Dependence* (London: Medical Research Council, 1994), pp. 1–96.

Minors, D. S. and Waterhouse, J. M. (1981) *Circadian Rhythms and the Human* (Bristol: John Wright).

Scott, E. M. and Waterhouse, J.M. (1988) *Physiology and the Scientific Method* (Manchester: Manchester University Press).

Waterhouse, J. M., Folkard, S. and Minors, D. S. (1992) 'Shiftwork, Health and Safety: An Overview of the Scientific Literature, 1978–1990', *HSE Contract Research Report*, no. 31 (London: HMSO, 1992).

Concluding Comments
Adrian Bonner

The various contributions in this book suggest that molecular, cellular, neurological, cognitive and social influences are involved in the development and maintenance of addictive behaviours. More extensive research into the links between these approaches will, one hopes, feed through into increasingly effective therapeutic outcomes. This is occurring to some extent already, with regard to our increased understanding of the neuropsychological processes, made possible by advances in brain-imaging technologies. However caution is needed because even in these scientific investigations there is a range of methodological pitfalls in the presently available neuropsychological assessment tools and also the application of, for example, magnetic resonance imaging (MRI). What appears to be a major step forward in our understanding of the neural substrates of the addictive process is based upon a still rather inexact science.

A major problem which often arises when multidisciplinary approaches are adopted is that of terminology. On the one hand, the jargon used by one speciality is not understandable by researchers in complementary fields of activity, or definitions and classification are inexact. An example of the latter is provided in Chapter 11, where the various meanings of the concept of 'craving' are explored.

It is likely that the level of harm to individuals and families will continue to increase and solutions to problems of minimising these risks should be pursued. Individual differences, at least in part, result from biological factors concerning the organisation of the nervous system, and the physiological and psychological vulnerability of the individual to acute and chronic use of addictive substances.

However, the events of childhood and an individual's relationships with others in complex human society will have a strong influence on his/her consummatory behaviours. Humankind is constituted from molecules but, in view of the multidimensional nature of the addictions, research into and management of these tragic human predicaments should be carried out within a multidisciplinary perspective in which clearly defined issues may be may identified and the appropriate questions asked. The Medical Research Council (MRC) *Field Review: The Basis of Drug Dependence* clearly indicates that UK research into the addictions is fragmented, and encourages multidisciplinary activities between basic and clinical scientists and social scientists. Whilst this is a necessary objective, appropriate methodology must be developed, as briefly commented on in Chapter 18.

FURTHER READING

Comings, D. E., 'Serotonin and the Biochemical Genetics of Alcoholism: Lessons from Studies of Attention Deficit Hyperactivity Disorder (ADHD) and Tourette Syndrome', in: P. V. Taberner and A. A. Badawy (eds), *Advances in Biomedical Alcohol Research* (Oxford: Pergamon Press, 1993), pp. 237–45.

MRC Field Review, *The Basis of Drug Dependence* (London: Medical Research Council, 1994) pp. 1–96.

Sergent, J., 'Brain-imaging Studies of Cognitive Functions', *Trends in Neuroscience*, 17(6)(1994): 221–27.

Appendix I: Recommendations for Sensible Drinking

In December 1995, prior to this book going to press, the UK Government (Department of Health) published a report on 'Sensible Drinking'.[1] This inter-departmental working-group report concluded that light to moderate consumption of alcohol provides some protection from coronary heart disease (CHD), ischaemic stroke and cholesterol gallstones for men older than 40 years and post-menopausal women. The report indicates the risks of long-term heavy drinking and suggests that 'all cause mortality' of moderate drinkers (1 unit a day for men and women) is similar to non-drinkers until consumption rises above 14 units per week for women and 21 units for men. Women are considered to be more at risk compared with men on the basis of physiological differences; weight, rate of alcohol metabolism, possible increased vulnerability to tissue damage, the possible link between alcohol consumption and breast cancer, risks to the fetus and early infant development.

In the development of 'bench marks' to guide individuals to sensible drinking, the report advocates the retention of the unit of alcohol (equivalent to 8g of ethanol) as the UK standard but suggests that, taking account of the risks attached to binge drinking, the guidelines should be related to daily rather than weekly consumption.

On the basis of the detailed evidence considered by the working group, which is briefly summarised above, the report sets out guidelines for sensible drinking as follows:

MEN

- The health benefit from drinking relates to men over 40 and the major part of this can be obtained at levels as low as one unit a day, with the maximum health advantage lying between 1 and 2 units a day.

- Regular consumption of between 3 and 4 units a day by men of all ages will not accrue significant health risk.

- Consistently drinking 4 or more units a day is not advised as a sensible drinking level because of the progressive health risk it carries.

WOMEN

- The health benefit from drinking for women relates to post-menopausal women and the major part of this can be obtained at levels as low as one unit a day, with a maximum health advantage lying between 1 and 2 units a day.

- Regular consumption of between 2 and 3 units a day by women of all ages will not accrue any significant health risk.

- Consistently drinking 3 or more units a day is not advised as a sensible drinking level because of the progressive health risk it carries.

THE DEVELOPMENT OF A 'SENSIBLE DRINKING' STRATEGY

Recommendations for sensible drinking were made in 1976 by means of a consultative document: *Prevention and Health: Everybody's Business*.[2] This was a response to the increasing number of hospital admissions for alcoholism, alcoholic psychosis and death rates due to liver cirrhosis. An example of this is seen in the standardised mortality ratios of a range of occupational groups (e.g. company directors: 2200; publicans: 773; armed forces: 350; civil engineers: 200). In 1984 the Health Education Council gave advice on 'safe limits'[3] to which individuals should limit their drinking, 18 'standard drinks' for men and 9 'standard drinks' for women (a 'standard drink' is equivalent to a 'unit'). Revised versions of this publication in 1987 and 1989 suggested the 'sensible limits' should be 21 and 14 per week for men and women, respectively.

These recommended limits were endorsed by the Royal College of General Practitioners, the Royal College of Psychiatrists, and the Royal College of Physicians in reports in 1986/7.[4,5,6] This advice of the Royal Colleges was used to inform the report 'Action Against Alcohol Misuse' in 1991[7] which was used to set the targets to reduce alcohol misuse in *The Health of the Nation*[8] and related national health strategies. The targets set at this time included reducing the number of men drinking more than 21 units per week from 28 per cent to 18 per cent, and reducing the number of women drinking above 14 units from 11 per cent to 7 per cent. These targets were to be achieved by the year 2005.

The recent government report 'Sensible Drinking' is significant because it attempts to adjust the recommended levels of alcohol for men from 21 to 28 and women from 14 to 21 units per week and also supports the health benefits of drinking alcohol by certain groups in the population.

The evidence used in 'Sensible Drinking' is based on data from drinking habits of the population in the UK and other countries, epidemiological, mortality and toxicological studies. These approaches are undoubtedly valid from a 'medical model' perspective of alcohol abuse but do not (indeed cannot) take into account individual vulnerability linked to the interplay of biological, psychological and social forces which have been discussed in this book. This is understandable because the data relating to this multidimensional description of alcohol abuse are not yet as scientifically robust as the data which have been used in the report. However, problems of regarding alcoholism and other addictions as unitary diseases have been discussed in Chapter 17 of this book.

Not surprisingly considerable public debate has been generated which has been fuelled by sensationalism in the press at the more 'professional level'. This move has been vehemently criticised by the three Royal Colleges not least because, although there are some slight benefits to health in a limited part of the population, alcohol consumption has a significant influence on cirrhosis of the liver, cancer (squamous carcinomas of the upper aerodigestive tract, and cancers of the oral cavity, pharynx, larynx and oesphagus), hypertension, reproduction (including pregnancy and infant development), mental illness and neurological disorders. The recommendations are perceived as being influenced by other factors also, and this illustrates the difficulty in devising a set of guidelines for the population as a whole but which, ultimately, must be applied to an individual – for all the differences in physiology, psychology, sociology that this entails. Some of these points are made cogently by Michael Marmot in Appendix II.

The recommendations, and any others which might be produced, merit close scrutiny in the light of the problems outlined in Chapter 17. We stress that setting benchmarks for sensible drinking is fraught with ethical, methodological and conceptual problems and reiterate the need for integrated research across a range of disciplines as has been outlined by the Medical Research Council.[9]

NOTES

1. 'Sensible Drinking: The Report of an Inter-Departmental Working Group', December, 1995 (London: Department of Health).
2. Department of Health and Social Security (1976), *Prevention and Health: Everybody's Business. A Reassement of Public and Personal Health* (London: HMSO).
3. Health Education Council (1984), 'That's the Limit', alcohol information pamphlet, with subsequent updates.
4. Royal College of General Practitioners (1987), *Alcohol: A Balanced View* (London: Royal College of General Practitioners).
5. The Royal College of Psychiatrists (1986), *Alcohol: Our Favourite Drug* (London: Tavistock).
6. Royal College of Physicians (1987), *A Great and Growing Evil: The Medical Consequences of Alcohol Abuse* (London: Tavistock).
7. *The Lord President's Report on Action Against Alcohol Misuse* (London: HMSO, 1991).
8. Department of Health (1992) *The Health of the Nation: A Strategy for Health in England* (London: HMSO).
9. Anonymous (1994), *MRC Field Review of the Basis of Drug Dependence.* (London: Medical Research Council) pp. 1–96.

Appendix II: A Not-so-Sensible Drinks Policy

Letter to *The Lancet* From Professor Michael Marmot

The British Government's policy on alcohol, as stated in *The Health of the Nation*, has been to reduce the proportion of people drinking above the sensible limits (21 units a week for men and 14 for women). Yet if it were possible to divine government policy by government action, one would conclude that this same government's policy is to increase alcohol consumption in the population. It has lately increased opening hours of public houses and, in last month's budget, the Chancellor of the Exchequer played his part in keeping the rise in alcohol prices below inflation by reducing the tax on whisky and holding steady, in absolute amounts, the tax on other alcoholic drinks. Evidence suggests that both these actions will lead to an increase in consumption.[1] On 12 December, a third step was taken in the same direction, with the issue of a government report that, in its own words, aims to redefine the benchmarks for sensible drinking.[2] It has been widely reported as overturning the previous consensus, and government policy, on sensible limits of alcohol consumption by expanding them to 4 units a day for men and 3 for women.

This report comes less than 6 months after the Royal Colleges of Physicians, Psychiatrists, and General Practitioners jointly concluded that low to moderate alcohol consumption protected against coronary heart disease but confirmed that the sensible limits of 21 and 14 units should continue because to increase them would be to do more harm than good.[3] Is this yet another example of the health experts disagreeing? No. This latest report was not the result of expert deliberations. In a famous episode of the television comedy *Yes Prime Minister*, senior civil servants observe that you should not have a doctor as minister of health because he is biased by human suffering. The members of the government interdepartmental working group, all civil servants, were not chosen for their expertise in the area of alcohol and health. Rather, they solicited advice. As inspection of the 89 submissions to the group reveals, it is a pity they ignored much of the advice they received.

Setting thresholds of consumption above which harm accrues is an inexact science. First, units are defined as containing 8 g of alcohol but standard drinks may contain 9–12 g. Second, the point at which risk takes off varies among studies. For example, the American Cancer Society study of 276,000 men shows a steady increase in mortality risk from 1 drink a day,[4] whereas the British Doctors Study concluded that mortality risk rises above about 3 units (2 American units) a day.[5] Third, the risk curve differs for different health endpoints. The level of consumption at which risk becomes significant may be higher for cirrhosis, for example, than it is for blood pressure, drink driving, being in trouble with the police, being involved in an assault,

307

and, possibly, breast cancer.[6] It is surprising that this working group felt that the data were precise enough to warrant a rise in the recommended sensible levels of drinking. That their confidence was less than total is shown by the contorted wording of their conclusions. Between 3 and 4 units a day is safe for men, they conclude, and between 2 and 3 units safe for women. Yet they go on to say, in agreement with the Royal Colleges' report, that 4 units a day in men and 3 units a day in women are associated with progressive health risk. What can they mean? Are 4 (and 3) units safe or unsafe? If the working group is saying that one cannot distinguish precisely a safe level, why did they go public in a way that predictably led to the headlines that the British government is encouraging higher levels of consumption?

If such change in policy were to lead to an increase in consumption it could damage the public health. The Royal Colleges' group, which I chaired, was convinced by the evidence that an increase in the mean population level of alcohol consumption will lead to an increase in the prevalence of heavy drinking – the population theory. We were therefore concerned that changing the sensible limit guidelines for individuals would result in net harm to the population. The interdepartmental working group acknowledges that this is a position held by 'most experts'. Indeed, their report cites evidence that some indices of harm are correlated with mean population levels of consumption. With little justification, they then go on to hope that perhaps the population theory may not apply in the UK – a blithe dismissal of the experts' view that allows them to suggest that men over 40 and post-menopausal women who drink infrequently might consider drinking more and imply that people drinking near the current sensible limits might increase their consumption without harm.

Why the fuss? Does anyone take any notice of guidelines? The main effect seems sometimes to give ammunition as if they needed it, to those who find agents of the nanny state hiding under every bed. There is little evidence that health education will, by itself, change consumption, although advertising might. The importance of the report may not be because of a direct influence on alcohol consumption but because of the stimulus it gives to those promoting their product. That, taken together with the failure to adjust prices and the liberalisation of opening hours, may well lead to an increase in alcohol-associated problems – and to the obvious conclusion that the health of the nation is but one small consideration to this government.

Professor Michael Marmot (University College, London) is Chairman of the Committee on Sensible Levels of Drinking, a committee of the three Royal Colleges of Medicine, 1995.

NOTES

1. G. Edwards, F. Anderson, T. F. Babor et al., *Alcohol Policy and the Public Good* (Oxford: Oxford University Press, 1994).
2. Sensible Drinking: The Report of an Inter-department Working Group (London: Department of Health, 1995).
3. The Royal Colleges Report, *Alcohol and the Heart in Perspective: Sensible Limits Reaffirmed* (London: Royal Colleges of Physicians, Psychiatrists, and General Practitioners, 1995).
4. P. Bofetta, L. Garfinkel, 'Alcohol, Drinking and Mortality among Men Enrolled in the American Cancer Society Prospective Study', *Epidemiology* (1990) **1**: 342–8.
5. R. Doll, R. Pero, E. Hall, K. Whatley, and R. Gray, 'Mortality in Relation to Consumption of Alcohol: 13 Years' Observations on Male British Doctors', *BMJ* (1994) **309**: 911–18.

Index

absenteeism, *see* work
abstinence, 7, 11, 58, 59, 122, 123,
    126, 158–60, 165–73, 182, 234
accidents
    due to drugs, 57, 58, 296
addiction, xv, xvi, 3–12, 41, 43, 45, 47,
    51, 52, 58, 59, 90–102, 158–75,
    194–6, 223–5, 299, 302, 303
    see also bingeing; chocolate; food;
        gambling; stealing; tobacco; work
    see also specific drugs:
        amphetamines; analgesics;
        barbiturates; caffeine; cocaine,
        ecstasy; endorphins; hallucinogens;
        heroin; LDS; marijuana; opiates;
        tobacco; tranquillizers
adrenaline, *see* catecholamines
affective state, 41, 45, 47, 48, 52,
    59–65, 69, 70, 100–4, 108–11,
    125, 145, 147, 186, 193, 196, 197,
    201–5, 234, 241, 251, 254, 255,
    268, 271, 281, 282
age, 22–56, 58–61, 267–1
alcohol, 3–6, 8, 9, 13–16, 18–20, 22,
    26, 42–53, 56–65, 69–74, 77, 79,
    87, 90–111, 122–8, 130, 139–57,
    168, 179–81, 183, 195, 196, 203,
    213–26, 233–91
    metabolism, 44, 46, 48, 65, 214–16,
        247, 248, 268, 274
    see also memory
amnesia, *see* memory
amphetamines, 4, 8, 27, 42, 62, 64, 69,
    71, 74, 78, 107
analgesics, 47
animal models, *see* experimentation
anxiolytics, *see* tranquillizers
aspartate receptor, 45, 64, 217–19
aversion, 41
    see also avoidance
avoidance, 41, 97–9, 104–8

barbiturates, 7, 27, 44, 45, 47, 58–65,
    69, 71, 107, 111, 148, 180, 218, 281
behaviour, 159–75
    see also abstinence; addiction;
        aversion; avoidance; compulsion;
        dependence; reinforcement; reward;

sensitization; sex; tolerance;
    vulnerability
benzodiazepines, *see* barbiturates
bingeing, 58, 59, 286, 289, 290
    see also food
brain damage, 245–52
    effect of drugs, 56–68

caffeine, 4–6, 69, 71, 77, 78, 94, 111,
    124, 185, 186
cannabis, 3–6, 26–9, 42–4, 58, 59, 62,
    69, 71, 78, 110
cardiovascular system, 69–84, 131, 234,
    241, 249, 250, 268, 278, 280, 281
catecholamines, 43, 75–9, 106, 149,
    182, 198, 219
    see also dopamine
causality, *see* experimentation
central nervous system, 7, 142, 145–9,
    214, 215, 220–2, 268
    see also brain damage
chocolate, 3, 9, 185–7
    see also food
cirrhosis, *see* liver
classical conditioning, 9, 159, 160
    see also operant conditioning
cocaine, 4–8, 11, 20, 27, 30, 34–6, 42,
    45, 57, 60–4, 69, 71, 74–7, 79,
    90–102, 107, 110–12, 179
    see also opiates
cocoa, *see* caffeine
coffee, *see* caffeine
compulsion, 11, 89, 90, 97–9, 104–8
conditioning, *see* classical conditioning;
    operant conditioning
correlation, *see* experimentation
crack, *see* cocaine
craving, 9, 10, 43, 91, 165, 168–70,
    179–90, 302
crime, 26–37, 96, 100, 111, 130, 245,
    255, 256

death
    due to drugs, 56, 60, 61, 69, 70, 76,
        79
dependence, 6, 7, 17, 41–8, 53
diet, 57, 58, 60, 62, 65, 70, 74, 142,
    247, 250, 278–80

310